T0195505

Practical General Practice
NURSING

For General Practice Nurses everywhere, who work so hard to care for their communities with their expertise and hearts.

Practical General Practice
NURSING

Marion M. Welsh, EdD, MSc, PgCLTHE, FHEA, RNT, BSc, SPGP, SCM, RGN
Independent Educational Consultant

Susan F. Brooks, MSc, BSc (Hons), Registered Nurse, PGCE, Independent Prescriber (V300)
Director of Studies for Advanced Clinical Practice
and Teaching Fellow
University of Surrey

ELSEVIER

Elsevier
3251 Riverport Lane
St. Louis, Missouri 63043

PRACTICAL GENERAL PRACTICE NURSING   ISBN: 978-0-702-08028-9
Copyright © 2022 by Elsevier, Ltd. All rights reserved.

No part of this publication may be reproduced or transmitted in any form or by any means, electronic or
mechanical, including photocopying, recording, or any information storage and retrieval system, without
permission in writing from the publisher. Details on how to seek permission, further information about the
Publisher's permissions policies and our arrangements with organizations such as the Copyright Clearance
Center and the Copyright Licensing Agency, can be found at our website: www.elsevier.com/permissions.

This book and the individual contributions contained in it are protected under copyright by the Publisher
(other than as may be noted herein).

Notice

Practitioners and researchers must always rely on their own experience and knowledge in evaluating
and using any information, methods, compounds or experiments described herein. Because of rapid
advances in the medical sciences, in particular, independent verification of diagnoses and drug dosages
should be made. To the fullest extent of the law, no responsibility is assumed by Elsevier, authors, editors
or contributors for any injury and/or damage to persons or property as a matter of products liability,
negligence or otherwise, or from any use or operation of any methods, products, instructions, or ideas
contained in the material herein.

Director, Content Development: Laurie K Gower
Content Strategist: Poppy Garraway
Content Development Specialist: Denise Roslonski
Senior Project Manager: Manchu Mohan
Designer: Brian Salisbury
Illustration Manager: Teresa McBryan

Printed in India

Last digit is the print number: 9 8 7 6 5 4 3 2 1

Working together
to grow libraries in
developing countries

www.elsevier.com • www.bookaid.org

CONTENTS

CONTRIBUTORS

Kirsty Armstrong, RGN, BSc (Hons), NPDip, MA (Ed)
Advanced Nurse Practitioner/Lecturer/Independent
  General Practice Nurse Adviser

Susan F. Brooks, MSc, BSc (Hons), Registered Nurse, PGCE, Independent Prescriber (V300)
Director of Studies for Advanced Clinical Practice
  and Teaching Fellow
University of Surrey

Edwin Tapiwa Chamanga, Masters in Skin Integrity Skills and Treatments (Tissue Viability), BSc in District Nursing, Dip HE Adult Nursing
Head of Nursing - Tissue Viability and Continence
  Care
Epsom and St Helier University Hospital
Surrey

Jane Chiodini, MSc (Trav Med) RGN, RM, FFTM, RCPS (Glasg)
Queen's Nurse
Travel Health Specialist Nurse and Dean of the Faculty
  of Travel Medicine of the Royal College of Physicians
  and Surgeons of Glasgow

Kirsteen Marie Coady, Queen's Nurse (QN)
BA Professional Studies, Advanced Practice with RCN
  Nurse Practitioner award 2009
BA Community Nursing (General Practice Nursing)
  with Specialist Practice 2005
Nurse consultant, NHS Grampian House of Care
  trainer, NHS Education for Scotland Advisor and
  Supervisor for General Practice Nurses

Pat Colliety, PhD, MA, BSc RHV, RN (child)
Former Principal Teaching Fellow
School of Health Sciences
University of Surrey
Guildford

Alison MacLeod Craig, Bachelor of Nursing (BN Commend), Master of Science (MSc) Public Health - Health Promotion and Education, Postgraduate Award in Medical Education (PGA Med Ed), Nurse Diploma of Sexual and Reproductive Health
Nurse Consultant Sexual Health
NHS Lothian

Jacqueline Ann Dale, RGN, DN, MA, FHEA, Non-Medical Prescriber
University Teacher
The University of Sheffield

Deborah Louise Duncan, BSc, PGCAP, PGDIP, MSc, FHEA, AKC, ARNS, RGN, RM, NT, QN
Lecturer in Nursing
School of Nursing and Midwifery
Queen's University
Belfast

Colette Henderson, RN, NISP, RNT, BSc (Hons) NP, PgCert NP, MSc, FHEA
Lecturer in Nursing, Programme Lead MSc Advanced
  Practice
School of Nursing and Health Sciences
University of Dundee
Kirkcaldy, Fife

IVANO MAZZONCINI, BA, Dip, Professional Studies Community Psychiatric Studies
Registered Mental Nurse (R.M.N.)
Team Leader/CPN (Retired)
Esteem Early Intervention Psychosis Services
Staff Nurse RMN
Nurse Bank
NHS Greater Glasgow and Clyde
Glasgow

CAROL MCALANEY, BSc, Dip. Higher Education Nursing (Mental Health)
Registered Mental Nurse (R.M.N)
Charge Nurse
Esteem Early Intervention 1st Episode Psychosis
NHS Greater Glasgow and Clyde
Glasgow

EVELYN MCELHINNEY, PhD, MSc, BSc SPQ, PgC LTHE, FHEA, RN
Senior Lecturer
Programme Lead MSc Advancing Nursing
Glasgow Caledonian University

ALAN R. MIDDLETON, MSc, BSc, DipCHN, PgCLTHE, RNLD, RGN, FHEA
Senior Lecturer
Glasgow Caledonian University
Glasgow

EILEEN P. MUNSON, RD, VR, Queen's Nurse, MSc ANP, BSc (Hons) SPQ GPN, RGN, RM, RNT, V300 Non-Medical Prescriber
Senior Lecturer for Advanced Clinical Practice
University of South Wales
Pontypridd

JOANNE POWELL, BSc (Hons), MSc, FHEA
Senior Lecturer
Kingston University and St George's University London
Sunbury

NICKI WALSH, MSc, BSc (Hons) DN, BSc (Hons), SPQDN, RNT, FHEA, RN, MIHPE
Programme Lead BA (Hons) in Health & Social Care, MA in Health & Social Care Leadership, PG Cert in General Practice Nurse and MSc Primary and Community Care
Bishop Grosseteste University
Lincoln

EVELYN WALTON, PGCE, MSc, BSc (Hons), RN
Nurse Lecturer
Ulster University

MARION M. WELSH, EdD, MSc, PgCLTHE, FHEA, RNT, BSc, SPGP, SCM, RGN
Independent Educational Consultant

FOREWORD

Sue Brooks and Marion Welsh are esteemed colleagues of mine who have drawn on the expertise of UK-wide academia and practice to develop a much-needed practical overview of the key concepts of general practice nursing. This collaboration provides insight into the key areas addressed within general practice nursing, including initial consultations; screenings; immunisations; holistic, personalised care; population health and the most pressing issue of health inequalities.

The period of 2020–2021 proved to be an unprecedented time of uncertainty with devastating effects on all parts of society as the COVID-19 pandemic took hold. This had a significant effect on all health and social care services, including primary care, and it has had a particular impact on general practice nurses (GPNs), who have been pivotal in helping to deliver the national vaccination programme. Thus, it is timely to reflect on and re-evaluate the role of the GPN and consider the key facets that underpin the role, as the following chapters of this book address.

It is not only time for reflection but an opportunity to articulate the value of the GPN, who plays a vital role in the new age of primary care with the evolution of primary care networks (PCNs). As more GPNs become clinical leads, clinical directors of PCNs and leaders within the wider integrated care system (ICS), the voice of the GPN will be louder and more influential in demonstrating the value of the GPN role. This, in turn, will influence and ensure that the education needs of new GPNs are consistent and future-proofed to safeguard best practice and to promote public safety.

This book offers pragmatic insight into the key attributes of general practice nursing, with a balance of theory and contemporary practice. It explores the inception of the GPN role, recognises the GPN role within the wider healthcare system and provides robust contemporary resources to inform nurses new to general practice nursing, as well as useful revision resources for established GPNs. It is a guiding principle of mine that practical guidance is made explicit in the first instance in terms of setting the scene for practitioners, as this publication illustrates in rich detail.

Enjoy, be loud and be proud to be a general practice nurse!

ANGIE HACK

PREFACE

The opportunity to contribute to nursing practice, in whatever form that emerges, is something that remains irresistible. More so, when from a practice nursing perspective, we were keenly aware of how few books there are that celebrate and advance nursing knowledge within the community nursing discipline of practice nursing.

We set about constructing this first edition of *Practical General Practice Nursing* with the 'early career' general practice nurse in mind, aiming to produce a resource that truly captures the scope of what is a complex and ostensibly unique nursing role. Throughout this book we have endeavoured to outline the practical expectations of working within the general practice setting using evidence-based guidance to optimise the standard of care provided. Signposting to this guidance has included frequent references to what we feel is a valuable 'companion text' by Staten and Staten (2020), which covers step-wise guidelines for effective clinical management in general practice.

Producing *Practical General Practice Nursing*, which is wide ranging in its content and context, has not been without its challenges. In making this resource relevant for practice nurses across the UK, we purposefully enlisted contributors from front-line practitioners and nurse educators from England, Northern Ireland, Scotland and Wales. Whilst this approach highlighted their passion and commitment to nursing, it also illuminated the nuances of healthcare provision being a devolved issue across the UK's constituent Governments, with variances obvious in how systems, structures, and processes operate under the construct of the National Health Service.

A further challenge has been the relentless pace of change within healthcare, which can render a book of this nature becoming dated very quickly; however, the unassailable commitment to art and craft of caring, which seeps from these chapters, does not change. With this in mind, within this text, some authors have opted to use the word *patient* to identify individuals within the practice population receiving direct care. The use of the word *patient* in this context is not intended to imply passiveness on behalf of individuals or a position of power exercised by the general practice nurse but to represent the provision of safe and effective person-centred care.

This book celebrates the advancement and contribution of general practice nursing in caring for the practice populations they serve and, amid a global pandemic, their dedication in the face of unrelenting pressure is applauded. We hope this book provides a valuable 'go-to book' for practice nurses beginning their journey, and we would like to express our thanks to each of the contributors who has worked with us to produce this text.

MARION M. WELSH
SUSAN F. BROOKS

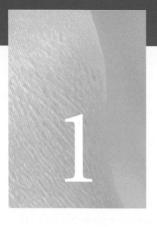

1

CONTEMPORARY GENERAL PRACTICE NURSING

NICKI WALSH

INTRODUCTION

General practice lies at the heart of first-contact primary care and is regarded as the bedrock of the National Health Service (NHS) in responding to the holistic healthcare needs of individuals, families and communities. In providing over 90% of care provision and consultations that greatly exceed the 300 million per year noted by NHS England in 2017, general practice provides a diverse range of healthcare services that includes access to individualised care and treatment, care co-ordination, and public health interventions, as well as referral to other NHS healthcare and social care services. This demonstrates not only the strengths and unique position general practice occupies in contributing to primary care but also the challenges it faces in remaining sustainable and responsive to the emergent demands of healthcare.

This chapter provides a contemporary overview of general practice and the essential role of general practice nursing in the provision and shaping of general practice services. This chapter introduces the key topics that will be contextually considered and expanded upon within the discrete chapters of this text.

IMPACT FACTORS AFFECTING HEALTHCARE PROVISION

The NHS is subject to perpetual change as it endeavours to provide safe, cost-effective, high-quality healthcare. Different ways of working, service reform, redesign and modernisation are just some of the watchwords used by the UK's constituent governments of England, Northern Ireland, Scotland, and Wales to convey change and establish fit-for-purpose healthcare. Whilst the impact of change on the NHS as an organisation, its constituent parts and its workforce should not be underestimated, inherently, change also envisions improvement and advancement.

A significant change experienced by general practice has been the paradigm shift in the provision of healthcare and social care services from a secondary care, hospital-based system to primary care. The catalyst for this change is rooted in contemporary healthcare provision being appreciably complex and diverse that the NHS's 'one-size-fits-all' approach has become outmoded. Consequently, transformational change has ensued to reform the NHS and associated social care services to ensure these are appropriate and sustainable to meet the emerging healthcare needs of the UK population.

Demographic Impact Factors

The structure, quality and utilisation of healthcare services within the NHS, and by default, general practice, are significantly influenced by a range of societal impact factors, which means the dynamics underpinning care provision are under perpetual review. Prominent amongst these is the ability of the NHS to cope with the increasing and challenging demands of caring for a rapidly ageing population and global migration.

This is evidenced by figures from 2018, when the net UK population was 66.4 million, the largest ever according to the Office for National Statistics (ONS, 2019), with predictions for the increase to continue and reach over 74 million by 2039. The ONS also confirms that 18% of the population is 65 or over, with 2.4% being over 85 years (ONS, 2017). This indicates that in 2016, there were 285 people aged over 65 for every 1000 aged between 16 and 64 years, this being the traditional working-age range, although this is changing. Whilst these data are based on a number of influencing factors, including birth, migration and mortality rates, they also show that the actual and potential impact of caring for an ageing population has significantly challenged the provision and sustainability of healthcare services and will continue to do so moving forward. Furthermore, the predictions around the health needs of individuals older than age 90 will have an impact. According to the ONS (2019), in 2018 there were 584,024 people in the UK aged over 90, including 13,170 centenarians (aged 100 years and over), reflecting a net increase of 0.7% in what is now classed as the 'very old' population.

Whilst greater life expectancy is seen as a positive health outcome, the paradox is that that living longer correlates with the risk of developing a long-term condition (LTC), such as cardiovascular disease, chronic respiratory conditions and diabetes. Moreover, the advancements in scientific knowledge and medical technologies that enable people to live longer also mean they may experience the development of multiple conditions and multiple morbidities (NHS England, 2014). This adds to the complexities in caring for a subgroup of the population who are more likely to experience poorer health outcomes, resulting in more intense packages of care and management. In a similar vein, meeting the social needs of ageing and frail populations can be inherently complicated and places a significant strain on delivery systems that are perpetually overextended and financially challenged (Robertson et al., 2017). These impact factors present unprecedented challenges and demands for service delivery across all areas of health and social care and require provider responses that are dynamic, safe, effective, and person centred to meet the expectations of individuals, families, and carers (Charles et al., 2018; Oliver et al., 2014).

Shaping Healthcare Provision

One model of care that has been mooted to address the aforementioned impact factors is 'moving care closer to home' (NHS England, 2014), which, as far as practicable, focuses on the wholesale provision of community-based integrated care. This model of transitional care entails general practice as the focal point

for care, the avoidance of unnecessary hospital admissions, effective hospital discharge planning and the efficient use of technology-enabled care provision, such as telehealth. Similar policies and reports that address transitioning healthcare provision from secondary to primary care have been produced by NHS Scotland (2016 (Health and Social Care Delivery Plan)), NHS Wales (2018 (Wales Planning Framework)), and the Department of Health of Northern Ireland (2016 (Systems Not Structures)).

These strategies do, however, require system-wide engagement, for example, buy-in via local sustainability and transformation plans (STPs; Alderwick et al., 2016), and signal the need for continued financial investment in the NHS and the social care sector to alleviate concerns regarding the increasing cost of delivering care (Robertson et al., 2017). Moreover, these strategies also highlight the need to proactively address workforce shortages, especially within general practice, where recruitment and retention are failing to keep pace with the demand for services (Ham et al., 2016; Queen's Nursing Institute, 2016).

ENVISAGING AN NHS FIT FOR PURPOSE

In 1948, the NHS was founded on the principle of providing excellent healthcare to society, and although fiscally funded, such care would be universally free at the point of delivery. Whilst this ideal remains steadfast, over the decades, it has become apparent that the NHS's generic approach to healthcare, as being "one size fits all," is neither practical nor sustainable. It is clearly recognised that the original 1948 model was created to manage the acute healthcare needs of a post-war society but has for several decades struggled to fully meet the complex and evolving needs of the UK population. These needs are reflected in the context of differing clinical priorities, primarily the healthcare burden associated with managing long-term conditions. However, despite the perceived deficits, there is a quintessential desire by the British public that the NHS should not only be maintained but also enhanced to ensure its responsiveness, capability, and capacity (Ham et al., 2016); this has been acutely sensed in the NHS's valiant response to the 2019 coronavirus (COVID-19) pandemic.

Successive UK governments have attempted to improve service provision by offering varying service models, such as those that support the improvement and integration of health and social care services. However, because of the nuanced complexities of care provision and limited resources, both human and financial, these do not always manage to keep pace with the ebb and flow of requirements. It could be contended that rather than continually developing new models, contemporary models need to be more adaptable to permit creative thinking and new ways of working to future-proof the provision of quality care and therein support dynamic leadership in driving sustainable change.

In some areas of the UK, healthcare solutions have seen the introduction of business-orientated models, with tight governance and quality-assurance measures that stem from industry and marketplace commissioning. This has resulted in variations in care provision and arguably resulted in a postcode lottery within some localities. It could be further argued that general practice has been propelled to the forefront of these redesign strategies, with little consideration of the consequences for the delivery of care, the workforce, or the practice population. The dissatisfaction this provokes raises important issues regarding the delivery of a sustainable and equitable healthcare system, one that needs to focus on the context of delivery rather than attempting a system-wide fix.

Landscape of General Practice

Any alteration in paradigm thinking regarding models of care needs to be supported by investments in people, places and provision (costs) and take account of attitudinal and cultural shifts around expectations. With this vision in mind, a number of policy directives have attempted to clarify the roles and responsibilities of general practice and professionals, for example, within England, the General Practice Forward View (NHS England, 2016) and Confidence, Capability and Capacity: A Ten Point Action Plan for General Practice Nursing (NHS England, 2018; see the Resources section). These strategies, as noted throughout this text, aim to support 'shifting the balance of care' to the general practice setting whilst simultaneously ensuring seamless care transitions, which still need to exist between the traditional silos of primary and secondary care.

A recent plan by NHS England, the NHS Long Term Plan (NHS England, 2019), details healthcare priorities and funding for the next decade and was developed through work with frontline professional groups, patient groups, and a range of other experts in the field and beyond. Similar policy developments have emerged in Scotland (NHS Scotland, 2016 (Health and Social Care Delivery Plan)), Wales (NHS Wales, 2018 (NHS Wales Planning Framework)), and Northern Ireland (Department of Health of Northern Ireland, 2019 (Systems Not Structures)). Ostensibly, the NHS Long-Term Plan does not bring anything new to the table in endorsing general practice as a pivotal part of a sustainable healthcare system, maintaining a holistic vision when 'doing things differently' and seeking engagement from all stakeholders. However, the Long-Term Plan does elevate the central importance of giving control back to the patient whilst simultaneously addressing public health priorities in protecting health, preventing ill health and the wider impact of eliminating health inequalities.

GENERAL PRACTICE – CONTRIBUTION AND STRUCTURE

The World Health Organisation (WHO) acknowledges the global importance of primary healthcare services in providing better access to services to enable better health outcomes and reduce hospitalisation, with a focus on personal healthcare and continuity of care rather than the curative 'disease model' (WHO, 2018, p. 4). Within the UK, the strengths of general practice lie in it being an 'expert medical specialist' model that provides high-quality holistic care in the context of sustained contact with local populations. General practice also evidences the extensive remit of professionals and the associated wider primary care workforce. With over 90% of care in the UK being delivered in community settings (Innes, 2019), the essential role general practice plays, and the equally indispensable role of the general practice nurse (GPN), is uncontested within the raft of healthcare policies, strategies, and frameworks that detail the structural context of general practice. Although these documents will adopt differing formats in the articulation of healthcare provision across the four UK countries, familiarity and understanding by the GPN are of critical importance as they provide the route map for care delivery, service provision, and importantly, the evolving role dimensions of the GPN. Equally important are the key nursing documents that complement the policy stance, such as the 10-point plan for general practice nursing (NHS England, 2018), which identifies the need to deliver more convenient access to care, more personalised care in the community and a stronger focus on prevention and population health, driving better outcomes and experiences for individuals.

The General Medical Services Contract

Although working mainly within partnerships, general practitioners (GPs) occupy an unparalleled position within the NHS in being self-employed independent contractors who provide services for NHS Trusts/ Boards in accordance with the General Medical Service (GMS) contract. In broad terms, the GMS contract is multifunctional in representing the mechanism for health improvement in community settings and details how GPs' services will be delivered and how they will be paid. The contract is nationally agreed; that is, it takes account of healthcare being a devolved issue across the four UK countries. The contemporary processes that secure the agreement of the contract, as it relates to England, Northern Ireland, Scotland and Wales, are similar in that NHS employers/governments negotiate with the General Practitioners Committee (GPC), which is part of the British Medical Association (BMA), on revisions, changes, and updates to the GMS contract.

Historically, the contracting of GP services existed before and after the inception of the NHS; however, it was not until the mid-1960s that the first GMS contract emerged. This contract remained largely unchanged until 1990, when the Conservative government imposed upon GPs a new contract outlining radical changes, such as GPs becoming fundholders; GP income based on treatment tariffs; clinical target setting; and stipulation of service to be provided, such as public health and chronic disease management initiatives. As a result, this contract was the catalyst for the expansion of the GPN role and resulted in a significant increase in the number of GPNs.

In April 2004 the 'new' GMS contract was implemented, bringing further reform with the introduction of renewed governance arrangements and financially incentivised payments based on a Quality Outcomes Framework (QOF), to which most general practices became signatories, although participation was voluntary. The justification for the introduction of the QOF lay in the delivery of quality, evidence-based care and improvements in the delivery of clinical care and services to local communities. The structure of the 2004 GMS contract remains contemporary and covers three main areas:

- **The Global Sum** – This covers the costs of running a general practice, including some essential GP services.
- **The QOF** – A financially incentivised scheme that covers the two areas of clinical and public health, and general practices can choose to provide these services. It should be noted, however, that as of 2016, the QOF was abolished in Scotland because practitioners found this system to be overtly bureaucratic and a tick-box exercise, which did not align with principles of general practice provision; this has now been replaced with the provision of a consolidated Global Sum. In Wales, the QOF has been replaced with the Quality Assurance and Improvement Framework (QAIF), and although the QAIF retains the incentivised point accumulation for financial remuneration, it is detailed under differing domains of quality assurance, quality improvement, and access.
- **Enhanced Services (ES)** – This covers additional services that practices can choose to provide, such as 24-hour ambulatory blood pressure monitoring, anticoagulation services, complex leg ulcer treatment and ear irrigation. ES can be commissioned nationally or locally to meet the population's healthcare needs.

Since 2004, the GMS contracts have been subject to review and updates based on the direction and priorities set by the sitting devolved governments across the four home countries, and although bespoke differences exist, the overarching themes offer consensus. For example, the 2018 GMS contract in Scotland articulates GPs as being 'expert medical generalists' who will work with an expanded general practice/multidisciplinary team in providing services and functions, many of which were traditionally the providence of GPs (Scottish Government, 2018). The contract indicates significant investment in the redesign of service models to better facilitate the delivery of the spectrum of care needs, from simple to complex. This investment also includes the development of the general practice workforce to extend its capability and capacity, examples of which relate to the continued development of general practice clusters. The role of the GPN is specifically highlighted within the Scottish GMS contract, endorsing the significant role GPNs play in the management of long-term conditions and minor illness; however, importantly, it is noted as a role that entails supporting the GP in the delivery of care planning.

In aligning with the Long-Term Plan (BMA, 2019), the English GMS contract, published in 2019, with a subsequent update in 2020, has been hailed as a 'game changer' with similar themes and ambitions regarding service improvement and significant financial investment. This includes establishing primary care networks and the wider recruitment of the general practice/primary care workforce. Also noted are planned enhancement for the patient experience, such as longer consultation times, the ability to book and attend online consultations, and direct access to other to frontline primary care professionals, all of which signal a sea-change in traditional structures and greater capacity for skill mix.

Although GMS contracts are nationally negotiated, those delivering the services need to be part of the process, especially when it comes to the assurance of professional competency. Any changes to contracts need to reflect support for professionals to attain and maintain competency.

GENERAL PRACTICE NURSING: MULTIFACETED, COMPLEX AND EVOLVING

The origins of general practice nursing can be traced back to the first GMS contract in 1966, which saw monies becoming available for ancillary staff to be employed in the general practice setting. In these early days, nurses were employed purely to work in treatment rooms to undertake fundamental nursing tasks, such as obtaining specimens, applying dressings, and administering injections. At this time, the range of skills required was not considered beyond that of any

registered nurse, and therefore GPNs did not require additional education or training to undertake these roles. However, with progressive changes to GP contracts in 1990 and in 2004 (as described earlier in the chapter), greater emphasis was placed on a diverse role for the GPN involving the management of long-term conditions, ill-health prevention and self-management techniques, which subsequently defined the need for additional education and training across the GPN workforce.

In 1998, the predecessor of the Nursing and Midwifery Council (NMC), the United Kingdom Central Council for Nursing and Midwifery (UKCC), published the standards for specialist education and practice and therein established the title of 'specialist practitioner' in relation to seven community nursing disciplines, including general practice. The NMC (2019, p. 2) articulates specialist practitioners as having a postregistration qualification relevant to their area of practice and therein being 'capable of exercising higher levels of judgement, discretion and decision making in clinical care in a specific practice area'. However, uptake of the Specialist Practitioner Qualification (SPQ) programme by some community disciplines, including general practice nursing, has been historically poor. A comprehensive stakeholder evaluation by the NMC (2019) identified a number of contributing factors, including perceptions of SPQ being unfit for contemporary practice. Furthermore, for the GPN, there is no requirement to undertake the SPQ qualification, unlike their district nursing peers. In 2020, the NMC indicated its intention to develop new standards of proficiency for SPQs, which includes general practice nursing.

The development of a new SPQ may address the QNI (2017) observations that the public still sees the role of the GPN as that of the traditional treatment room nurse. To ensure that the GPN role is both understood and valued, and to support career aspirations and succession planning, these perceptions must be challenged. To this end, the QNI plays a key role in articulating that the GPN role is multifaceted, complex, and evolving (Aldridge-Bent, 2017), as noted in Fig. 1.1.

This model identifies a role that exists beyond the provision of clinical tasks and captures the wide remit of professional knowledge, skills, and competencies needed by GPNs. In taking this work forward, the

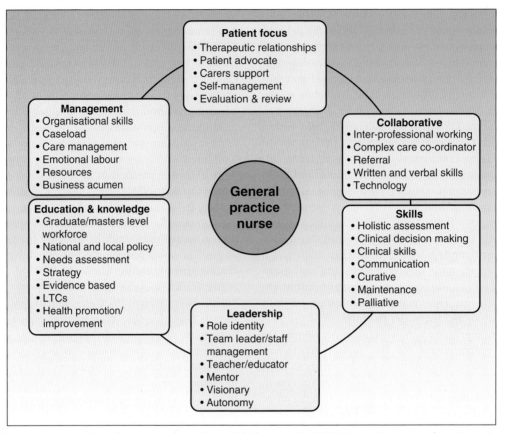

Fig. 1.1 ■ Contemporary vision of practice nursing. (From Aldridge-Bent, S. (2017). *In transition to general practice nursing.* Queen's Nursing Institute, p. 2.)

QNI has produced Voluntary Standards for Senior GPNs (QNI, 2017) and the QNI Standards of Education and Practice for Nurses New to General Practice Nursing (QNI, 2020). The Royal College of General Practitioners (RCGP) also developed a competency framework, which delineates a set of common core competencies and the range of skills, knowledge, and behaviours that align with being a proficient GPN (RCGP, 2015). However, it is recognised that this framework reflects an update of earlier work that commenced in 2012 and that service provision has changed considerably. Other organisations, such as Health Education England (HEE), have produced a career framework for GPNs that articulates with the NHS Knowledge and Skills Framework (see resources). The utility of these voluntary standards,

competencies, and frameworks lies in the opportunity they provide for illuminating role dimensions and allowing GPNs to reflect on and map their skills and knowledge against these to make further progress in professional development.

The aforementioned standards and competencies also provide valuable benchmarks in relation to recruitment to general practice nursing, where early-career GPNs may exhibit a significant level of nursing expertise and transferable skills (RCGP, 2015). However, the wide remit of the GPN role encompasses many areas of care provision that those new to the discipline may not have previously encountered, such as care of the child, management of long-term conditions and other preventative public health interventions, such as cervical screening and travel healthcare. To support recruitment and competency development, strategies such as the 10-point plan recognise the 'journey' for new and experienced GPNs and attempt to consolidate this by considering the variants that have an impact on and in practice. An example relates to caring for those living with diabetes (NHS England, 2015; Simmons et al., 2015; Walsh et al., 2011), who have traditionally been recipients of management packages that have been predominantly pharmacologically and medically focused, often losing sight of the individual, with the condition being central. Simmons et al. (2015) reference this in relation to a comprehensive set of competency statements developed by Training, Research and Education for Nurses in Diabetes (TREND-UK, 2015), which identify common clinical themes and align these with the requisite knowledge and skills required of the practitioner, on a level that ranges from unregistered to nurse consultant. These authors assert that whilst useful, this framework does not reference person-centred approaches or detail the requirements surrounding initial education and learning.

Multidisciplinary Teamwork in General Practice

For the GPN, multidisciplinary teamwork is imperative and contingent on developing a clear understanding of the structure and processes associated with general practice services, interprofessional working and service integration, and importantly, an appreciation of the roles and responsibilities of the wider team. The functionality of the multidisciplinary team (MDT) enables change to occur to improve the health and wellbeing of practice populations and meet the real-world expectations of patients, families, and carers. The MDT is an essential component in delivering quality care whose prominence has advanced within the general practice setting. NHS England (2014, p. 12) cites MDT as follows:

drawing appropriately from multiple disciplines to explore problems outside of normal boundaries and reach solutions based on a new understanding of complex situations.

They believe this can be achieved by:

Multidisciplinary and Multiagency working involves appropriately utilising knowledge, skills and best practice from multiple disciplines and across service provider boundaries, e.g. health, social care or voluntary and private sector providers to redefine, re scope and reframe health and social care delivery issues and reach solutions based on an improved collective understanding of complex patient need(s).

Charles et al. (2018) envision MDTs metaphorically wrapping around service users and their family/support network and emphasise the need to transcend professional boundaries and overcome 'silo working'.

Supporting the General Practice Workforce

The strategies outlined by the NHS in envisioning care, such as those detailed within the Five Year Forward View (NHS England, 2014), the General Practice Forward View (NHS England, 2016) and Next Steps in the Five Year Forward View (2017), are examples of consensus across the UK that identify that the healthcare workforce is critical to the success of moving care as close to the patient as possible; however, this is contingent on the development of effective recruitment and retention strategies. The General Practice Forward View (NHS England, 2016), in addressing concerns in this area, indicates key investments and improvements to support the workforce, such as a reduction in the bureaucratic burdens that affect general practice to release 'time' for care, care design, and the development of primary care estates. Equally important is the detail that aligns with developing the future workforce, which is particularly significant for succession planning within practice nursing (Walsh & Mason, 2018). Galvanising support and actively progressing interest in practice nursing as a career option is imperative, and across the UK, several initiatives have endorsed general practice as an appropriate learning environment for undergraduate nurses (Donley & Norman, 2018). The NMC (2019) standards also provide welcome opportunities for experienced GPNs to develop their roles as supervisors and assessors of nurse learners.

Enhancement of the GPN role in the delivery of safe and effective quality care delivery must also be supported via continuous professional development (CPD), which, as discussed in significant detail in Chapter 20, should be tailored to meet role expectations and the diversity of skills required within general practice. It is essential that the evidence-based knowledge, skills, and attributes of all staff working in general practice be maintained through effective and quality-assured education and training (Simmons et al., 2015; Walsh et al., 2011).

SUMMARY

General practice represents the focal point of care within the UK's healthcare system. The contemporary demands placed on general practice are evident in the shifting dimensions of care and service provision, coupled with the need to deal with increasingly complex healthcare and social care needs. GPNs have a pivotal role in shaping the effective provision of quality care to meet these challenges. Their role has progressed dramatically over the past decades and evolved in response to service developments, patient expectations and technological and clinical advancements. From these standpoints, general practice nursing has shown great adaptability and responsiveness, which are important attributes in progressing professional identity and the contribution GPNs make to care within the general practice setting.

RESOURCES

General Practice Forward View (NHS England, 2016): https://www.england.nhs.uk/wp-content/uploads/2016/04/gpfv.pdf

General Practice—Developing Confidence, Capability and Capacity: A Ten Point Action Plan for General Practice Nursing (NHS England, 2018): https://www.england.nhs.uk/wp-content/uploads/2018/01/general-practice-nursing-ten-point-plan-v17.pdf

The QNI Standards of Education and Practice for Nurses New to General Practice (QNI, 2020): https://www.qni.org.uk/wp-content/uploads/2020/05/Standards-of-Education-and-Practice-for-Nurses-New-to-General-Practice-Nursing.pdf

Royal College of General Practitioners (RCGP) General Practice Nurse Competencies: https://www.rcgp.org.uk/membership/practice-teams-nurses-and-managers/,/media/Files/Membership/GPF/RCGP-GPF-Nurse-Competencies.ashx

REFERENCES

Alderwick, H., Dunn, P., McKenna, H., Walsh, N., & Ham, C. (2016). *Sustainability and transformation plans in the NHS: How are they being developed in practice?* King's Fund.

Aldridge-Bent, S. (2017). *In transition to general practice nursing.* Queen's Nursing Institute.

British Medical Association. (2019). *Investment and evolution: A five-year framework for GP contract reform to implement the NHS Long Term Plan.* https://www.england.nhs.uk/wp-content/uploads/2019/01/gp-contract-2019.pdf

Charles, A., Ham, C., Baird, B., Alderwick, H., & Bennett, L. (2018). *Re-imagining community services.* King's Fund.

Department of Health of Northern Ireland. (2016). *Systems not structures—Changing health and social care.* https://www.health-ni.gov.uk/publications/systems-not-structures-changing-health-and-social-care-full-report

Donley, C., & Norman, K. (2018). Nursing student perspectives on a quality-learning environment in general practice. *Primary Health Care, 28*(4), pp. 36–42. https://doi.org/10.7748/phc.2018.e1388

Ham, C., Berwick, D., & Dixon, J. (2016). *Improving quality in the English NHS: A strategy for action.* King's Fund.

Innes, L. (2019). General Practice Nurse education in Scotland—now and in the future. *Education for Primary Care, 30*(5), 236–266. https://doi.org/10.1080/14739879.2019.1626771

NHS England. (2014). *Five year forward view.* https://www.england.nhs.uk/wp-content/uploads/2014/10/5yfv-web.pdf

NHS England. (2016). *General practice forward view: Workforce plan.* https://www.england.nhs.uk/gp/gpfv/workforce/

NHS England. (2017). *Next steps in the five year forward view.* https://www.england.nhs.uk/wp-content/uploads/2017/03/NEXT-STEPS-ON-THE-NHS-FIVE-YEAR-FORWARD-VIEW.pdf

NHS England. (2018). *Confidence, capability and capacity: A ten point action plan for general practice nursing.*

NHS England. (2019). *NHS long term plan.* https://www.longtermplan.nhs.uk/

NHS Scotland. (2016). *Health and social care delivery plan.*

NHS Wales. (2018). *NHS Wales planning framework 2019/22.* http://www.wales.nhs.uk/sitesplus/documents/862/Item%205.1.1%20NHS%20Wales%20Planning%20Framework%202019-22.pdf

Nursing and Midwifery Council. (2019). *Evaluation of post-registration standards of proficiency for specialist community public health nurses and the standards for specialist education and practice standards.*

Office for National Statistics. (2017). *Overview of the UK population: July 2017.* https://www.ons.gov.uk/releases/overviewoftheukpopulationjuly2017

Office for National Statistics. (2019). *Overview of the UK population: August 2019.* https://www.ons.gov.uk/releases/overviewoftheukpopulationjuly2019

Oliver, D., Foot, C., & Humphries, R. (2014). *Making our health and care systems fit for an ageing population.* King's Fund.

Queen's Nursing Institute. (2016). *General practice nursing for the 21st century: A Time of Opportunity.*

Queen's Nursing Institute. (2017). *Voluntary standards for nurses working in general practice.* https://www.qni.org.uk/nursing-in-the-community/practice-standards-models/general-practice-nurse-standards/

Queen's Nursing Institute. (2020). *The QNI standards of education and practice for nurses new to general practice.* https://www.qni.org.uk/wp-content/uploads/2020/05/Standards-of-Education-and-Practice-for-Nurses-New-to-General-Practice-Nursing.pdf

Robertson, R., Wenzel, L., Thomson, J., & Charles, A. (2017). *Understanding NHS financial pressures: How they are affecting patient care?* King's Fund.

Royal College of General Practitioners. (2015). *RCGP general practice nurse competencies.* https://www.rcgp.org.uk/membership/practice-teams-nurses-and-managers/,/media/Files/Membership/GPF/RCGP-GPF-Nurse-Competencies.ashx

Scottish Government. (2018). *The 2018 General Medical Services contract in Scotland.* https://www.gov.scot/binaries/content/documents/govscot/publications/advice-and-guidance/2017/11/2018-gms-contract-scotland/documents/00527530-pdf/00527530-pdf/govscot%3Adocument/00527530.pdf?forceDownload5true

Simmons D., Deakin, T., Walsh, N., Turner, B., Lawrence S., Priest, L., George, S., Vanterpool, G., McArdle, J., Rylance, A., & Terry, G. (2015). Diabetes UK position statement: Competency frameworks in diabetes. *Diabetic Medicine, 32*(5), 576–584. http://onlinelibrary.wiley.com/doi/10.1111/dme.12702/epdf

Training, Research and Education for Nurses in Diabetes (TREND-UK). (2015). *An integrated career and competency framework for diabetes nursing.*

Walsh, N., George, S., Priest, L., Deakin, T., Karet, B., Vanterpool, G., & Simmons, D. (2011). The current status of diabetes professional educational standards and competencies in the UK—A position statement from the Diabetes UK HCP Education Competency Framework Task and Finish Group. *Diabetic Medicine, 28*(12), 1501–1507. https://doi.org/10.1111/j.1464-5491.2011.0341

Walsh, N., & Mason, R. (2018). "Hitting the ground running": An evaluation of management placements for student nurses with UK general practice. *Primary Health Care, 28*(7), 34–41. https://doi.org/10.7748/phc.2018.e1443

World Health Organisation. (2018). *Primary health care: Closing the gap between public health and primary care through integration.*

2

PRACTICE NURSING: RESPONDING TO THE PUBLIC HEALTH CHALLENGES

MARION M. WELSH

INTRODUCTION

Despite the medical and social advancements that, over the decades, have resulted in population longevity and health improvement, contemporary public health activities remain dynamic in responding to the multitude of diverse challenges that currently exist within the UK. These challenges are primarily associated with protecting populations against environmental hazards and infectious diseases/viruses and the improvement of poor health outcomes that emerge as a consequence of complex health and societal problems.

The public health challenges faced by healthcare professionals are unquestionably serious, and whilst these challenges have never been greater, opportunities exist to make a positive impact to safeguard the public's health. Whilst the activities carried out by specialist public health professionals and the wider National Health Service (NHS) and social care workforce are diverse, they are purposefully driven towards protecting and promoting health and wellbeing and preventing ill health within populations, communities and individuals (Faculty of Public Health, 2018).

This chapter explores the contemporary context of public health and the significant contribution made by the general practice nurse (GPN). Consideration is given to the practical aspects of promoting health and applying contemporary theories, strategies and models to guide practice.

At the point of writing this chapter, the 2019 coronavirus (COVID-19) outbreak dominates the public health agenda, and whilst a raft of public health measures have been instigated to deal with this pandemic, detailed commentary is justifiably unavailable at this juncture. Nonetheless, the unprecedented challenges of COVID-19 reinforce the critical public health role played by public health specialists, practitioners, the NHS, the voluntary sector and the public.

CONTEMPORARY PUBLIC HEALTH

Formulating a contemporary understanding of public health acknowledges that the concepts and practices concerning its evolution are not new. Measures aimed at protecting the public's health can be dated much earlier than the public health movement of the 19th century, which sought to address unsanitary living conditions and communicable diseases triggered by industrialisation and social upheaval (Donaldson & Rutter, 2018), culminating in the first Public Health Act in 1848. Today's public health challenges are no less complex and pivot on the enduring issues of providing safe environments, reducing the number of years individuals spend in poor health caused by noncommunicable diseases, preventing infectious diseases and, importantly, reducing health inequalities (Institute of Health Equity, 2020). These challenges capture the broader environmental, societal and behavioural focus that defines public health in its quest to protect and improve the health of entire populations and communities to benefit individuals. This standpoint is reflected within the UK's continued uses of Acheson's (1988, p. 1) classic definition of public health as 'the science and art of promoting and protecting health, well-being, preventing ill-health and prolonging life through the organised efforts of society'.

However, establishing a contemporary understanding of public health must include consideration in a global context (Bloom & Caderette, 2019) to effectively prepare and respond to the worldwide threats posed by virulent infectious diseases that sporadically and rapidly emerge to present a serious risk to worldwide health (e.g., sudden acute respiratory syndrome (SARS), avian flu, Ebola, Zika, influenza (type A H1N1) and COVID-19).

Donaldson and Rutter (2018) clarify public health as having a clear remit in providing population-level interventions, thus differentiating it from clinical medicine's one-to-one, treatment-orientated engagement with patients presenting with a condition/problem. However, the synergy between these discrete health disciplines is being intentionally blurred to align with meeting the contemporary public health challenges, which are often the catalysts for ill-health presentations. Donaldson and Rutter (2018) also argue that the public health role is no longer the sole providence of those trained in the speciality (i.e., public health specialists and practitioners) but core for all healthcare and social care professionals/workers and as such requires collaborative multidisciplinary, multiagency and cross-sectoral working. This ethos is being reflected in the educational preparation of healthcare professionals, with the Faculty of Public Health's (2016) core domains of *Health Protection*, *Health Improvement* and *Healthcare Public Health* (quality service development and delivery) being evidenced within medical, nursing and some allied health professions curricula (Public Health Educators in Medical Schools/Faculty of Health 2019; Nursing and Midwifery Council (NMC), 2018b, 2019).

Tackling the persistent public health challenges facing the UK places a strong focus on wellness and therein synergy with these aforementioned core domains. However, the language used to explain and expand on these domains is often interchangeably used to identify subcategories and areas of practice, within which specific population health interventions are detailed. For example, *health protection* is associated with ill-health prevention by identifying and eradicating/reducing risk factors. *Health improvement*, used synonymously with *health promotion*, is associated with strategies that enable and empower individuals to adopt healthy behaviours. Table 2.1 provides some examples of activities that would align with the Faculty of Health (2016) core domains.

TABLE 2.1		
Examples of Public Health Activities Within Core Public Health Domains		
Health Protection	**Health Improvement**	**Healthcare – Public Health**
Screening and surveillance	Epidemiology; monitoring prevalence, incidence and patterns of disease and other variables impaction on health	Evidence-based interventions
Pathogenesis and immunology		Contemporary models
Immunisation, vaccination and herd immunity		supporting behaviour change
Infection prevention and control	Global health – patterns of health and wellbeing outcomes	Skills development for service users
Communicable disease surveillance	Determinants of health, illness and wellbeing	Risk assessment and assessment tools
Antimicrobial stewardship and resistance	Health literacy; information accessibility	Policy awareness and influencing; health and safety legislation/regulation
Responding to potential hazards	Inequalities in health outcomes	Health economics
National screening	Promoting healthy behaviours and living across the life span	Informatics, data analytics, interpretation and management
Emergency responses	Child development and adverse childhood experiences (ACEs)	Research and audit
	Violence, abuse and safeguarding	Commissioning, planning
	Empowerment	Integrated assessment, care planning and evaluation
		Communication and advocacy skills, partnership and collaborative working
		Cultural competence

SOCIAL DETERMINANTS OF HEALTH AND HEALTH INEQUALITIES

The persistent public health challenges of preventing poor health, keeping people safe and enabling people to live longer are well versed across a wide spectrum of UK policies, strategies and professional literature (Craig & Robinson 2019; Public Health England (PHE), 2016). These challenges are also clearly described across a variety of clinical contexts, in particular, in caring for the increasingly older population and addressing the exponential increase in long-term conditions and multimorbidity (Mercer & Wang, 2020). However, a consistent thread permeating these aspects of the public health agenda is the necessity to acknowledge the impact of social determinants of health to narrow the gap in health inequalities.

Targeting the social determinants of health remains at the crux of efforts to improve public health outcomes by conveying the social conditions that affect how individuals live and thrive (Marmot & Bell, 2019). The social determinants of health are multifactorial and associated with key variables, such as early-years experiences, environments, education, employment, housing and supportive networks/communities (Institute of Health Equity, 2020). As a complex set of interrelated circumstances that has the potential to positively or negatively influence health outcomes, the determinants of health generally lie beyond the remit of NHS healthcare provision. However, knowledge of their impact is important because these determinants are largely responsible for health inequalities, where the root cause lies in the relationship between poverty and ill health and therein limits people's knowledge and sense of control in shaping health choices.

The World Health Organisation (2007 p3) indicates that 'Social inequities in health are systematic differences in health status between different socio-economic groups. These inequities are socially produced (and therefore modifiable) and unfair'. Braveman et al. (2017, p. 4) provide a contemporary definition of the term *health inequity,* more commonly used within North America to pinpoint determinants that are deemed socially unjust:

Health equity means that everyone has a fair and just opportunity to be as healthy as possible. This requires removing obstacles to health such as poverty,

discrimination and their consequences, including powerlessness and lack of access to good jobs with fair pay, quality education and housing, safe environments and health care.

McCartney et al. (2019, p. 28) debate the context and meaning of *health inequalities,* including whether these inequalities, in contrast to the NHS Health Scotland (2015) stance, occur by chance, and contemporaneously offer the following definition:

Health inequalities are the systematic, avoidable and unfair differences in health outcomes that can be observed between populations, between social groups within the same population or as a gradient across a population ranked by social position.

Irrespective of the debate points, experiencing health inequalities represents living in circumstances that inflict more years spent in ill health and limit life expectancy (Institute of Health Equity, 2020). The differences in people's health status across the population, and population subgroups, emerges as a loss – a loss of personal potential, reduced earning capacity, opportunities and privileges (NHS Health Scotland, 2015).

Whilst there have been, over previous decades, notable improvements in healthcare and social care provision, resulting in better health outcomes and increased life expectancy, the last decade has not maintained this trend. Life expectancy, recognised as a measure of health, has, for the UK's most affluent 10%, continued to improve; however, this sharply contrasts with the most deprived 10%, where life expectancy has either stalled or fallen (Institute of Health Equity, 2020). In real terms, PHE (2019) translates this as a difference of 19 years between the poorest and most affluent in society, meaning health inequalities within society remain a serious threat to population health and wellbeing. Consequently, the publication *Health Equity in England: The Marmot Review 10 Years On* (Institute of Health Equity, 2020) is damning in its criticism of the lack of progress towards health attainment based on the continued expansion of the health divide, resulting in deprived populations experiencing longer periods in poor health, diminishing life expectancy and increased mortality rates at an earlier age. Moreover, the report highlights the impact of austerity, particularly in relation to regional and gender variables, such as the declining life expectancy of women living in northern England. Whilst the findings of this report concern England, the findings are transferable to populations within Scotland, Northern Ireland and Wales. Consequently, the report challenges the government's policy makers to recognise that healthcare has less of an impact on people's health than the wider social determinants, with routes to improvement needing to align with political action and social change to improve the public's health.

PUBLIC HEALTH PRIORITIES

Against this backdrop, the UK's constituent governments' respective healthcare policies and strategies continue to pinpoint public health imperatives to drive forward actions to optimise health outcomes, reduce health inequalities within communities and increase life expectancy. Underpinned by the need for responsive, progressive, cohesive and integrated healthcare and social care strategies, public health agencies (PHE, Public Health Agency for Northern Ireland, Public Health Scotland, Public Health Wales) demonstrate broad consensus in conveying overarching priorities that reflect improving health and tackling inequalities:

1. Environments: Protection from environmental hazards and infections to provide healthy, safe communities
2. Promote population health: Living well, eating well, healthy weight, physical activity
3. Early years: Securing the health of future generations
4. Improving mental health and wellbeing: Reducing suicide and self-harm; building resilience
5. Healthy behaviours: Harm reduction; reduced use of alcohol, tobacco, and other recreational drugs
6. Strengthen public health systems and function: Developing and mobilising knowledge and skills to improve health and wellbeing
7. Promoting staff health and wellbeing: Healthy working environments

Whole-Systems Approaches and Primary Care

An overarching concept within contemporary public health is the development of whole-systems approaches to support the attainment of nationally set priorities (Department of Health/PHE, 2014; Public Health Agency for Northern Ireland, 2014; PHE, 2019; Public Health Scotland, 2019; Public Health Wales, 2019), which in some regions of the UK have been developed in conjunction with local authorities. An example of this type of partnership agreement exists between the Scottish government and the Convention of Scottish Local Authorities (COSLA), which, following a major review of public health function in Scotland (Scottish Government, 2015), triggered a programme of reform to improve healthy life expectancy and reduce health inequalities within communities.

The essence of a whole systems approach involves communities, people and professionals working collaboratively to tackle real-life public health challenges and in doing so develop shared understandings of how local systems need to operate to bring about sustainable change in the short, medium and long terms to benefit individuals (PHE, 2019). This captures the complexity of threading together multiple variables that benefits the whole of the healthcare system and entails the crosscutting involvement of all stakeholders, including patients. As part of this whole-systems approach, primary care remains the bedrock of accessible first-contact care provision, and in this context, general practice nursing's contribution to protecting health, promoting health and preventing ill health is significant. The GPN's unique scope of practice across the age span provides sustained opportunities to engage with individuals, families, carers and communities to positively contribute to public health strategies.

NURSING AND THE GPN CONTRIBUTION TO PUBLIC HEALTH

Operating across a wide variety of health settings, nurses and midwives make a significant contribution to improving health outcomes and reducing inequalities as part of their contact with individuals, communities and populations (NMC, 2018b, 2019). Although public health activities are historically within nursing practice (Donovan & Warner, 2017), the extent to which therapeutic interventions actually and potentially occur is generally contingent on the types of roles and responsibilities and the level of engagement. These are reflective of specialist public health roles, for example, specialist community public health nurses (health visitors, school nurses, occupational health nurses, family health nurses), health protection nurses and infection prevention and control nurses, and those with a less specialised and intensive focus but a nonetheless critical role, such as GPNs. The contributions of the wider nursing workforce are captured within several contemporary publications, such as the Royal College of Nursing (2016) report *The Value and Contribution of Nursing to Public Health in the UK* and the Royal College of Midwives' (2017) 'Stepping Up to Public Health: A New Maternity Model for Women and Families, Midwives and Maternity Support Workers'.

Whilst the aforementioned publications relate to post-qualifying roles, a recurring theme within the nursing literature is the need to prepare the undergraduate nursing and midwifery workforce to meet the real-world public health challenges and therein ensure the sustainability of healthcare provision (Clark et al., 2016; Lasater et al., 2020). These authors argue that preregistration educational curricula based solely on an illness model are untenable. Taking cognisance, the NMC's Standards of Proficiency for Registered Nurses (NMC, 2018b) now require nurse learners to demonstrate knowledge, skills and attributes to address population health in 11 public health–orientated proficiencies (Platform 2, 'Promoting Health and Preventing Ill Health'). Similarly, the new Standards of Proficiency for Midwives (NMC, 2019) also indicate 10 proficiencies that must be successfully achieved. The GPN is ideally placed to assist learners in achieving these proficiencies under the new NMC arrangements for placement learning (NMC, 2018a).

In occupying a unique and privileged position in having sustained contact with individuals, families and carers, the GPN has significant capability to drive forward public health interventions. Although the GPN does not currently have a direct role in the strategic shaping of public health provision at a population level, this being the providence of specialists, GPNs have a clear remit at the individual and community levels:

■ Individual level: Holistic person-centred care, which may entail enabling and empowering patients to assume greater control over their health outcomes via health promotion strategies; providing information to patients, families and carers on a range of public health topics; signposting to evidence-based information; and delivering health surveillance, screening and immunisation programmes.

■ Community level: Undertaking needs assessment of local practice population and developing services to meet needs, which may range from smoking cessation for discrete population groups (Ross, 2020) to domestic abuse (Smickle et al., 2020) to engaging with community issues, engaging in advocacy and being a community resource for health improvement.

More pragmatically, the GPN's role in contributing to 'Making Every Contact Count' (PHE, 2016) as part of everyday interactions with individuals is of crucial importance and involves utilising strategies and behaviour-change interventions to support and empower people to make positives changes in their lifestyles. Health Education England has developed a repository of practical resources and examples for practitioners, teams and organisations. Similarly, GPNs will find the Department of Health/PHE (2014) *Framework for Personalised Care and Population Health for Nurses, Midwives, Health Visitors and Allied Health Professionals: Caring for Populations Across the Life Course* a useful resource (see Resources section).

PROTECTING HEALTH, PROMOTING HEALTH, PREVENTING ILL HEALTH

Whilst the public health agenda provides the direction and vision for population health, within the primary care setting, the GPN's role is bounded by interventions in which the theoretical basis remains firmly fixed on promoting health and wellness for the patients, families and communities they serve. These interventions may take place opportunistically or intentionally and, depending on the nature of the consultation, will unquestionably be wide ranging.

The confines in which specific *health protection* interventions occur are most likely, depending on local arrangements, to be associated with national population-based immunisation and health screening programmes. Consequently, the GPN requires a sound knowledge of the UK immunisation schedule (Gov. UK, 2019) and the various screening programmes (UK National Screening Committee, 2018), irrespective of whether these may take place on-site within the general practice setting (e.g., cervical screening), at a central/mobile location (breast screening and abdominal aortic aneurism screening) or are self-administered (bowel screening). The GPN occupies a critical role in supporting patients to uptake vaccinations and participate in screening programmes because misinformed perceptions of risk and the fear associated with procedures and result outcomes are commonplace. The GPN may also have responsibilities, which include immunisation for travel (see Chapter 19) and employment (hepatitis B) as well as promoting screening associated with the management of long-term conditions, with some practices providing additional services, such as retinopathy screening for their patients with diabetes.

Healthcare Screening

As a well-established public health strategy, the key purpose of screening is to detect the absence or presence of disease indicators in individuals who are currently asymptomatic to prevent the onset of disease and/or delay its progression. At a fundamental level, screening differs from clinical medicine by intentionally targeting apparently healthy people who may be at risk of developing a particular disease and instigating screening at a preclinical stage to change the disease trajectory and prognosis (UK National Screening Committee, 2018). However, it is important to recognise that, per se, screening is not a diagnostic tool but the mechanism by which the identification of a 'positive' screening test triggers a referral to a clinician for further investigation to refute or confirm diagnosis, and in respect of the latter, instigate treatment.

The increasing priority to optimise health outcomes across the life span and tackle the health burden associated with long-term conditions means that screening activities across the UK are wide ranging and currently overseen by the UK National Screening Committee (UKNSC). The UKNSC, as an independent body, continuously evaluates current evidence and recommends population screening for an extensive range of clinical conditions (see Resources section). A primary function of the UKNSC is to ensure that screening improves health outcomes and does not introduce unacceptable risks, which could result in doing more harm than good. For these reasons, national screening programmes for a number of major diseases do not exist, for example, for type 2 diabetes, where there is insufficient evidence to indicate that screening is more effective than opportunistic case finding, and for lung cancer, where screening would save lives but with testing procedures that would carry significant risk and be expensive to conduct at a population level. These issues are evident in the seminal criteria set out by Wilson and Junger (1968), which are still used to inform the development and implementation of screening programmes:

1. The condition being screened for should represent an important health problem.
2. There should be treatment available for those with a confirmed diagnosis.
3. There should be facilities available to diagnose and treat the disease.
4. There should be a recognisable latent or early symptomatic stage of the disease.
5. A suitable evidence-based test/examination should be available.
6. The test/examination should be acceptable to the population.
7. The natural history of the disease should be understood.
8. There should be policies in place that identify whom to treat as patients.
9. The cost of screening should be economically viable as part of the total cost of healthcare.
10. Screening should be a continuous process to support refinement of the methods, processes, and outcomes of screening.

Wilson and Junger's (1968) criteria are indicative of tests/examinations, which require demonstrating they are safe, easy to perform, easy to interpret, and importantly, accurate, reliable, sensitive and specific. The latter emphasises that whilst 'no test is 100% effective' in detecting the presence of disease indicator(s), a test does need evidence of the extent to which is it highly reliable and valid:

■ **Reliability** means that if the same test was repeated on the same person time after time, the same results would consistently occur.

- **Validity** means the screening test demonstrates a high level of sensitivity and specificity.
  - **Sensitivity** is the ability of the test/examination to identify 'true positives' (i.e., a disease indicator is present).
  - **Specificity** is the ability of the test/examination to identify 'true negatives' (i.e., a disease indicator is not present).

The ability of a test/examination to exhibit high 'specificity' and 'sensitivity' is not always possible, with the potential for 'false-positive' and 'false-negative' results to occur. However, whilst there is some tolerance for false positives in the context of screening, which further diagnostic investigation will address, any potential for high rates of false negatives for screening tests/examinations is untenable.

Promoting the engagement of health screening with patients is also contingent on an awareness of the ethical dimensions, which, beyond the necessity for beneficence, entails respect for patient autonomy in terms of patients' right to decline health screening. Common reasons for nonengagement are often associated with fear, anxiety or phobia of the screening procedure or receiving positive test results. To this must be added the ethical and legal practical dimensions of screening within vulnerable groups, such as adults with incapacity and those with a learning disability who will require support in engaging with mainstream services (see Chapter 16).

Along with the UK's national screening programmes and the ongoing secondary and tertiary surveillance screening of patients diagnosed with long-term conditions, the GPN may be involved in local screening initiatives and campaigns that focus on major causes of mortality and morbidity, such as cardiovascular and kidney disease, diabetes and dementia. In aligning with anticipatory care (see Chapter 4), these initiatives often take the form of risk-based assessment, awareness raising and management 'health checks' (England: NHS Health Check Ages 40–74, NHS Health Scotland: Keep Well Ages 40–64, Northern Ireland Chest, Heart and Stroke (NICHS) Public Well Checks, NHS Wales Health Check) that in some localities are specifically targeted within populations experiencing health inequalities. These health checks involve history taking and the assessment of lifestyle and biometric risk factors associated with particular conditions, for example, physical activity, smoking status, blood pressure, body mass index (BMI), blood glucose and cholesterol level. NHS England indicates that evaluation of the efficacy of health checks remains challenging due to a lack of randomised controlled trials; however, Cambridge University (2017), on behalf of PHE, provided evidence that these types of public health–focused screening initiatives save lives.

The GPN has a substantial role in operationalising health screening, and the numerous barriers that prevent patients from engaging with screening emphasise the importance of health improvement strategies to increase knowledge and understanding to enable health choices. More practical measures may entail consideration of how local screening services are communicated, delivered and supported to address personal issues relating to time, childcare and travel to attend screenings. Consequently, the GPN, in having sustained contact with target and at-risk groups, needs to be well versed not only in the practical and ethical parameters influencing screening but also in the legal issues that relate to dealing with defined population subgroups.

Health-promoting activities are a broad and complex field of practice but focus on enabling people to make lifestyle choices and adopt behaviours that prevent the onset of disease and disability where the impact can be overwhelming, physically, mentally and socially. For the GPN, health promotion mainly resonates with reducing alcohol consumption, smoking cessation, healthy diet and physical activity in the context of supporting patients' self-management of long-term conditions. However, in being distinct from clinical medicine, where the priority centres on treatment, the effort to promote health and prevent ill health occurs at the primary, secondary and tertiary levels. For example, the correlation between smoking and chronic obstructive pulmonary disease establishes primary intervention as dissuading individuals from starting smoking to minimise the risk of disease occurrence; secondary prevention occurs after diagnosis and aims to prevent further decline in lung function and to reduce physical incapacity, social isolation and depression (Global Initiative for Chronic Obstructive Lung Disease, 2019); and tertiary prevention focuses on minimising acute exacerbations via anticipatory care

to hospital admissions. These levels of intervention equally apply to the spectrum of public health issues the GPN may encounter, such as sexual health consultation where risk-taking behaviour is a threat to health (see Chapter 15) and mental health wellbeing (see Chapter 12).

The GPN's ability to promote health and support patients in making behaviour changes requires knowledge, skill and familiarity with strategies and models, which are practical and applied in reference to the UK government's health policies, public health priorities and the NMC Standards of Proficiency (NMC, 2018b). Whilst the latter details the proficiencies to be demonstrated by nurse learners in 'promoting health and preventing ill health' (Platform 2; NMC, 2018b), these standards, as Thompson (2020) notes, equally apply to the registered nurse underpinned by knowledge of current public health drivers, epidemiology and use of public health information and intelligence (informatics, data analytics, interpretation).

THEORIES, MODELS AND STRATEGIES

As components of public health, strategies aimed at promoting health are rooted within behavioural sciences and employ models of health promotion aimed at positively influencing people's knowledge, attitudes and behaviours, enabling them to take control of their health outcomes. However, the variables that influence individuals' behaviours are multifactorial, and GPNs need to sensitively take account of patients' priorities based on their real-world social and environmental lived experiences (Thompson, 2020); to do otherwise negates the science of nursing practice. This caution resonates with the sentiment expressed within the Ottawa Charter (World Health Organisation, 1986, p. 4), which indicates, 'Health is created and lived by people within the settings of their everyday life; where they learn, work, play and love'.

Whilst challenges for the GPN exist in triggering health-promoting discussions as part of a consultation, not the least of which is based on the inherent time constraints, a range of evidence-based health promotion strategies and models exist to support and manage consultations. Primarily, these strategies and models serve as frameworks to guide practice

and structure interventions; however, the real-world application will undoubtedly exhibit limitations, and any foray into the literature will provide a critique on which to base an evaluation of their utility. Another variable that the GPN must consider is that not every patient they encounter will have the same willingness or capacity for behaviour change. However, therapeutic communication, and the forum this provides, can be a potent tool for promoting behaviour change. Communication will be used in varying formats, be these verbal (brief intervention, motivational interviewing, health promotion models) and often in conjunction with other strategies and resources, which may include the use of technology/social media as forms of positive reinforcement. However, as considered in the following discussion, communication also involves consideration of health literacy.

Brief Intervention

Brief intervention involves communication and negotiation skills to initiate and structure meaningful conversation on health issues, such as smoking, alcohol use and physical activity. Brief intervention is based on the Ask, Advise, Act model (National Institute for Health and Care Excellence (NICE), 2018) and is highly applicable within the general practice setting because it represents a cost-effective and evidence-based approach that has been successfully used in addressing a range of lifestyle issues. The premise of brief intervention, whether used in a shortened 'stand-alone' form as 'very brief advice' (VBA) or as part of longer 'extended' sessions, is to explore with patients their motivations and provide support to them as they contemplate risk reduction by changing their behaviour. For example, VBA can be used to raise the issue of cigarette smoking, which still remains the UK's primary cause of preventable morbidity and premature death. Ross (2020) indicates that VBA represents a rapid and practical approach to recording smoking status and triggering discussions with patients who may have moved beyond a precontemplative state (Prochaska & DiClemente, 1982) and are perhaps ready to take proactive steps towards stopping smoking (Fig 2.1).

Ross (2020) further indicates that practitioners should not be deterred from making repeated annual inquiries about smoking status, and for those patients attending annual/interim reviews for long-term conditions, this provides an appropriate opportunity to make this contact count. The use of VBA concurs with evidence-based guidelines produced by NICE (2018) for smoking cessation, which are deemed to be more successful if patients are in receipt of support and guidance. GPNs are well placed to initiate discussions using VBA, which may eventually entail referral to local specialist smoking cessation services, where interventions may include the use of e-cigarettes, nicotine replacement therapy (NRT), CO_2 monitoring, motivational interviewing and coaching. The

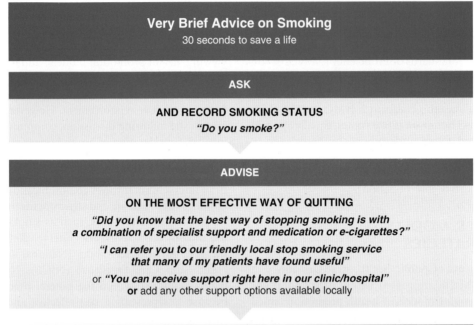
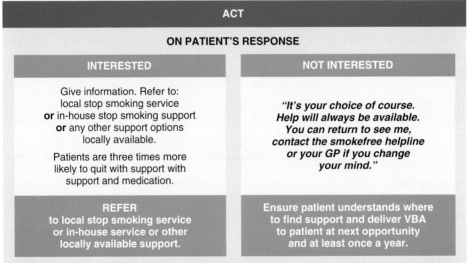

Fig. 2.1 ▪ Very brief advice on smoking. (From Ross L. (2020). Smoking cessation 1: Interventions to support attempts at quitting. Nursing Times, 16(3), 30–33.)

Tailoring VBA to match available local support

Identify hierarchy of locally available stop smoking support
The list of stop smoking interventions below are ranked in order of effectiveness.

Identify which interventions are **readily available locally.** The highest ranked interventions should inform the ADVISE and ACT components of *Very Brief Advice on Smoking.*

Support	Available ✓
1. Local Stop Smoking Service: behavioural support from a trained specialist stop smoking practitioner + medication (combination NRT, varenicline, burpropion) or e-cigarette	
2. In-house stop smoking service: behavioural support from trained stop smoking practitioner + medication (combination NRT, varenicline, burpropion) or e-cigarette	
3. Medication (combination NRT, varenicline, burpropion) prescribed by a doctor, or use of an e-cigarette	
4. Behavioural support alone from a trained stop smoking practitioner	
5. Medication (combination NRT) *over the counter* from a pharmacist, on general sale or use of an e-cigarette	
6. A proactive telephone helpline staffed by trained stop smoking practitioners	
7. A single episode of smoking cessation advice in addition to delivery of VBA	
8. Provide contact information for Smokefree National Helpline	
9. Printed self-help materials	
10. Stand alone text messaging service	
11. Other (specify):	

Fig. 2.1, cont'd

National Centre for Smoking Cessation and Training (NCSCT) provides evidence-based e-learning resources for practitioners to develop skills in deploying brief interventions (see Resources section).

Motivational Interviewing

Another viable strategy is motivational interviewing, defined as 'a collaborative, person-centred form of guiding to elicit and strengthen motivation for change' (Miller & Rollnick 2009) that adopts a non-confrontational empathetic counselling style to develop and strengthen an individual's motivation for behaviour change. Originally developed to mediate changing behaviour for substance misuse and addiction disorders, this evidence-based intervention has developed wider applicability in the context of promoting health. Motivational interviewing involves a therapeutic communication about change, which involves using open questions and reflection to clarify an individual's aspirations, ability and plans to change. The premise of motivational interviewing is to persuade rather than coerce, using communication to strengthen the motivation for and movement towards a specific goal by eliciting and exploring the person's own arguments for change through the following strategies:

1. **Express empathy through reflective listening:** This indicates particular attention being paid to the type of language used by practitioners within the discussion, this being equally as important as the content.
2. **Develop discrepancy between clients' goals or values and their current behaviour:** This indicates exploring with patients how their current behaviour differs from what they would like this to look like.
3. **Avoid argument and direct confrontation:** This indicates that behaviour change will only occur when people feel ready to do so, not when 'told to'.
4. **Adjust to client resistance rather than opposing it directly:** This indicates accepting that patients may/will hold competing views or ambivalence about their behaviours and signals the need to work from and respect their position.
5. **Support self-efficacy and optimism:** This indicates that the solutions patients may identify for themselves are more likely to be the most effective and ones they can sustain.

In recognising that the advanced communication and counselling skills needed to instigate conversations using motivational interviewing may influence its success, training in this medium has been recognised as a necessary starting point. Consequently, a number of programmes are available, such as that offered by the Royal College of Nursing, which further indicates that motivational interviewing provides an additional resource to support 'Making Every Contact Count' and provides an online training module to develop practitioner skills (see Resources section).

Contemporary Health Promotion Models

Other traditional approaches to promoting health, using well-established models, which, within the healthcare arena, continue to be utilised as valid contemporary frameworks on which to structure interventions, include the following:

- Health belief model (Rosenstock, 1966; later adapted by Becker, 1974)
- Theories of reasoned action (Fishbein & Ajzen, 1975)
- Transtheoretical stages of change model (Prochaska & DiClemente, 1982)
- Social learning theory (Bandura, 1977)
- Self-determination theory (Deci & Ryan, 1991)

These models, rooted within behavioural sciences to motivate behaviour change, entail differing perspectives in clarifying the variables that influence lifestyle choices and explore approaches to promoting change. The use of these models typically demands sustained interactions with patients to explore, review and provide support over weeks and months. Thompson (2020) provides very clear depictions of the health belief model (Fig. 2.2) and the stages of change model (Fig. 2.3) that could be pragmatically applied by the GPN in a range of situations.

Health Literacy

Health literacy has clear linkage with health protection and promotion in the context of public health. It is defined as the 'degree to which individuals have the capacity to obtain, process, and understand basic health information and services needed to make appropriate health decisions' (Ratzan & Parker, 2000), which, along with age and the range of social determinants, has been shown to be a strong predictor of individuals' health status.

A significant proportion of the population suffers from poor health literacy and particularly those with lower socioeconomic status, and in having a correlation with behavioural risk factors, limited use of healthcare systems results in poorer healthcare outcomes. Patients with long-term conditions, physical and mental, have also been noted as having poor literacy skills, which has implications for the GPN in remaining cognisant of the potential existence of poor literacy skills.

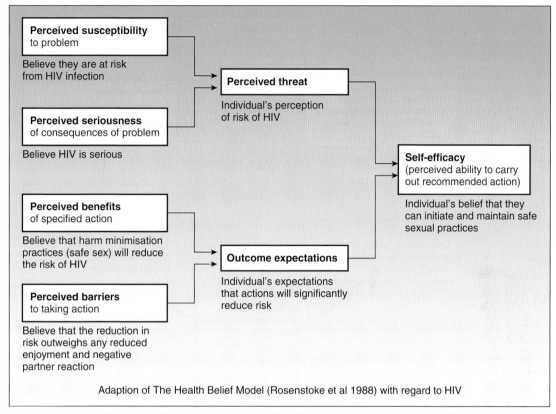

Fig. 2.2 ■ The health belief model. (From Thompson, S. R. (2019). Supporting patients to make lifestyle behaviour changes. Nursing Standard, 35(12). https://doi.org/10.7748/ns.2019.e11338)

Health literary reflects language development relative to oral literacy, involving speech and speech comprehension; print literacy, determined by the ability to read, write and understand written language; and finally, functional literacy, involving literacy to perform a specific task. In promoting health, the GPN, other members of the multidisciplinary team and administration staff may become aware of patients exhibiting difficulty with health literacy in relation to those who, for example, do not uptake screening invites, have difficulty in understanding treatment/concordant regimens, have frequent hospitalisations and generally exhibit poorer overall health. Key indicators of poor health literacy may also include failure to complete documents such as patient registration questionnaires, frequently missed appointments and follow-up referrals and failure to take or errors in self-administration of medication because they cannot read the labels. These important indicators have obvious links to medication mismanagement, delayed diagnosis and more patients more likely to engage in risk-taking behaviours. The UK's constituent governments have sought to address health literacy needs via a range of strategies and resources, including the use of technologies to effect better health outcomes, and have produced a range of resources for population groups and clinical conditions (see Resources section). Improving patients' knowledge, understanding and skills to use health information is a fundamental aspect of the GPN's role in and contribution to improving the public's health.

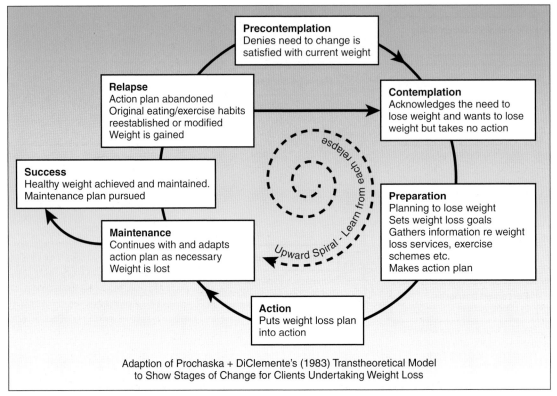

Fig. 2.3 ■ The stages of change. (Adapted from Prochaska, J. O., & DiClemente, C. (1982). Trans- theoretical therapy: Toward a more integrative model of change. Psychotherapy Theory Research and Practice, 19(3), 276–288.)

SUMMARY

The key challenges associated with the public health agenda present the GPN with a raft of opportunities to support the health and wellbeing of the practice population. Having an understanding of the contemporary facets of what drives public health and utilising tools to enable pragmatic deployment are fundamental aspects of the GPN role and the contribution GPNs make.

RESOURCES

A range of valuable generic and bespoke resources exist to support GPNs in developing their public health role; the following are of particular relevance to the primary care setting:

CPD Practice Nursing – NHS Education for Scotland: https://learn.nes.nhs.scot/24328/nursing-cpd/general-practice-nurse-continuing-professional-development-cpd-learning-resource

Framework for Personalised Care and Population Health for Nurses, Midwives, Health Visitors and Allied Health Professionals: Caring for Populations Across the Life Course: https://assets.publishing.service.gov.uk/government/uploads/system/uploads/attachment_data/file/377450/Framework_for_personalised_care_and_population_health_for_nurses.pdf

Gov.UK Immunisation Schedule 2019: https://assets.publishing.service.gov.uk/government/uploads/system/uploads/attachment_data/file/855727/Greenbook_chapter_11_UK_Immunisation_schedule.pdf

Health Literacy for All; Assistive Technology for Patients and Staff in Northern Ireland: https://www.texthelp.com/en-gb/sectors/workplace/healthcare/ni/

Motivational Interviewing: https://www.rcn.org.uk/clinical-topics/supporting-behaviour-change

National Centre for Smoking Cessation and Training: https://www.ncsct.co.uk/publication_very-brief-advice.php

NHS Education for Scotland – The Health Literacy Place: http://www.healthliteracyplace.org.uk/

NHS England Health Literacy Toolkit: https://assets.publishing.service.gov.uk/government/uploads/system/uploads/

attachment_data/file/377450/Framework_for_personalised_
care_and_population_health_for_nurses.pdf

Public Health England: Making Every Contact Count (MECC):
https://www.gov.uk/government/publications/making-every-
contact-count-mecc-practical-resources

Public Health Agency Northern Ireland: https://www.publichealth.
hscni.net/

Public Health Scotland: https://publichealthscotland.scot/

Public Health Agency for Northern Ireland – Corporate Plan
2017–2021: https://www.publichealth.hscni.net/sites/default/files/
directorates/files/PHA%20Corporate%20Plan%202017-2021.pdf

Public Health Wales: https://phw.nhs.wales/

Public Health Wales – Our Strategic Plan 2019–2022: https://
phw.nhs.wales/about-us/our-priorities/long-term-strategy-
documents/public-health-wales-strategic-plan-2019-22/

Royal College of Nursing: Motivational Interviewing: Video
Scenarios: https://www.rcn.org.uk/clinical-topics/supporting-
behaviour-change/motivational-interviewing-video-scenarios

Royal Society for Public Health – Everyday Interactions Tool Kit:
https://www.rsph.org.uk/static/uploaded/2c2132ff-cdac-4864-
b1f1ebf3899fce43.pdf

UK National Screening Committee – Guidance for the Development,
Production and Review of Information to Support UK Population
Screening Programmes: https://assets.publishing.service.gov.uk/
government/uploads/system/uploads/attachment_data/file/730598/
UK_NSC_screening_information_development_guidance.pdf

REFERENCES

Acheson, D. (1988). *Acheson report: Independent inquiry into
inequalities in health report.* The Stationery Office.

Bandura, A. J. (1977). *Social learning theory.* Prentice Hall.

Bloom, D. E., & Cadarette, D. (2019). Infectious disease threats in
the 21st century: Strengthening the global response. *Frontiers in
Immunology, 10,* 549. https://www.frontiersin.org/arti-
cles/10.3389/fimmu.2019.00549/full

Braveman, P., Arkin, E., Proctor, D., Acker, J., & Plough, A. (2017).
What is health equity? https://behavioralpolicy.org/wp-content/
uploads/2018/12/What-is-Health-Equity.pdf

Cambridge University. (2017). *NHS Health Check Programme rapid
evidence synthesis.* https://www.healthcheck.nhs.uk/
seecmsfile/?id=306?

Clark, M., Raffay, M., Hendricks, K., & Gagon, A. J. (2016). Global
and public health core competencies for nursing education: A
systematic review of essential competencies. *Nurse Education
Today, 40,* 173–180.

Craig, A., & Robinson, M. (2019). Towards a preventative approach
to improving health and reducing health inequalities: a view
from Scotland. *Public Health, 169,* 195–200.

Deci, E. L., & Ryan, R. M. (1985). *Intrinsic motivation and self-
determination in human behavior.* Plenum.

Department of Health/Public Health England. (2014). *Framework
for personalised care and population health for nurses, midwives,
health visitors and allied health professionals: Caring for
populations across the life course.* https://assets.publishing.service.

gov.uk/government/uploads/system/uploads/attachment_data/
file/377450/Framework_for_personalised_care_and_
population_health_for_nurses.pdf

Donaldson, L. J., & Rutter, P. D. (2018). *Donaldson's essential public
health* (4th ed.). CRC Press.

Donavan, H., & Warner, J. (2017). Nurses' role in public health and
integration of health and social care. *Primary Health Care, 27*(8),
20–24.

Faculty of Public Health. (2016). *Good public health practice
framework.*

Faculty of Public Health. (2018). *Role of the NHS in prevention:
Discussion paper.*

Global Initiative for Chronic Obstructive Lung Disease. (2019). *Global
strategy for the diagnosis, management, and prevention of chronic
obstructive pulmonary disease 2020.* https://goldcopd.org/wp-
content/uploads/2019/11/GOLD-2020-REPORT-ver1.0wms.pdf

Gov.UK. (2019). *Immunisation schedule 2019.* https://assets.
publishing.service.gov.uk/government/uploads/system/uploads/
attachment_data/file/855727/Greenbook_chapter_11_UK_
Immunisation_schedule.pdf

Institute of Health Equity. (2020). *Health equity in England: The
Marmot Review 10 years on.*

Lasater, K., Kyle, R. G., & Atherton, I. M. (2020). Population health
as a platform for nurse education: A qualitative study of nurse
leaders. *Nurse Education Today, 86,* 1–6.

Marmot, M., & Bell, R. (2019). Social determinants and noncommunicable disease: Time for integrated action. *British
Medical Journal, 365,* 10–12.

McCartney, G., Popham, F., McMaster, R., & Cumbers, A. (2019).
Defining health inequalities. *Public Health, 172,* 22–30.

Mercer, S. W., & Wang, H. H. (2020). Long-term conditions. In A.
Staten & P. Staten (Eds.), *Practical general practice: Guidelines for
effective clinical management.* Elsevier, pp. 7–10.

Miller, W. R., & Rollnick, S. (2009). Ten things MI is not. *Behavioural and Cognitive Psychotherapy, 37,* 129–140.

National Institute for Health and Care Excellence. (2018). *NICE
guideline NG92: Stop smoking interventions and services.* https://
www.nice.org.uk/guidance/ng92/chapter/Recommendations

NHS Health Scotland. (2015). *Health inequalities: What are they?
How do we reduce them?* Scottish Government.

Nursing and Midwifery Council. (2018a). *Standards for student
supervision and assessment.*

Nursing and Midwifery Council. (2018b). *Standards of proficiency
for registered nurses.*

Nursing and Midwifery Council. (2019). *Standards of proficiency
for midwives.*

Prochaska, J. O., & DiClemente, C. (1982). Transtheoretical therapy: Toward a more integrative model of change. *Psychotherapy
Theory Research and Practice, 19*(3), 276–288.

Public Health Agency for Northern Ireland. (2017). *Corporate
plan 2017–2021.* https://www.publichealth.hscni.net/sites/de-
fault/files/directorates/files/PHA%20Corporate%20Plan%20
2017-2021.pdf

Public Health Educators in Medical Schools/Faculty of Health.
(2019). *Undergraduate public health curriculum for UK medical
schools 2019: A consensus statement.* https://www.fph.org.uk/

media/2685/phems-updated-consensus-statement-2019-with-foreword_final.pdf

Public Health England. (2016). *Public health skills and knowledge framework.* https://www.gov.uk/government/publications/public-health-skills-and-knowledge-framework-phskf

Public Health England. (2016). *Making every contact count (MECC): Consensus statement.*

Public Health England (2019). *PHE strategy 2019–2025.* https://assets.publishing.service.gov.uk/government/uploads/system/uploads/attachment_data/file/830105/PHE_Strategy__2020-25__Executive_Summary.pdf

Public Health England. (2019). Whole systems approach to obesity: A guide to support local approaches to promoting a health weight. https://assets.publishing.service.gov.uk/government/uploads/system/uploads/attachment_data/file/820783/Whole_systems_approach_to_obesity_guide.pdf

Public Health Scotland. (2019). *The reform programme.* https://publichealthreform.scot/the-reform-programme/scotlands-public-health-priorities

Public Health Wales. (2019). *Our strategic plan 2019–2022.* https://phw.nhs.wales/about-us/our-priorities/long-term-strategy-documents/public-health-wales-strategic-plan-2019-22/

Ratzan, S. C., & Parker, R. M. (2000). Introduction. In C. R. Selden, M. Zorn, S. C. Ratzan & R. M. Parker (Eds.), *National Library of Medicine current bibliographies in medicine: Health literacy* (NLM Pub. No. CBM 2000–1). National Institutes of Health.

Ross L. (2020). Smoking cessation 1: Interventions to support attempts at quitting. *Nursing Times, 16*(3), 30–33.

Royal College of Midwives. (2017). *Stepping up to public health: A new maternity model for women and families, midwives and maternity support workers.*

Royal College of Nursing. (2016). *The value and contribution of nursing to public health in the UK.*

Scottish Government. (2015). *Review of public health in Scotland: Strengthening the function and re-focusing action for a healthier Scotland.*

Smickle, M., Woods, J., & Lee, M. (2020). Development of a nurse-led domestic abuse service for general practice. *Nursing Times, 116*(3), 20–23.

Thompson, S. R. (2020). Supporting patients to make lifestyle behaviour changes. *Nursing Standard, 35*(12). https://doi.org/10.7748/ns.2019.e11338

UK National Screening Committee. (2018). *Guidance for the development, production and review of information to support UK population screening programmes.* https://assets.publishing.service.gov.uk/government/uploads/system/uploads/attachment_data/file/730598/UK_NSC_screening_information_development_guidance.pdf

Wilson, J. M., & Junger, Y. G. (1968). *Principles and practice of mass screening for disease.* World Health Organisation.

World Health Organisation. (1986). *Ottawa charter for health promotion.* https://www.who.int/healthpromotion/conferences/previous/ottawa/en/

World Health Organisation 2007. Concepts and principles for tackling social inequities in health: Levelling up Part 1. Denmark: World Health Organisation. https://www.euro.who.int/__data/assets/pdf_file/0010/74737/E89383.pdf

3

DELIVERING QUALITY HEALTHCARE IN GENERAL PRACTICE

MARION M. WELSH

INTRODUCTION

General practice nursing is characterised by a role that is complex, varied and highly autonomous and therein carries with it clear expectations that the care provided will be of the highest quality (Scottish Government, 2018). For the general practice nurse (GPN), this entails demonstrating the professional knowledge and skills that culminate in delivering safe, effective, compassionate patient-centred care. Notably, this requires of the GPN the ability to articulate the evidence base on which quality care is provided to justify clinical decision-making and care planning and to involve patients in the delivery of such care.

The dimensions that drive the provision of quality care in the general practice setting represent a plethora of interrelated activities, which necessitates having a clear understanding of the concept, dimensions and dispositions of quality healthcare, in terms of what it means, what drives it, how it is measured, and finally, how it is developed and sustained. Quality, as it relates to healthcare, nonetheless represents a vast and complex topic arena, and consequently, a wealth of detailed literature exists, representing differing and varied perspectives, from organisational, professional and clinical standpoints. This chapter, however, seeks to provide a strategic overview of key concepts associated with delivering high-quality healthcare as a forerunner to discussions on its discrete application, which are contextually applied within the subsequent chapters of this book.

DEFINING QUALITY IN HEALTHCARE

The maxim for high-quality care has become common parlance within successive governments' healthcare policies and the National Health Service (NHS) and has initiated numerous programmes for change, redesign and improvements to meet public expectations (Jabbal, 2017). However, capturing the practical meaning of 'high-quality healthcare' to achieve a universally acceptable definition remains both challenging and elusive, and a wide array of definitions exists, influenced by differing stakeholder perspectives, be these organisations, regulatory bodies, professionals or patients.

The Department of Health's (2008) expression of quality healthcare continues to hold sway, centring on three core concepts: patient safety, clinical effectiveness, and importantly, the experience of patients. These concepts have come to represent the contemporary understanding of quality healthcare, not only at the legislative and healthcare policy level across the four UK countries (where the responsibility for healthcare delivery is devolved) but also professionally, as reflected in the Royal College of General Practitioners' (2016, p. 9) articulation of quality healthcare as a

commitment to continually improving the quality of healthcare focusing on the preferences and needs of the people who use services. It encompasses a set of values (including self-reflection, shared learning, partnership, leadership, the use of theory, and understanding of context) and a set of methods (including measurement, understanding variation, cyclical change, benchmarking and a set of tools and techniques).

Whilst definitions of quality healthcare seek to convey an outline of its meaning and expectations, its practical application is contingent on the use of a quality framework, such as Donabedian's (1980) classic model, which provides the basis for practitioners to consider care delivery in terms of the following:

- Structure: In determining how care is strategically organised
- Process: The actions undertaken/discrete elements of care provision that will be addressed
- Outcomes: Evaluating/measuring the impact

These concepts become a practical reality when aligned with six key performance quality indicators originally proposed by the internationally renowned Institute of Medicine (2001) as being safe, timely, effective, efficient, patient centred and equitable. Whilst these quality indicators provide a global framework for quality healthcare provision, their implementation, relative to discrete clinical presentations and care pathways, needs to be practically detailed to comply with expectations associated with evidence-based clinical standards. This permits the general practice team to establish structures and processes on which subsequent patient outcomes will be evaluated and therein demonstrate good clinical governance.

CLINICAL GOVERNANCE PRIORITIES

At a strategic and organisational level, quality healthcare remains highly politicised, and the need to visibly deliver and measure the quality of healthcare has, over the past few decades, continued to gather momentum. This sharply contrasts the early days of the NHS where the quality of care was implicitly regarded as good due to the public's trust in the NHS and professionals, by virtue of their education and training. However, between 1980 and 2000, politically driven modernisation of the NHS witnessed significant change with the recognition of patients' legal rights (the Patient's Charter of 1991, now subsumed within documents such as the NHS Constitution for England 2015 (NHS England, 2015) and the Patient Rights (Scotland)

Act 2011), benchmarking clinical standards and professionalism. In parallel with these activities, the National Institute for Health and Care Excellence (NICE) and the Scottish Intercollegiate Guidelines Network (SIGN) emerged and were charged with overseeing the publication of evidence-based clinical guidelines, and accountability became a watchword embedded in the concept of clinical governance.

Less auspiciously, the origins of clinical governance were also fuelled by failings within the NHS, firstly witnessed with the unacceptably high mortality rates for paediatric cardiac surgery (Bristol Royal Infirmary) and the retention of human organs without consent (Alder Hey Hospital) and then, secondly, with the heinous criminal acts perpetrated by Harold Shipman and Beverly Allitt. These events triggered numerous legislative acts across the four home countries, which imposed a statutory 'duty of quality' on care NHS organisations, which would thereafter be subject to monitoring and, where necessary, investigation to improve the quality of care provision. These emerged in the form of healthcare regulators within the four home countries (Care Quality Commission (England), Regulation and Quality Improvement Authority (Northern Ireland), Healthcare Improvement Scotland, Healthcare Inspectorate Wales) to oversee and report on the provision of quality care. However, despite the processes put in place, high-profile cases have continued to occur, such as the failings in 2013 of the Mid Staffordshire NHS Foundation Trust (Francis, 2013), demonstrating that clinical governance does not offer a panacea to offset serious professional and systems failures.

Clinical Governance Framework

Scally and Donaldson (1998, p. 61) classically defined clinical governance as

> *a framework through which NHS organisations are accountable for continuously improving the quality of their services and safe-guarding high standards of care by creating an environment in which excellence in clinical care will flourish.*

Whilst corporate responsibility for clinical governance lies with the NHS, responsibility and accountability for its implementation are devolved to individual NHS trusts/boards/organisations and individual practitioners.

Gray (2005) more meaningfully captured these actions as the 'right care, at the right time, by the right person', and since then, this phrase continues to be ubiquitously used to convey clinical governance. However, despite the conciseness of Gray's (2005) comments, these actions are contingent on the available best evidence; appropriately trained, competent and resourced practitioners/teams; and crucially, the involvement of the patient in decision-making processes. These elements are evident within the seven pillars of the clinical governance framework (Pearson, 2017), which, having synergy with the aforementioned key performance quality indicators, outlines a set of interrelated 'duty of quality activities', which seek to direct professionals and assure patients, via transparent structures, processes and outcomes, that the care they receive will be characterised by the following:

1. **Clinically effective:** Care/therapeutic interventions that are based on the best evidence available and have measurable outcomes – for example, use of evidence-based guidelines (NICE, SIGN) to inform the development of local/area practice protocols in the direct delivery of care that aim to eliminate wide variations in care.
2. **Risk managed:** Internally, within the organisation, the risk of harm is minimised within clinical settings via application of evidence-based clinical interventions and to inform local polices, which are subject to regular review, risk identification and reporting. Externally, professional risk is managed in the context of professional statutory regulatory bodies (Nursing and Midwifery Council, General Medical Council, Health Care Professions Council), self-regulation and validation/accreditation activities; practising within legal and ethical frameworks.
3. **Patient centred:** Care interventions that are based on patient preferences and culturally sensitive needs and values and involve the patient in decision-making processes.
4. **Cost effective:** Use of resources within care delivery and services that is effective and efficient and avoids waste.
5. **Organisationally effective:** Care delivery that aligns with the organisation's espoused strategic aims in providing quality care.

6. **Transparent:** A culture that supports open, transparent, high-quality communication, within and across NHS organisations and with partner agencies.
7. **Founded by a Learning Organisation:** Promoting and leading continuous improvement through reflection and organisational learning; professional development of individuals to support the delivery of high-quality care.

DELIVERING QUALITY CARE IN GENERAL PRACTICE

General practice has, since its inception, undergone significant change but nonetheless continues to demonstrate the provision of high-quality first-contact care (Care Quality Commission, 2017). The current challenges facing general practice are both diverse and numerous and currently predicate on effectively managing the shift in the balance of care from secondary to primary care, caring for ageing populations at increased risk of long-term conditions, multimorbidity and addressing health inequalities (Buck et al., 2019). To support these efforts, as detailed throughout the chapters of this book, evidence-based clinical standards, guidelines and models of care/service delivery aim to standardise and optimise the quality of care provided. From this standpoint, the GPN has a central role in supporting the implementation of evidence-based interventions.

Evidence-Based Practice

As a ubiquitous and well-established term, *evidence-based practice* (EBP) embodies a framework whose significance lies in the critical role it plays in supporting clinical decision-making. The World Health Organisation (WHO, 2017, p. 2) emphasises the important relationship between EBP and clinical decision-making in supporting the practitioner's ability to 'consider the feasibility, appropriateness, meaningfulness and effectiveness of health-care practices'.

Sackett et al.'s (2000, p. 1) updated seminal definition of EBP as 'the integration of best available evidence, clinical expertise and patient preferences and values' represents a relatively straightforward approach to conceptualising the tripartite elements. However, its application belies the complex set of interrelated processes and activities that align with the aforementioned seven pillars of clinical governance to support clinical decision-making processes.

The core elements of Sackett et al.'s (2000) original model continue to influence the array of contemporary EBP models, such as that offered by the Joanna Briggs Institute (JBI), an internationally recognised forum for nursing research. The JBI's updated model of evidence-based healthcare (Jordan et al., 2019) strategically details the multilayer elements of EBP and how these could be pragmatically used to guide real-world nursing practice. Noteworthy within the JBI model are activities associated with feedback and evaluation, which represent specific activities that resonate with joint decision-making with patients as part of real-world implementation. However, despite the aspirations of the model of care, the pursuit of delivering quality patient-centred care can be complex and challenging, particularly when current best evidence and practitioner knowledge indicate a specific course of action, but the patient does not concord – for example, in the management of venous leg ulceration, where the assessment and evidence clearly indicate treatment with four-layer compression bandaging but the patient is unwilling to accept or unable to tolerate. The reasoning for nonconcordance may become evident during the clinical consultation or at a later stage and necessitates sensitive communication inquiry. The implications are that in some instances, respecting patient autonomy (Valero, 2019) overrides the potential to maximise the opportunity to provide quality care, despite having the necessary resources.

Accessing Best Evidence to Inform Practice

Notable within many of the EBP models, including the one offered by the JBI (Jordan et al., 2019), is that the use of 'evidence' represents knowledge drawn from differing sources and differing types of evidence, which might be representative of the following:

1. **Empirical scientific research:** Such as that which is contributed to the production of clinical guidelines/standards by organisations, such as those produced by NICE, SIGN, and the British Thoracic Society for a range of conditions, such as asthma, diabetes, and chronic obstructive pulmonary disease (COPD).
2. **Data drawn from locally conducted audits and service evaluations:** Reports and recommendations based on data derived from evaluating clinical outcomes against benchmarked standards (local/national reporting).
3. **Professional expertise:** To inform decision-making.
4. **Individual patient preferences**

EBP is, however, an approach to practice and therefore is not synonymous with undertaking scientific research (Table 3.1), the former having a broader remit in supporting and informing decision-making in the delivery of quality care.

For the GPN, an array of clinical guidelines, such as those produced by SIGN and NICE, provide swift access to clinical evidence and standards to inform the development of bespoke practice-based protocols. The evidence-based guidelines produced by these organisations are compiled following robust scrutiny and ranking to establish their quality. This is reflected in the hierarchy of evidence (Ingham-Bloomfield, 2016), with expert opinion–based knowledge (e.g., case study or clinical reports, often produced by professional colleges/societies) being the least reliable form of evidence and robustly conducted randomised

TABLE 3.1	
Comparing Evidence-Based Practice and Research Approaches to Practice	
Evidence-Based Practice	**Research**
Systematic search for, and appraisal of, best *available* evidence	Systematic, planned scientific investigation determined by:
Use of evidence from a range of sources for making decisions; the evidence may be produced by research	Specifications of practice-based/clinical 'problem' to be investigated
Account taken of patient/client preferences, needs	Predetermined outcomes (i.e., results; recommendations)
Justifies or brings about a change in clinical practice	Contributes to understanding of the world – knowledge generation

controlled trials and systematic reviews/meta-analyses representing the cornerstone of evidence due to the scrupulous methodologies applied within these types of studies.

The reality of engaging with scientific research processes, whether as a consumer or investigator, can be daunting, but against the backdrop of safe and effective quality healthcare, nursing's historical propensity to solely rely on intuition and tradition to justify clinical decision-making is no longer tenable. Contemporary expectations of the GPN role indicate a skill set that includes the ability to appraise empirical healthcare research to examine, debate, initiate and support change in practice. Whilst an array of research-based texts exists to assist in developing critical appraisal skills, the GPN, in reviewing empirical research, needs to consider the following inquiry-based questions (Moule et al., 2017):

- Is the quality of the empirical evidence sufficiently convincing?
- Are the findings applicable/relevant in my professional setting/clinical context?
- What do the results/findings mean for my practice and my patients?

The presentation of research evidence normally emerges as either a qualitative- or quantitative-based study, formulated on the basis of a research question. The perspective offered by qualitative research is inquiry based on investigating real-life experiences by gathering narrative data to explore subjective meanings, perceptions and feelings. Conversely, quantitative research is objective and rooted in gathering numerical data to measure and conduct hypothesis testing (Robson & McCartan, 2016).

Technology has enabled the relatively easy search and retrieval of evidence-based literature via a range of relevant electronic bibliographic databases, such as MEDLINE (Medical Literature Analysis and Retrieval System Online), CINAHL (Cumulative Index to Nursing & Allied Health Literature), AMED (Allied and Complementary Medicine Database) and PsycINFO. Further, JBI and the Cochrane Collaborative also contribute to the range of resources and offer subject-specific systematic reviews. Engaging with NHS librarians, often located with local hospital libraries or continuing professional development facilities, can prove extremely useful for GPNs in their effort to develop expertise and confidence with database-searching skills.

To assist in the appraisal of research studies, be they individual research studies or systematic reviews, a number of critical appraisal tools exist, and amongst the most well known are those provided by the Critical Appraisal Skills Programme (CASP). These are essentially checklists, tailored to assess the specific methodological designs of research studies, presented as a set of questions specifically designed for evaluating the quality of research, allowing the practitioner to determine the trustworthiness and credibility of the findings presented (Robson & McCartan, 2016).

MEASURING QUALITY CARE – GENERAL PRACTICE

Clinical Audit

Within the general practice setting, the ability to measure quantifiable clinical outcomes, based on locally existing and available data sets, is relatively easy to achieve. Consequently, measuring quality in this way equates with conducting local clinical audits, which seek to benchmark current care provision against an established standard to evaluate and plan for service development and improvement. This would result in activities that, in line with Donabedian's model, would determine, for example, the following:

- Structure: The availability within the practice of a particular service; staffing and environmental considerations
- Process: Establishing the clinical and administrative elements of care that comprise this service
- Outcome: Impact, clinical or other, on the patient

In this context, the clinical audit represents a cyclical activity based on key stages, as follows:

- **Establish the benchmarked standard**: For example, consulting the evidence-based guidelines offered by NICE and SIGN.
- **Measure and compare current practice against benchmark:** Establish what is going to be measured by whom; comparison should be made in a nonjudgmental, transparent manner.
- **Reflect, plan, and implement change.**

- **Re-audit:** Within an appropriate time frame
- **Outcome:** Evaluation of the impact of changes using robust measures

A range of audit tools and templates exists to assist practitioners in becoming familiar with the audit principles, such as those provided by the Royal College of General Practitioners (RCGP; see Resources section).

Incentivised Schemes

Over the last 3 decades, a number of target-driven, financially incentivised voluntary schemes have been operationalised within the general practice setting and embedded within the successive renewal of the UK government's contract with general practitioners (GPs). Using quantifiable metrics, these pay-for-performance schemes have sought to drive and measure the quality of care by gathering information, primarily on process and clinical outcome indictors, benchmarked against national standards. For example, in managing type 2 diabetes, *outcome* measures would elicit the number of patients within the practice with this condition and how many of these patients attended for annual review, had their HbA1c measured within the last 6 months, had annual retinopathy screening performed and had their blood pressured measured. Outcome measurement would also include discrete clinical measurements, such as HbA1c, weight and blood pressure; however, Bampoe et al. (2018) suggest that these types of biophysical markers are poor discriminators in the delivery of quality care because they can be easily influenced by other extraneous variables that can affect their accuracy; in other words, a patient may be receiving exemplary care but exhibit poor clinical outcomes and, conversely, may experience poor care but demonstrate excellent clinical outcomes.

Acknowledging that healthcare delivery is a devolved issue, the mainstay of this incentivised information-gathering process is, for NHS England, NHS Northern Ireland and NHS Wales, and prior to 2016 for NHS Scotland, embodied within the Quality Outcomes Framework (QOF). This framework was universally introduced within England, Northern Ireland, Scotland and Wales as part of the General Medical Services (GMS) contract on 1 April 2004. As a pay-for-performance scheme, general practices are rewarded for achievement in a range of activities, which align with point accumulation resulting in financial payment in relation to the following:

- Clinical indicators
- Public health indicators (including the provision of additional services)
- Patient experience indicators
- Records and systems indicators

Whilst there is evidence that the quality of care delivered in general practice has undoubtedly improved, debate exists regarding the extent to which the QOF contributed to this effect. This is reflected in the contrasting views held about the relative merits of the QOF in contributing to and improving patient-centred quality care, particularly in responding to the contemporary challenges associated with managing long-term conditions and multimorbidity, as noted within Forbes et al.'s (2017) systematic review. Further criticism of the QOF sees this as being a reductionist tick-box exercise, highly selective in targeting specific conditions at the expense of others and poorly aligned in addressing health inequalities. Conversely, NHS England (2018) highlights the QOF's success in raising the standard of care by reducing the potential for variable suboptimal care and keenly argued this in relation to shifting the balance of care in respect to the management of long-term conditions, where more focus is being placed on localised primary care access and provision.

Despite the debate points, what does appear evident is that general practices have become more experienced and adept in assessment, care planning and supporting the patient's journey by developing skills in data handling, evaluation and prioritising services based on local needs. However, it is also clear the debate and ramifications of working within the QOF framework have, at national levels, witnessed and initiated divergent change. In NHS England, NHS Northern Ireland and NHS Wales, the QOF continues, with some concessionary modifications to structure and provide the basis for quality monitoring within primary care. In contrast, in 2016, Scotland opted to abolish the QOF in favour of a core global payment, which was triggered by concerns raised by professionals regarding the QOF's disproportionate focus on the biomedical model of care, the negative impact on patient consultations and its bureaucracy processes, which were inconsistent with the values of general practice and therein professionally unfulfilling. As detailed within the Scottish government publication *Improving Together* (Scottish Government, 2017), Scotland has developed, as part of reforming primary care provision, a National Monitoring and Evaluation Strategy for Primary Care in Scotland (Scottish Government, 2019) detailing a primary care outcomes framework, which will incorporate, from a range of sources, both quantitative and qualitative data to assess quality. A further quality strategy, which both Wales and Scotland are progressing, is the formation of GP clusters, which entails the grouping of five to eight GP practices within the same locality engaging in peer activities that promote the quality of care in general practice. This sense of collaboration and integration to deliver responsive, quality care within local communities has, within NHS England, emerged in the formation of sustainability and transformation plans.

CONTINUOUS QUALITY IMPROVEMENT

A critical element in the delivery of quality healthcare services is the commitment to continuous improvement, which entails maintaining a persistent focus on examining and optimising performance within the service. The practical aspects of continuous quality improvement involve people in real-world problem-solving activities, implementing change and evaluating outcomes in the pursuit of high-quality healthcare. A body of work exists on activities that support continuous quality improvement, and this includes sets of common principles that promote continuous improvement processes within NHS organisations, which Dawda et al. (2010, p. 5) outline as follows:

- **Culture:** A culture of quality should exist throughout the organisation. Quality should be prioritised over other issues, and every member of staff should be involved in delivering and improving quality.
- **Aims:** The needs of the patient are paramount, with the key aim being delivery of quality as perceived by the patient.

- **Collaboration:** Teamwork, evidenced by joint learning, planning and service delivery, is critical to the organisation's work.
- **Training:** Specific tools and techniques are employed to improve quality, rather than intuition and consensus alone. As with any science, there is a need to train staff to apply these.
- **Anti-perfectionism:** It is never assumed that ideas for service improvement will be perfect. Even seemingly excellent ideas are tested through practical implementation before being fully adopted. Similarly, care is never judged to have become perfect.

Models and Methodologies

To further assist practitioners in undertaking continuous quality-improvement activities, a range of contemporary methods, models and tools has emerged, exhibiting differences in their purpose and therefore worthy of appraisal regarding their discrete application. Amongst these are two that, despite having emerged from the industry sector, have gained increasing popularity within healthcare due to their focus on safety and quality enhancement (Kaplan et al., 2014):

- **Lean methodology:** This approach to continuous quality improvement seeks to eliminate practices that are wasteful and fail to add value to the service (Rotter et al., 2019). The ethos underpinning what is commonly referred to as 'lean thinking' centres on 'doing more with less' in the use of existing resources. Lean is founded on the principles of respect for people and the use of process mapping to identify deficiencies and the Plan–Do–Study–Act (PDSA) review cycle to implement and evaluate change. The benefits suggest improved efficacy and speed (NHS Institute for Innovation and Improvement, 2017). Within the general practice setting, case studies exist to show that this approach had a positive impact on service provision, particularly in relation to patient experience and empowering professions (Hung et al., 2015). Furthermore, as part of the ubiquitous Releasing Time to Care/Time to Care programmes that emerged across the NHS, the Productive General Practice Quick Start initiative has sought to develop the capacity and capability for quality improvement via a hands-on-site short-term support package (NHS Institute for Innovation and Improvement, 2017).

■ **Six sigma:** This is an organisational tool that aims to eliminate variable care, improve performance and promote capability (NHS Institute for Innovation and Improvement, 2017). This problem-solving tool seeks to identify the root causes of variable care by quantifying actual problems and improve effectiveness by reducing waste to promote consistent care. The six sigma model comprises actions that seek to do the following:

■ **Define** the problem.

■ **Measure** current performance with the use of statistical tools.

■ **Analyse** the issues/processes causing the problem.

■ **Improve:** Determine and implement the necessary improvements.

■ **Maintain:** Sustainable implementation of the improved processes.

The NHS Institute for Innovation and Improvement (2017) suggests that the use of such tools has provided early indications of favourable outcomes; however, the evidence base regarding their widespread use within healthcare and, more specifically, within the general practice setting/primary care setting remains limited. However, this area has spawned significant interest, with recent work within the NHS exploring the development of a hybrid version of lean and six sigma that incorporates the use of effective problem-solving tools to support a structured approach to continuous quality improvement. The implication for the GPN role is the need to be mindful of emergent processes and the variety of available tools, which, in light of the current challenges facing general practice, may prove valuable adjuncts to continuous quality-improvement activities.

SUMMARY

The delivery of high-quality care signals a complex field of endeavour for the GPN, a situation that has been intensified within the general practice as it attempts to respond to population health needs associated with shifting the balance of care. Despite the inherent clinical and organisational challenges of real-life practice, as part of the primary healthcare team, the GPN role demonstrates the capacity and capability to contribute to the development and delivery of evidence-based practice. This is, however, contingent on the GPN developing and maintaining the requisite knowledge base and skill set, which reflect an unequivocal understanding of the dimensions of quality healthcare relative to its meaning and discrete application in the delivery of patient-centred care. The following chapters provide the opportunity to consider the application of EBP to underpin quality care as it relates to the wide-ranging aspects of the GPN role.

RESOURCES

Care Quality Commission (England): https://www.cqc.org.uk/

Clinical Governance Practice Self-Assessment Tool: http://www.primarycareone.wales.nhs.uk/clinical-governance-practice-self-assess

Critical Skills Appraisal Programme (CASP): https://casp-uk.net/

Healthcare Improvement Scotland: http://www.healthcareimprovementscotland.org/

Healthcare Inspectorate Wales: https://hiw.org.uk/

National Institute for Health and Care Excellence (NICE): https://www.nice.org.uk/

Regulation and Quality Improvement Authority (Northern Ireland): https://www.rqia.org.uk/

Scottish Intercollegiate Guidelines Network (SIGN): https://www.sign.ac.uk/

Sustainability and Transformation Plans (STPs): https://www.england.nhs.uk/integratedcare/stps/faqs/

REFERENCES

Bampoe, S., Cook, T., Fleisher, L., Grocott, M. P. W., Neuman, M., Story, D., Myles, P., & Galler, G. (2018). Clinical indicators for reporting the effectiveness of patient quality and safety-related interventions: A protocol of a systematic review and Delphi consensus process as part of the international Standardised Endpoints for Perioperative Medicine initiative (StEP). *BMJ Open, 8*, Article e023427. https://doi.org/10.1136/bmjopen-2018-023427

Buck, D., Baylis, A., Dougall, D., & Robertson, R. (2019). *A vision for population health: Towards a healthier future.* https://www.kingsfund.org.uk/sites/default/files/2018-11/A%20vision%20for%20population%20health%20online%20version.pdf

Care Quality Commission. (2017). *The state of care in general practice 2014–2017.*

Dawda, P., Jenkins, R., & Varnam, R. (2010). *Quality improvement in general practice.* King's Fund.

Department of Health. (2008). *High quality care for all: NHS next stage review final report, department of health.* Crown Copyright.

Donabedian, A. (1980). *The definitions of quality and approaches to its assessment.* Health Administration Press.

Forbes, L. J. L., Marchand, C., Doran, T., & Peckham, S. (2017). The role of the Quality and Outcomes Framework in the care of long-term conditions: A systematic review. *British Journal of General Practice, 67*(664), e775–e784. https://doi.org/10.3399/bjgp17X693077

Francis, R. (2013). *Report of Mid Staffordshire NHS Foundation Trust public inquiry.* Stationery Office.

Gray, C. (2005). What is clinical governance? *British Medical Journal, 330,* Article s254. https://doi.org/10.1136/bmj.330.7506.s254-b

Hung, D., Martinez, M., Yakir, M., & Gray, C. (2015). Implementing a Lean management system in primary care. *Quality Management in Healthcare, 24*(3), 103–108.

Ingham-Bloomfield, R. (2016). A nurse's guide to the hierarchy of research designs and evidence. *Australian Journal of Advanced Nursing Online, 33*(3), 38–43.

Institute of Medicine. (2001). *Crossing the quality chasm: A new health system for the 21st century.* National Academy Press.

Jabbal, J. (2017). *Embedding a culture of quality improvement.* King's Fund.

Jordan Z., Lockwood, C., Munn, Z., & Aromataris, E. (2019). *The updated Joanna Briggs Institute model of evidence-based healthcare.* https://journals.lww.com/ijebh/FullText/2019/03000/The_updated_Joanna_Briggs_Institute_Model_of.8.as

Kaplan, G. S., Patterson, S. H., Ching, J. M., & Blackmore, C.C. (2014). Why Lean doesn't work for everyone. *BMJ Quality and Safety, 23*(12), 1–4.

Moule, P., Aveyard, H., & Goodman, M. (2017). *Nursing research* (3rd ed.). Sage.

NHS England. (2015). *The NHS Constitution (for England): The NHS belongs to us all.* Department of Health.

NHS England. (2018). *Report of the review of the Quality and Outcomes Framework in England.* https://www.england.nhs.uk/publication/report-of-the-review-of-the-quality-and-outcomes-framework-in-england/

NHS Institute for Innovation and Improvement. (2017). *Lean six sigma: Some basic concepts.* https://www.england.nhs.uk/improvement-hub/wp-content/uploads/sites/44/2017/11/Lean-Six-Sigma-Some-Basic-Concepts.pdf

Pearson, B. (2017). The clinical governance of multidisciplinary care. *International Journal of Health Governance, 22*(4), 246–250.

Robson, C., & McCartan, K. (2016). *Real world research* (4th ed.). Wiley.

Rotter, T., Plishka, C., Lawal, A., Harrison, L., Sari, N., Goodridge, D., Flynn, R., Chan, J., Fiander, M., Poksinska, B., Willoughby, K., & Kinsmanet, L. (2019). What is Lean management in health care? Development of an operational definition for a Cochrane systematic review. *Evaluation & the Health Professions, 42*(3), 366–390. https://journals.sagepub.com/doi/pdf/10.1177/0163278718756992

Royal College of General Practitioners. (2016). *Quality improvement for general practice: A guide for GPs and the whole practice team.*

Sackett, D. L., Straus, S. E., Richardson W. S., Rosenberg, W., & Haynes, R. B. (2000). *Evidence-based medicine: How to practice and teach EBM* (2nd ed.). Churchill Livingstone.

Scally, G., & Donaldson, L. J. (1998). Clinical governance and the drive for quality improvement in the new NHS in England. *British Medical Journal, 317*(7150), 61–65.

Scottish Government. (2017). *Improving together: A national framework for quality and GP clusters in Scotland.*

Scottish Government. (2018). *Paper 06: Developing the general practice nursing role in integrated community nursing teams.*

Scottish Government. (2019). *National monitoring and evaluation strategy for primary care in Scotland.*

The Patient Rights (Scotland) Act 2011. https://www.legislation.gov.uk/asp/2011/5/contents

Valero, A. I. (2019). Autonomies in interaction: Dimensions of patient autonomy and non-adherence to treatment. *Frontiers in Psychology, 10,* Article 1857. https://www.frontiersin.org/articles/10.3389/fpsyg.2019.01857/full

World Health Organisation. (2017). *Facilitating evidence-based practice in nursing and midwifery in the WHO European region.* http://www.euro.who.int/__data/assets/pdf_file/0017/348020/WH06_EBP_report_complete.pdf?ua=1

4

ANTICIPATORY CARE: PERSON-CENTRED MANAGEMENT OF LONG-TERM CONDITIONS IN PRIMARY CARE

KIRSTEEN MARIE COADY

INTRODUCTION

Long-term conditions (LTCs) are the most common reason for death and disability within populations worldwide and represent the greatest challenge facing healthcare systems as they endeavour to prevent early mortality and disability. Within the UK, general practice plays a crucial role in the evidence-based management of LTCs, with the general practice nurse (GPN) being the linchpin in managing and shaping care delivery.

This chapter explores the person-centred management of LTCs by initially defining LTCs, and against the backdrop of changing population demographics, it highlights the associated health burden and the clinical priorities in managing care within the UK. Key UK policy drivers for quality care are discussed and linked to strategic evidence-based interventions incorporating person-centred care and anticipatory care. The 'House of Care' model (Coulter et al., 2013) is explored as a structured approach to optimising the care, health and wellbeing of individuals cared for within general practice settings and the importance of cross-sector partnerships. The preferred terminology throughout is *long-term condition* as opposed to *chronic disease* because the former reflects contemporary use within healthcare settings, key documents and policy drivers. *Individual* is also the preferred terminology, as opposed to *patient*, because this recognises the individuals at the epicentre of their own experiences, not only within healthcare settings but also within the broader context of their own lives and the recognition of self. The word *patient* within the context of person-centeredness can denote a sense of vulnerability.

In establishing the principal approaches underpinning LTC management, this chapter provides the contextual backdrop to subsequent chapters that specifically detail the evidence-based management and self-management of specific LTCs and disabilities that are commonly managed within the general practice setting. The chapter concludes with a summary of the key concepts and incorporates a list of resources to enhance further learning.

CONCEPTUALISING LTC MANAGEMENT WITHIN GENERAL PRACTICE

Multiple definitions and explanations exist regarding the terminology associated with long-term physical health conditions or LTCs, but essentially, these terms represent illnesses whose pathology demonstrates slow progression and are therefore chronic in nature. The Department of Health (DOH, 2012b) defines an LTC as 'a condition that cannot, at present, be cured but is controlled by medication and/or other treatment/ therapies' (p. 3). LTCs are recognised as enduring non-communicable conditions that require ongoing medical care, such as diabetes, cardiovascular disease, chronic obstructive pulmonary disease, asthma, and dementia. Whilst these conditions commonly represent the UK's clinical priorities, LTCs also include a wide range of conditions and disabilities, such as coeliac disease, arthritis and some cancers, as well as physical and learning disabilities. Although the DOH (2012b) definition succinctly captures the clinical context of an LTC, a contemporary phenomenon is that many individuals are living with more than one LTC, termed *multimorbidity*. Whilst this adds to the complexity of care planning, the healthcare needs faced by individuals living with LTCs cannot be understated – they endeavour to cope with issues that include symptom management, medication regimes, accessing social care support, a sense of loss in health status and the impact on personal/family relationships.

The expertise and unique focus of the GPN in managing care and supporting individuals with LTCs are widely recognised as an intrinsic part of this professional role (Chowdhury et al., 2020). This necessitates a critical understanding of person-centred approaches and the application of service-delivery models that embrace collaboration, cooperation and enhanced communication with providers, professionals and individuals. A central tenet of LTC management is anticipatory care, which seeks to 'pre-empt' the potential for health problems emerging or actions to stymie further deterioration in health status. More specifically, managing LTC care demands a wide skill set to continuously improve the information, support, care and treatment of people living with LTCs, which will include the following:

- Assessment and consultation skills
- Health promotion
- Self-management
- Empowering individuals to be more actively involved in their own care
- Integrated care approaches
- Shared decision-making and care planning
- Partnership working
- Networking with third-sector, voluntary and community groups

DEVELOPMENT OF LTC MANAGEMENT AND THE GPN

Contemporary iterations of the General Medical Service (GMS) contract, as detailed in Chapter 1, have shaped the evolving role of the GPN in the management of LTCs. Most notably, the 1990 GMS contract paved the way for providing structured care for individuals suffering from LTCs and placed GPNs at the helm of managing this care (Queen's Nursing Institute (QNI), 2017), albeit these services being target driven and attracting monetary pay-for-performance incentives for general practitioners (GPs). The demands of

the GPN role also sparked the uptake of accredited and nonaccredited courses, initially in diabetes and asthma care, based on the enduring realisation that the GPN role carried a high level of professional accountability and autonomy. At this juncture, general practice provided the opportunity for the GPN role to flourish and develop, and contemporary research supports how effective and crucial the GPN has become in managing LTCs (Chowdhury et al., 2020).

The next major iteration of the GMS contract in 2004 saw the introduction of the Quality Outcomes Framework (QOF), a voluntary scheme that remains a salient feature of GMS contracts in England, Northern Ireland and Wales. In 2016, Scotland abolished the QOF and replaced this, in part, by implementing general practice clusters, which involve groups of six to eight practices with appointed leads who are responsible for assessing, managing and improving care quality. The QOF entails the acquisition of points, upon which finances are awarded based on the achievement of specific clinical and administrative indicators for specified LTCs, with the rationale that rewarding practices for providing an improved, evidence-based quality of care will lead to improved standardised healthcare (NHS England, 2019b). The QOF ultimately led to enhanced roles for the GPN and the onward development of the healthcare support worker (HCSW) roles, which, to this day, has increased the skill-mix capacity within general practice and delegation of tasks from the GPN to the HCSW (Primary Care One Wales, 2020). Although evidence based, the QOF has been widely criticised in being highly selective of the type of LTCs included, biomedical and having a 'tick-box' propensity rather than a person-centred approach (Forbes et al., 2017). Conversely, a positive feature of the QOF is the NHS digital platform, which publishes reports that are available to the public to view (see Resources section). People can see how their GP practice compares to others and are able to view disease prevalence in their locality. An example of QOF results is outlined in Fig. 4.1.

More recent iterations of the GMS contract, for example, 2018 within Scotland and 2019 within England, continue to place a high priority on effectively managing LTCs, endorsing the crucial role of general practice and the contribution of the GPN and the wider primary care team.

Percentage of total	10%	20%	30%	40%	50%	60%	70%	80%	90%	100%
Asthma ⑦ 4 indicators	100.0%									
All the 45 points: 1.2 percentage points above CCG Average, 2.6 above England average										
Atrial fibrillation ⑦ 3 indicators	100.0%									
All the 17 points: 0.6 percentage points above CCG Average, 1.5 above England average										
Cancer ⑦ 2 indicators	96.6%									
10.63 out of 11 points: 2.8 percentage points below CCG Average, 1.3 below England average										
Chronic kidney disease ⑦	98.6%									

Fig. 4.1 ■ Example of Quality Outcomes Framework (QOF) results. *CCG*, Clinical Commissioning Group. (From NHS England. (2019). *2019/20 General Medical Services (GMS) contract Quality and Outcomes Framework (QOF). Guidance for GMS contract 2019/20 in England April 2019.* https://www.england.nhs.uk/wp-content/uploads/2019/05/gms-contract-qof-guidance-april-2019.pdf)

PREVALENCE, DEMOGRAPHICS AND HEALTHCARE BURDEN

A well-established phenomenon is that the UK population is ageing, life expectancy has increased and mortality rates have declined, and although applauded, this correlates with the risk of living with an LTC or multiple LTCs and an increased need for future care (Office for National Statistics, 2019). Around 26 million people in the UK live with at least one LTC, with 10 million of those having two or more. The social impact of having an LTC indicates that only 59% of people with LTCs are in employed work in comparison to 72% of the general population. Box 4.1 details the service burden of LTCs.

BOX 4.1
SERVICE BURDEN OF LONG-TERM CONDITIONS

- 50% of all general practitioner appointments
- 64% of all hospital outpatient appointments
- 70% of all inpatient bed-days
- 50% emergency inpatient bed-days in the over-75 age group
- 25% of inpatient bed-days occupied by someone dying

Data from NHS England, Enhancing the quality of life for people living with Long term conditions, https://www.england.nhs.uk/wp-content/uploads/2014/09/ltc-infographic.pdf

Higher mortality rates for those with LTCs as well as stagnation of life expectancy occur in more deprived areas and demonstrate disparities across differing communities (Public Health England, 2018). In 2012, individuals in the poorest social class (class V) had a 60% higher prevalence of LTCs than those in the richest social class (class I), and 30% of people living with poverty experienced greater severity of disease (DOH, 2012b). LTCs accounted for about 50% of all GP appointments, 64% of all outpatient appointments and over 70% of all inpatient bed days (DOH 2012b). Whilst capturing contemporary data on a national level remains challenging, the implications of providing LTC care, which takes account of an aging population, the escalation in multimorbidity and managing the expectations of individuals, have resulted in increasing demand and therein a considerable challenge to healthcare provision (Institute for Government, 2019). In 2016, the UK population at age 65 could expect to live another 20 years, with just under a half of these years involving living with one or more LTCs (Organisation for Economic Co-operation and Development, 2019). People are living longer, but many of these years are spent living with significant health problems. By 2035, the number of those aged over 85 is projected to double that of the previous 2 decades, with the majority of people living with four or more LTCs (Kingston et al., 2018), thus placing an immense burden on healthcare systems. Given the prevalence of LTCs (Kingston et al., 2018) and the current unknown aftermath of the 2019 coronavirus (COVID-19) pandemic, the care and management of those with LTCs are a major challenge not only in the UK but globally.

HEALTH INEQUALITIES AND LTCS

Health inequalities represent the unjust preventable differences in people's health across the population and between specific population groups, particularly for those living in the most deprived communities (Williams et al., 2020). There is well-documented evidence confirming that individuals suffering health inequalities are at higher risk of developing LTCs, including multimorbidity, which occurs at least 10 to 15 years earlier and, as previously indicated, with greater severity in comparison to those living in the most affluent communities (Institute of Health Equity, 2020).

LTCs can also adversely affect the individual's social perceptions of self, affecting the individual's quality of life and spawning further inequality – for example, in relation to employment (a social determinant of health), where over 50% of people consider their health status an impediment to the type and quantity of work they can reasonably manage. Moreover, this perception rises to 80% when an individual has three or more LTCs (Williams et al., 2020). The impact of living with an LTC reflects an increased risk of developing anxiety and depressive illnesses that adversely affect the underlying illness and mental health status, leading to poorer outcomes triggered by aetiology, which often remains unrecognised (Chew-Graham et al., 2014).

As emphasised in Chapter 2, the need to address the burgeoning problem of health inequalities to minimise the impact of LTCs and multimorbidity is imperative, and government policies must pave the way forward. NHS England's *Improving Access for All: Reducing Inequalities in Access to General Practice Services* (2017) is a key resource that can support GPNs in working towards maximising equality so that those who need care receive the right care, at the *right place, right time* and by the *right person*.

DRIVERS FOR LTC HEALTHCARE DELIVERY

Although the NHS exists as a UK-wide organisation, its governance is devolved to the UK constituent

governments of England, Scotland, Northern Ireland and Wales, which have created key government policy drivers to address health inequalities within populations and provide a basis for healthcare providers to tackle the burden of managing LTCs. Although there are policy variations across the four nations, they all seek to promote the principles of self-management within populations, prevent hospital admissions and improve individuals' quality of life. The landmark *Improving the Health and Well-Being of People With Long-Term Conditions,* published by the DOH in 2010, perceptively recognised that personalised care planning underpins the excellent management of LTCs and end-of-life care. The paper outlined that care for those with LTCs should be

- more individualised,
- focussed on prevention of disease and complications,
- aligned to support people in making healthier and more informed choices,
- aimed to reduce health inequalities, and
- closer to home.

Furthermore, adding to these principles, the NHS Long-Term Plan (NHS England, 2019a) states that the NHS will be

- more joined up and co-ordinated in its care,
- more proactive in the services it provides, and
- more differentiated in its support to offer individuals.

Other key drivers include the Scottish government's National Clinical Strategy, published in 2016 (Scottish Government, 2016a). This is a high-level visionary paper for healthcare and social care services that addresses the need for change over a 15-year period to ensure sustainability and that the care is right for every individual. Because the majority of healthcare is delivered within primary care, this paper highlights the need for person-centred change and supported self-management strategies to address health inequalities. Furthermore, the paper recognises the worth of GPNs, establishing that 'the rise in the number of practice nurses in the last ten years has shown that they are able to take on a great deal of care and treatment, with particular benefit to people requiring ongoing management of long-term conditions' (Scottish

Government, 2016a, p. 45). The Health and Social Care Delivery Plan (Scottish Government, 2016b) presents a programme that is focused on prevention, early intervention and support for self-management within communities. The aim is to enable those living in Scotland to live longer, healthier lives with the highest standard of care, be this at home or in a homely setting. In progressing this agenda, *Practising Realistic Medicine: Chief Medical Officer for Scotland Annual Report* (Scottish Government, 2018) outlines ways to support the translation of the principles developed within the previous 2017 report *Realising Realistic Medicine and Tackling Sustainability of NHS Service Provision*. The 2018 report examines the ways in which the principles of realistic medicine can be applied to positively influence the social determinants of health, such as childhood experiences, social support and access to health services. NHS England's Long-Term Plan (2019a) seeks to address concerns about funding, staffing levels, inequalities and the pressures that are emerging from an ageing and growing population. The plan looks ahead to responsively redesign care, including integrated GP teams, and to offer patients the right to digital consultations, which could revolutionise LTC care and access to meet demand. The extent to which the potential of digital consultations has been realised has been accelerated in the UK by the COVID-19 pandemic.

HEALTH SCREENING AND SURVEILLANCE

As detailed in Chapter 2, health screening and surveillance are fundamental public health components of the GPN's role, with the aims of early detection of disease and prevention of complications of existing disease. Despite the current variances in the operationalising of the QOF across the UK, it does provide a framework for health screening and surveillance within general practice. The QOF, as an incentive payment scheme, as opposed to a performance management tool, aims to improve patient care by rewarding practices for the quality of care they provide to individuals with LTCs, based on the best available research evidence (NHS England, 2019b). The quality of the care provided is assessed against a range of evidence-based clinical indicators across a number of key

performance areas. However, as Forbes et al.'s (2017) systematic review indicated, the QOF entails disease-focussed management, which may arguably lead to 'disabling' rather than 'enabling' individuals and, as a consequence, may prohibit the opportunity to explore what really matters to people living with LTCs. Furthermore, with routine LTC review consultations focusing on the assessment of biomedical markers, the healthcare professional undeniably assumes the role of 'expert'; this may add to the treatment burden, with the individual becoming overwhelmed, their agenda being unheard and feeling unable to confidently participate in shared decision-making about their health (Chew-Graham et al., 2013). Chew-Graham et al. (2013) are amongst many who report that practitioners experience the LTC consultation as perfunctory disease surveillance and the QOF agenda and protocols as unresponsive in identifying unmet needs. As a consequence, target-driven approaches that focus on disease-management metrics can unwittingly ignore the individual's needs and have the potential to cause harm if health screening/surveillance becomes regimented and ignores individual needs. This situation is heightened in working with vulnerable population groups, for example, in caring for individuals with dementia, where anxiety, distress and pain may be encountered by the individual during venepuncture for a QOF measurement, which could be particularly traumatic. *Practising Realistic Medicine* (Scottish Government, 2018) provides direction for the application of person-centred care that places the individual at the centre of shared decision-making. The ethos of realistic medicine is about exploring the individual's preferences regarding what is most important to them and developing a shared understanding of how healthcare might realistically contribute to this using open, authentic and meaningful conversations. Providing a good experience of care for people living with LTCs is a fundamental aspect of *Practising Realistic Medicine* and is contingent on the values and behaviours of professionals to underpin communication approaches. The concepts outlined within *Practising Realistic Medicine* regarding individuals exercising choice and assuming greater control of decisions that affect them align with the expectations of the Nursing and Midwifery Council (NMC) for the registered nurse, as detailed within *The Future Nurse: Standards of*

BOX 4.2
REALISTIC MEDICINE – ENHANCING DECISION-MAKING

1. Is this test, treatment or procedure really needed?
2. What are the potential benefits and risks?
3. What are the possible side effects?
4. Are there simpler, safer or alternative treatment options?
5. What would happen if I did nothing?

From Scottish Government. (2018). *Practising realistic medicine: Chief Medical Officer for Scotland annual report.*

Proficiency for Registered Nurses and the seven platforms of care therein (NMC, 2018).

Box 4.2 provides a summary of five crucial questions within the realistic medicine concept that GPNs and other care professionals should consider using to enhance decision-making. Indeed, individuals with LTCs can be encouraged to ask these questions themselves to help make informed choices within a partnership approach with a healthcare professional, and they are encouraged by Choosing Wisely UK (2020), which is part of a global initiative to improve the conversations between people and healthcare professionals and has simplified the questions to the following:

1. What are the benefits?
2. What are the risks?
3. What are the alternatives?
4. What if I do nothing?

Within the general practice setting, this approach could assist the individual with hypertension, for example, in deciding whether to opt for statin treatment for primary prevention and aids shared decision-making, as delineated within the DOH's (2012a) 'no decision about me, without me'. This framework also supports health literacy, which, as indicated in Chapter 2, refers to the personal and relational factors that affect an individual's ability to acquire, understand and use information about health and health services. The importance of health literacy is considerable; it can improve individual care and access to services and contribute to reducing inequalities (Batterham et al., 2016).

PERSON-CENTRED MODELS OF CARE FOR LTCS

- The cornerstone of LTC care is the provision of person-centred care, where the emphasis is placed on 'who' the person is, rather than 'what disease or condition' they are presenting with. This perspective challenges traditional paternalistic, top-down approaches to managing consultations that place an overt focus on biomedical markers by health professionals adopting 'expert' positions (Chew-Graham et al., 2013). Person-centred care supports people to develop the knowledge, skills and confidence to manage their conditions and, importantly, give voice to their agenda to make informed choices about their own health (Health Foundation, 2016). The term *person centred* is more appropriate than *patient centred* because the onus is on an individual person and not a focus on disease. The four principles of person-centred care are as follows (Health Foundation, 2016):
- Care is PERSONALISED.
- Care is CO-ORDINATED.
- Care is ENABLING.
- Each person is treated with DIGNITY, COMPASSION and RESPECT.

Consultation styles that solely focus on discussing the disease or condition can alienate the unprepared individual and what matters to them within their lives in living with the condition. The 'What Matters to You?' health improvement initiative (Healthcare Improvement Scotland, 2019), which originated in NHS England in 2016 and has been widely adopted across the UK, with a designated 'What Matters to You?' day each year, encourages more meaningful conversations between healthcare professionals and those they care for. The initiative's mantra of 'ask what matters, listen to what matters and do what matters' promotes safe, effective person-centred care.

The structuring of care for LTC management has, over the decades, shifted from a biomedical model to person-centred anticipatory approaches. Numerous models have emerged, many based on Wagner's (1998) seminal chronic care model, and these reflect the healthcare systems and processes in which they operate. Contemporary models that have been developed

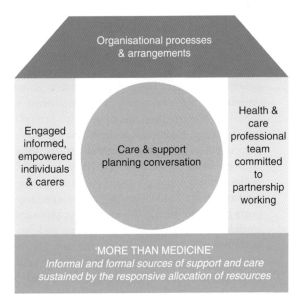

Fig. 4.2 ◼ House of Care analogy. (Health and Social Care Alliance Scotland 2016: The House of Care Model. Section: Health and Social Care Integration. Last accessed 28/08/2020. https://www.alliance-scotland.org.uk/health-and-social-care-integration/house-of-care/house-of-care-model/.)

within the UK reflect the aspiration to deal with LTCs holistically and seek to convey the structure, values and intentions of quality care. One such model that has gained prominence is the 'House of Care', which is a person-centred, powerful model capable of contributing to supporting individuals to self-manage LTCs in community settings. The House of Care model was developed by the Year of Care partnership, originally for a diabetes programme in England, and was specifically adapted for UK primary care settings to pave the way for collaborative relationships to help people self-manage their LTCs (Coulter et al., 2013, 2016). It uses the metaphor of a house, centres on individuals as the focal point rather than their specific 'disease', carries the philosophy of being 'more than medicine' and truly embraces person-centeredness. The house metaphor, as detailed in Fig. 4.2, delineates a whole-systems approach with interdependency between the structural components of the 'house', which need to be in place and functional to support each other in co-ordinating the care for those with LTCs. The interdependent structures are crucial to the House of Care's stability; a weakness in one area could result in the

metaphorical collapse of the house, which, in practical terms, could lead to ineffective care.

Key elements of the House of Care model are as follows:

- People with LTCs feeling engaged in decisions about their treatment and being able to act on these decisions
- Professionals being committed to working in partnership with individuals
- Systems being in place to organise resources effectively
- Having a whole-systems approach to commissioning health and care services

Whilst the clinical monitoring of LTCs is a crucial aspect of care management, such as the serological monitoring for particular diseases, the House of Care model also encompasses psychological health and social care. The use of a holistic model seeks to empower individuals, who can manage their conditions with improved emotional, physical and mental health (Williams et al., 2020). The model can also promote equality within consultations because individuals registered at the practice receive their test results before attending a protected appointment for a meaningful 'care and support planning' (CSP) consultation/conversation, which can take many forms, such as via video consultations, as outlined within NHS England's (2019a) Long-Term Plan. CSP reflects a structured process whereby individuals set their own aims and goals to address their concerns and aligns with the 'What Matters to You?' initiative (Healthcare Improvement Scotland, 2019). CSP represents a viable forum that supports a balance of agendas and partnership approaches leading to formulating person-led, as opposed to nurse-led, care planning. CSP is structured around SMART objectives (Specific, Measurable, Achievable, Realistic, and Time bound) to respond to individuals' needs and explore their perception of, readiness for and confidence towards change. Furze (2015) provides excellent practical examples that can act as a framework during person-led CSP conversations and goal-setting sessions.

The impact of CSP conversations can help change the lives of others if they are person-focussed rather than disease orientated or dominated by a nursing/medical agenda. GPNs are perfectly placed within primary care to demonstrate professionalism in partnerships working to enhance CSP conversations, whether via face-to-face meetings, video consultation or telephone. GPNs are also in a prime position to help identify a multitude of problems that often arise in the context of living with an LTC, such as uncovering social isolation and networking with services/agencies that may help support individuals (such as third-sector services), signifying the 'more than medicine approach' (Williams et al., 2020).

CSP aligns with other strategies, such as 'Making Every Contact Count' (MECC), if the focus is on the individual themselves and their needs. As identified in Chapter 2, MECC is an evidence-based approach to improving health and wellbeing (NHS Health Education England, 2020) that has a significant affinity with LTC management and can be used in tandem with CSP. However, the key concerns in exploring what really matters to people may be multifactorial, and CSP conversations are person-led, but if lifestyle change is what really matters, then MECC is an appropriate strategy. A key consideration at this juncture is that what really matters to individuals may not directly align with their LTCs, and in this context, third-sector agencies may able to bridge the gap in meeting needs and enabling individuals. The GPN has a fundamental role in signposting those in their care to voluntary-sector agencies, which may help them to achieve their full potential or help meet an unmet need.

ANTICIPATORY CARE PLANNING AND LTCS

Taking the time to listen and have a truly shared conversation is an invaluable aspect of shared decision-making, which lies at the heart of CSP. However, this process may be impeded in those suffering social isolation, which, although more common in the elderly, does affect younger adults and children. Reduced social contact and feelings of loneliness are associated side effects of living with an LTC; for example, having a chronic and debilitating dermatological condition, such as psoriasis, induces a reduced quality of life. GPNs are in a unique position to identify people who may be at particular risk of social isolation, and this includes consideration of the impact of COVID-19 and the necessary escalation in social distancing, self-isolation and shielding for individuals with LTCs who may be at higher clinical risk.

Anticipatory care planning can be a powerful tool for facilitating 'thinking-ahead' conversations with individuals, and if conducted in a person-centred manner, this can help individuals and carers set personal goals to ensure that the *right thing* is done at the *right time* by the *right person*, ultimately leading to the *right outcome* so that personal choices are heeded (Cumming et al., 2017). The anticipatory care 'thinking-ahead' ideology is supported by a key information summary (KIS) that contains accurate information about the individual and has been found to reduce the risk of hospital admission by 30% to 50% (Cumming et al., 2017). A person-centred app entitled 'Let's Think Ahead' has been developed to support anticipatory care planning and can be recommended to those living with LTC, where appropriate, who have access to smart technology.

Anticipatory care planning should not be a strategy reserved for individuals facing end-of-life care or overtly complex health needs but for anyone who could potentially benefit, including those living with multiple LTCs. The evidence suggests that the early intervention of anticipatory care planning can, irrespective of age, optimise health outcomes, improve the quality of life and contribute to appropriate care provision (Cumming et al., 2017). Anticipatory care planning and the formation of the KIS within a person's primary care record should be seen as a powerful, commonplace tool to enhance and optimise care. Anticipatory care planning's aim is to address individual needs whilst simultaneously increasing safety netting by sharing information between primary and secondary care and reducing unnecessary hospital admissions. The emergence of the COVID-19 pandemic has hastened the formation of the KIS and anticipatory care planning by healthcare professionals. Arguably, the complex change processes triggered by the COVID-19 pandemic promoted the implementation of the principles of anticipatory care planning.

KEY LEARNING POINTS

- LTCs are a major health and economic burden within the UK and globally.
- Those living with LTCs are more likely to live in deprived areas.
- Care for those with LTCs should be *people* focussed and not *disease* focussed.

- Powerful 'What Matters to You?' conversations are at the heart of person-centeredness.
- GPNs/primary care teams are ideally placed to support those living with LTCs.
- The realistic medicine five questions are crucial to enable work in partnerships.
- The House of Care is a model of care to promote CSP within primary care.
- CSP can support individuals towards self-management and fulfilled lives.
- Anticipatory Care Planning should be commonplace for those living with LTCs.
- The COVID-19 pandemic has accelerated anticipatory care planning and the use of technology.

SUMMARY

The management of LTCs is complex and involves partnerships within a culture of person-centeredness. In essence, individuals with LTCs are reliant upon care driven by service providers, and this chapter has focussed on the need for care to be structured in a person-centred manner and the need for health inequalities to be addressed to maximise healthcare provision.

The House of Care model, which incorporates CSP, has been identified as a model of care that paves the way for person-centeredness and equality within consultations, and GPNs are in a privileged position to establish what really matters to people. The challenge is to provide *people-focussed* care rather than *disease-focussed* care. Person-centred conversations have the power to lead to self-managing populations, individuals living their lives to the best they can. Third-sector organisations are central to helping individuals with LTCs to live more fulfilled lives if underlying needs are met.

The global pandemic of COVID-19 has affected the management of LTCs and has driven forward the use of technology and anticipatory care planning. Anticipatory care planning can ensure that needs are met and individual wishes are known at all stages of living with an LTC. The challenge for policy makers and professionals alike is to collaborate and share in decision-making to ensure that the values of those living with LTCs bring about a self-managing, more fulfilled population. The challenge lies within.

RESOURCES

Addressing Loneliness: https://patient.info/doctor/social-isolation-how-to-help-patients-be-less-lonely

Health and Social Care Alliance Scotland: https://www.alliance-scotland.org.uk

House of Care: http://www.kingsfund.org.uk/blog/2013/10/supporting-people-long-term-conditions-what-house-care

NHS Digital – Quality Outcomes Framework Reports: https://www.ons.gov.uk/

Royal College of General Practitioners – Care and Support Planning: http://www.rcgp.org.uk/clinical-and-research/clinical-resources/collaborative-care-and-support-planning.aspx

Scottish Government – Realistic Medicine: https://www.gov.scot/publications/summary-practising-realistic-medicine/

The Coalition for Collaborative Care and NHS England – Handbook for Care and Support Planning: http://coalitionforcollaborativecare.org.uk/news/personalised-care-and-support-planning-hand book-launched/

The Health Foundation – Person-Centred Care and Self-Management: http://personcentredcare.health.org.uk/

The Year of Care Partnership – House of Care Model and Person-Centred Care: http://www.yearofcare.co.uk/

REFERENCES

Batterham, R., Hawkins, M., Collins, P., Buchbinder, R., & Osborne, R. (2016). Health literacy: Applying current concepts to improve health services and reduce health equalities. *Journal of Public Health, 132,* 3–12.

Chew-Graham, C., Hunter, C., Langer, S., Stenhoff, A., Drinkwater, J., Guthrie, E., & Salmon, P. (2013). How QOF is shaping primary care review consultations: A longitudinal qualitative study. *BMC Family Practice, 14,* Article 103.

Chew-Graham, C., Sartorius, N., Cimino, L. C., & Gask, L. (2014). Diabetes and depression in general practice: Meeting the challenge of managing comorbidity. *British Journal of General Practice, 64*(625), 386–387. https://doi.org/10.3399/bjgp14X680809

Choosing Wisely UK. (2020). *About Choosing Wisely UK.* https://www.choosingwisely.co.uk/about-choosing-wisely-uk

Chowdhury, S., Stephen, C., McInnes, S., & Halcomb, E. (2020). Nurse-led interventions to manage hypertension in general practice nursing: A systematic review protocol. *Collegian, 27,* 340–343.

Coulter, A., Kramer, G., Warren, T., & Salisbury, C. (2016). Building the House of Care for people with long-term conditions: The foundation of the House of Care framework. *British Journal of General Practice, 66*(645), 288–290. https://doi.org/10.3399/bigp16X684745

Coulter, A., Robert, S., & Dixon, A. (2013). *Delivering better services for people with long-term conditions: Building the House of Care.* King's Fund. https://www.kingsfund.org.uk/sites/default/files/field/field_publication_file/delivering-better-services-for-people-with-long-term-conditions.pdf

Cumming, S., Steel, S., & Barrie, J. (2017). Anticipatory care planning in Scotland. *International Journal of Integrated Care, 17*(3), 1–8.

Department of Health. (2010). *Improving the health and well-being of people with long term conditions.* https://www.yearofcare.co.uk/

sites/default/files/pdfs/dh_improving%20the%20h&wb%20 of%20people%20with%20LTCs.pdf

Department of Health. (2012a). *Liberating the NHS: No decision about me, without me.* https://assets.publishing.service.gov.uk/ government/uploads/system/uploads/attachment_data/ file/216980/Liberating-the-NHS-No-decision-about-me-without-me-Government-response.pdf

Department of Health. (2012b). *Long-term conditions compendium of information: 3rd edition.* https://www.gov.uk/government/ publications/long-term-conditions-compendium-of-information-third-edition

Forbes, L., Marchland, C., Doran, T., & Peckham, S. (2017). The role of the Quality and Outcomes Framework in the care of long-term conditions: A systematic review. *British Journal of Medical Practice,* e775–782. https://bjgp.org/content/ bjgp/67/664/e775.full.pdf

Furze, G. (2015). Diabetes Evidence based Management 79 Goal setting: a key skill for person centred care. *Practice Nursing,* 2015, 26(5), 241–244.

Health Foundation. (2016). *Person-centred care made simple. What everyone should know about person-centred care.* https://www.health. org.uk/sites/default/files/PersonCentredCareMadeSimple.pdf

Healthcare Improvement Scotland. (2019). 'What matters to you?' Supporting more meaningful conversations in day-to-day practice: A multiple case study evaluation. https://www.whatmatterstoyou. scot/wp-content/uploads/2020/02/20200217-WMTY19-report-FINAL.pdf

Institute for Government. (2019). *Performance tracker 2019 – General practice.* https://www.instituteforgovernment.org.uk/ publication/performance-tracker-2019/general-practice

Institute of Health Equity. (2020). *Health equity in England: The Marmot Review 10 years on.* Institute of Heath Equity.

Kingston, A., Robison, L., Booth, H., Knapp, M., & Jagger, C. (2018). Projections of multi-morbidity in the older population in England to 2015: Estimates from the Population Ageing and Care Simulation (PACSim) model. *Age and Ageing, 47*(3), 374–380. https://doi.org/10.1093/ageing/afx201

NHS England. (2017). *Improving access for all: Reducing inequalities in access to general practice services.* https://www.england.nhs.uk/ publication/improving-access-for-all-reducing-inequalities-in-access-to-general-practice-services/

NHS England. (2019a). *NHS long term plan.* https://www.longterm plan.nhs.uk/

NHS England. (2019b). *2019/20 General Medical Services (GMS) contract Quality and Outcomes Framework (QOF). Guidance for GMS contract 2019/20 in England April 2019.* https://www. england.nhs.uk/wp-content/uploads/2019/05/gms-contract-qof-guidance-april-2019.pdf

NHS Health Education England. (2020). *Making every contact count frameworks.* https://www.makingeverycontactcount.co.uk/ evidence/frameworks

Nursing and Midwifery Council. (2018). *Future nurse: Standards of proficiency for registered nurses.*

Office for National Statistics. (2019). *Overview of the UK population: August 2019.* https://www.ons.gov.uk/releases/ overviewoftheukpopulationjuly2019

Organisation for Economic Co-operation and Development. (2019). *United Kingdom: Country health profile 2019, state of health in the EU.* OECD Publishing, Paris/European Observatory on Health Systems and Policies. https://doi.org/10.1787/744df2e3-en

Primary Care One Wales. (2020). *Primary and community care nursing.* http://www.primarycareone.wales.nhs.uk/pc-community-nurses

Public Health England. (2018). *A review of recent trends in mortality in England.* PHE Publication Gateway.

Queen's Nursing Institute. (2017). *Transition to general practice nursing.* https://www.qni.org.uk/wp-content/uploads/2017/01/ Transition-to-General-Practice-Nursing.pdf

Scottish Government. (2016a). *A national clinical strategy for Scotland.* https://www.gov.scot/publications/national-clinical-strategy-scotland/

Scottish Government. (2016b). *The health and social care delivery plan.* https://www.gov.scot/publications/health-social-care-delivery-plan/

Scottish Government. (2018). *Practising realistic medicine: Chief Medical Officer for Scotland annual report.*

Wagner, E. H. (1998). Chronic disease management: What will it take to improve care for chronic illness? *Effective Clinical Practice, 1*(1), 2–4.

Williams, E., Buck, D., & Babaloa, G. (2020). *What are health inequalities?* https://www.kingsfund.org.uk/publications/what-are-health-inequalities?gclid=EAIaIQobChMIxa6_8L7e6gIVQuv tCh1j7g0yEAAYASAAEgJ3rfD_BwE

5

LEGAL, ETHICAL AND PROFESSIONAL PRACTICE: FRAMEWORKS FOR CARE DELIVERY

COLETTE HENDERSON

INTRODUCTION

On a daily basis, the general practice nurse (GPN) is required to make highly complex care decisions that necessitate working within legal, ethical and professional frameworks to ensure quality outcomes for the patients they care for, their employers and wider society are met. This chapter aims to build on GPN core knowledge of ethical practice and values (Nursing and Midwifery Council (NMC), 2018) by discussing the legal frameworks governing and informing the delivery of health and social care within the UK. The role of the GPN and the challenges associated with powerful relationships, autonomy, ethical decision-making, advocacy and accountability will also be discussed. In concluding, this chapter will discuss the Royal College of General Practitioners and Royal College of Nursing (RCGP/RCN, 2015) GPN competencies and the Queen's Nursing Institute/Queen's Nursing Institute Scotland (QNI/QNIS, 2017) voluntary Standards for General Practice.

LEGAL FRAMEWORKS FOR HEALTHCARE AND SOCIAL CARE DELIVERY ACROSS THE UK

Global austerity, increasing demand and expectations, ageing populations and issues with sustaining the current workforce have commanded that countries consider more sustainable, cost-effective ways of delivering healthcare. Across the UK, one of the key progressions to enable this has been the integration of healthcare and social care. The ethos of integration of care is to concentrate on prevention and early intervention whilst ensuring

high-quality care and seamless access to the services and care required (Department of Health and Social Care (DHSC), 2015; Scottish Government (SG), 2015). Although an integrated healthcare and social care system operates in Northern Ireland, policy review has ensured alignment with healthcare policy across the UK in terms of high quality, community-led, person-centred care (Thompson, 2016).

England

In England, the Health and Social Care Act (Department of Health (DOH), 2012) established the obligations for healthcare and social care services, and the 2014 Care Act (DOH, 2014) provided the legal framework for the integration of healthcare and social care (DHSC, 2015). The Health and Social Care Act (DOH, 2012) created clinical commissioning groups whose aim was to commission services for local populations. The 2014 Care Act (DOH, 2014) established Health Education England (HEE) as a nondepartmental public body whose role as a national organisation is to ensure educational development for the healthcare workforce in England (HEE, 2017). Collectively, this legal framework aimed to transform the provision of care to ensure high-quality, person-centred and community-based care led by general practitioner (GP) practices (DOH, 2012).

HEE published a General Practice Workforce Development plan in 2017. The plan covered four main sections. Section 1 considered preregistration nursing and raising the profile of general practice nursing as a viable career option, whilst section 2 highlighted educational and support requirements for newly qualified nurses. Section 3 outlined recommendations for maximising the development of the established GPN, including educational requirements and career-development opportunities. The fourth section outlined recommendations for expanding the general practice workforce, with a focus on the role of the healthcare assistant. Recommendations from this workforce development plan led to the development of a 10-point action plan (Fig. 5.1) by National Health Service (NHS) England (2017). This action plan provides a strategic national direction to ensure the development of the general practice nursing workforce.

Northern Ireland

Healthcare was devolved to the Northern Ireland government in 1999. The DOH maintains responsibility for providing the strategic and legal framework for the provision of healthcare and social care in Northern Ireland. The 2009 Health and Social Care (Reform) (Northern Ireland) Act stipulates specific roles for service commissioners and service providers in Northern Ireland. Commissioning of services is the responsibility of the Health and Social Care Board (HSCB) and the Public Health Agency (PHA). Feeding into the HSCB are the five local commissioning groups established by the act whose responsibility is to assess local healthcare and social care needs. The 2009 act also established five healthcare and social care trusts and one ambulance trust to provide the requisite healthcare and social care services for the population of Northern Ireland.

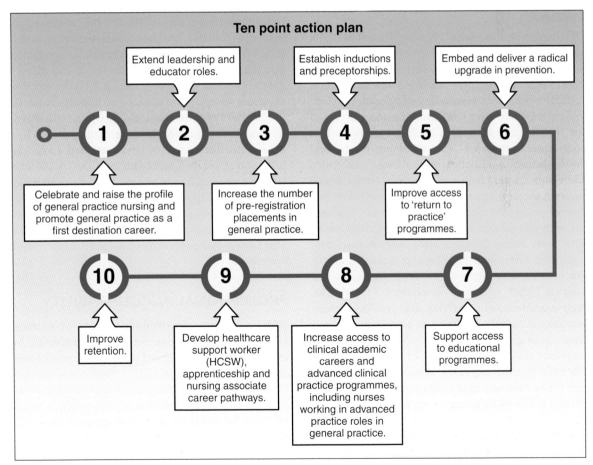

Fig. 5.1 ▪ A 10-point action plan for general practice nursing. (From NHS England. (2017). *General practice – Developing confidence, capability and capacity.* https://www.england.nhs.uk/wp-content/uploads/2018/01/general-practice-nursing-ten-point-plan-v17.pdf)

In 2016 the PHA and HSCB produced a framework for general practice nursing, required as a result of the key drivers indicated earlier in this chapter. This framework provides detail on the systems, governance, competencies and role requirements for nurses working in general practice and primary care in Northern Ireland to ensure standardised and sustainable care. The framework provides recommendations within four key areas:

- Workforce review
- Core competency framework
- Education
- Professional governance

These recommendations have been utilised to inform work reviewing GP-led services in Northern Ireland.

Scotland

The Public Bodies (Joint Working) (Scotland) Act (2014) provides the legal framework for the integration of healthcare and social care in Scotland (SG, 2019). One approach to achieving the integration agenda, which also provided professional development opportunities for GPNs, was the introduction of the *Transforming Roles* (SG, 2015) programme. This programme promoted role development beyond the traditional whilst assuring national uniformity. There was a strong focus on integrated teams, which required the development of nursing roles, including that of the GPN. Subsequently, national guidance has been created that seeks to refresh and refocus the GPN role. Policy directives, role competencies and significant investment have been provided to enable this Scottish development (SG, 2018). A number of Scottish higher education institutions (HEIs) have been commissioned to develop and provide relevant educational modules, focusing on areas such as minor illness management, long-term conditions, asthma, telephone triage and mental health in primary care. The SG's *Transforming Roles,* Paper 6 (2018, p. 3) details the key features of the refocused general practice nursing role, concentrating on the following:

- Public health, including primary and secondary prevention and addressing health inequalities
- Care and support planning, including anticipatory care

- Assessing illness and injury
- Supporting management of long-term conditions
- Supporting people with complex conditions or who are frail as part of integrated community teams
- Promoting mental health and wellbeing
- Providing nursing care across the life cycle

Wales

In 2014 the Welsh government set the direction for primary care services, with an aim of providing a 'social' model of health. This stipulated that the focus of care should encompass physical health and mental health and wellbeing. The policy directive aimed to ensure the development of the general practice workforce. It included funding the development of advanced nurse practice. The Health and Social Care (Quality and Engagement) (Wales) Bill (2019) sets the legal direction for healthcare and wellbeing within Wales. The bill supports the ethos of integration of care discussed earlier in this chapter. It also places a duty of candour on NHS bodies in Wales in an effort to ensure an open and honest environment, with the ultimate aim of providing assurance to service users.

A number of key economic and policy drivers have necessitated the review of healthcare and social care provision across the four countries of the UK. This has led to an appreciation of the substantial role provided by GPNs and supports the transformation of service provision within general practice and primary care. This transformation ensures the development of GPNs, who form a vital component of the primary care workforce in the UK.

PROFESSIONAL ACCOUNTABILITY

NMC registrants are required to work at all times within their scope of practice and are responsible for all acts or omissions carried out in the course of their professional duty (NMC, 2018). *Professional accountability* denotes that registrants are responsible for their practice and are required to justify this practice; that is, they may be called to account for this. Consequently, registrants should be able to provide a rationale for their decision-making, acts or omissions regardless of any advice or input they may have had from another healthcare professional. As an NMC registrant, nurses working in a general practice setting are required to make decisions in a variety of circumstances for patients. A GPN will often work as an autonomous practitioner, but there will be times when seeking advice from colleagues is essential. It is therefore imperative that the GPN comprehend accountability as it relates to the professional, legal, employment and ethical dimensions.

Duty of Care and the Law

Implicit within the NMC Code (2018) is the legal requirement that nurses have a duty of care for any patient whose care they are involved in or are responsible for (Dowie, 2017). A 'duty of care' refers to the legal obligation to safeguard the health and wellbeing of others. Dimond (2015) advises that the test of the existence of a duty of care originates from case law, the case being the 1932 landmark case of *Donoghue v. Stevenson* (Dimond, 2015). In this case, Mrs. Donoghue drank from a bottle of ginger beer that contained a decomposing snail. Subsequently, Mrs. Donoghue became unwell and sued the manufacturer for negligence, winning the case. The judge ruled that the manufacturer had failed to foresee that its actions or omissions could result in harm to the complainant (Mrs. Donoghue) and ruled that care should be taken to avoid acts or omissions that may cause harm. For a case to prove negligence, three key factors have to be ascertained:

- There was a duty of care.
- There was a breach in that duty of care.
- As a result of that breach in the duty of care, reasonably foreseeable harm occurred.

This requirement to establish all three key factors is highlighted in the 1968 case of *Barnett v. Chelsea & Kensington Hospital Management Committee* (Dimond, 2015). In this case a patient unwittingly took a fatal dose of arsenic and attended the local emergency department. The nurse called for the duty doctor to assess the patient, but she was directed to send the patient home and advise him to see his own GP; the man consequently died. In this case, however, the doctor was *not* deemed to be negligent because the dose of arsenic was fatal, and it was ruled that the patient would have died anyway (Dimond, 2015). Nevertheless, Dowie (2017) emphasises that although nurses may not be found guilty of negligence, they could still be held to account by the NMC.

Employment

As an employee, the GPN is responsible for their practice and may be asked by their employer to account for their practice. The contract of employment and the job description seek to detail the professional roles and responsibilities, and the GPN should ensure these documents are current. Vicarious liability ensures that the employer is responsible for any negligent acts or omissions of the employee, providing the employee is working within the terms and range of their employment. Whilst any approval from the employer for the GPN to change role ensures that the employer is vicariously liable, an updated contract and job description should be requested and provided if there are any significant role changes (Dimond, 2015).

The standard of care required for any role or intervention a GPN provides will be judged against that of the ordinary competent practitioner under the same or similar circumstances and must be evidence-based (Dimond, 2015). To ensure GPNs are practising as accountable employees, they should ensure they have the requisite knowledge and skills to practise in an evidence-based, competent manner at an appropriate standard.

The GPN also needs to be aware that dependent on their employment location within the UK, differences may exist between the UK countries in terms of the legal systems and jurisdictions, such as those that exist between English and Scottish law. For example, in reference to the standard of care, where a duty of care has already been established, should a case for negligence emerge, under English law, the Bolam test would prevail (*Bolam v. Friern Barnet HMC,* 1957). Under Scots law, the slightly different test of *Hunter v. Hanley* (1955) applies.

Ethical Practice

To align with NMC requirements and contemporary healthcare policies, nurses are required to have an understanding of and concern for ensuring the provision of ethically appropriate care in all encounters. Milliken and Grace (2017) argue that awareness of and sensitivity towards ethical nursing care are required to ensure individualised acceptable outcomes for patients. This supports current national healthcare policies of person-centred care (DOH, 2012; SG, 2010; Thompson, 2016; Welsh Government, 2014). Milliken and Grace (2017) state that this ethical awareness requires nurses to recognise their responsibilities and accountability in providing ethically appropriate care. The authors continue to elucidate this point in discussing known quandaries, such as withholding diagnoses from patients, but argue that all actions are essentially ethical in nature, and nurses should ensure ethically sensitive daily practice. Inaccurate documentation, for example, could have adverse outcomes for patients in terms of the management of their care. GPNs must continually reflect on practice and ensure they provide ethically appropriate care and account for their decisions.

ETHICAL DECISION-MAKING

Decision-making is a fundamental component of the nurse role (Barlow et al., 2018; QNI/QNIS, 2017). As indicated previously, GPNs should strive to provide care that is ethically appropriate, and this will require decisions to be taken in concert with patients about their individualised care, which could lead to ethical dilemmas. To consider this more fully, it is important to have a clear understanding of the concept of ethics and ethical principles and reflect on some of the dilemmas a GPN might be faced with.

Butts and Rich (2020) advise that ethics is essentially a philosophical approach to comprehending and differentiating human actions that are deemed to be right from human actions that are deemed to be wrong. The authors indicate that to make a sound ethical decision, those involved should aim to ensure their emotions are controlled or detached from the decision to be made. This will be challenging for GPNs, who, by the nature of their role, are required to share decision-making in applying a personalised approach to care to ensure patients are at the centre of their care (DOH, 2012; SG, 2010). Conversely, Barlow et al. (2018) indicate that they think emotions are positive aspects when considering ethical decision-making. Although the topic is clearly controversial, in providing individualised, person-centred care, the GPN must be cognisant of the potential emotional conflict in ethical decision-making.

Paulsen (2011) advises that conversations about ethics usually involve principles, and principles are required to provide some protection to the individuals involved, particularly in healthcare, where some interventions may be open to interpretation. Beauchamp and Childress (2013) identified and articulated the ethical principles of beneficence, nonmaleficence, autonomy and justice. Beneficence aligns with representing the best interest of the other person. Nonmaleficence means doing no harm but, within healthcare, pragmatically requires consideration of risks and minimisation of any potential harm. Polit and Beck (2017) concur and argue that harm may not be visible and in some cases would be difficult to predict, such as distress or anxiety, and although this was discussed in relation to research, it is still a relevant consideration for the GPN. Autonomy is the right of an individual to make their own choice without fear of prejudice or penalty, and justice requires impartial and equitable treatment (Beauchamp & Childress, 2013).

Aiming to put the patient at the centre of decisions made about their care is fundamental to the role GPNs have with people in their care and aligns with current healthcare policy. Shared decision-making and a personalised approach to care are key elements of ensuring people are at the centre of their care (SG, 2010). Coulter and Collins (2011) advise that shared decision-making ensures there are two experts, the professional who has the specialised knowledge, skills and expertise, and the individual, who is an expert in their own life and knows the impact of their condition and their priorities. Shared decision-making is particularly important when choosing between alternative interventions, when there is uncertainty or conflict and in problematic situations such as ethical dilemmas (Coulter & Collins, 2011).

Barlow et al. (2018) advise that concerns about patient safety are in some part due to highly publicised healthcare failings that have subsequently led to an increased focus on ethical decision-making by professionals. They argue that key areas of consideration with regard to ethical decision-making are the role of the patient advocate, which will be discussed further later, and the power balance in both nurse and patient relationships and nurse and doctor relationships.

The role of the nurse and GPN is rapidly changing and developing (Barlow et al., 2018; DOH, 2012;

SG, 2015). These developments required nurses to become more involved in decision-making and clearly signal that contemporary practice remains evidence-based, supported by the use and application of current clinical guidelines. However, Barlow et al. (2018) indicate that with current healthcare policy directives ensuring patients are partners in their care, contemporary practice cannot rely solely on evidence but will be driven in part through ethically sensitive practice. Conflict can arise when the evidence base is at odds with the provision of what is thought by the nurse to be quality care or when ethical principles are at odds with the best interests of the patient. Conflict can also arise when the care identified by a doctor does not align to what a nurse might view as quality care. These potential dilemmas could occur in general practice. Barlow et al. (2018) argue that cognisance and comprehension of ethical principles and strong professional relationships are key to resolving ethical dilemmas in practice.

NURSING ROLES – RIGHTS AND ADVOCACY

Explicit within the NMC Code (2018) is the requirement for nurses to act as advocates for patients. Contemporary healthcare policy and practice across the UK require the delivery of cost-effective, person-centred care, with the additional challenges of increasingly complex nursing roles for a digitally literate population. Smith and Mee (2017) report from evidence that nurses struggle at times to undertake an advocacy role. Choi (2015) argues that advocacy as a concept is not well understood, and to function effectively as an advocate, nurses are required to possess qualities such as professional competence, empathy, resilience and accountability. Choi (2015) concurs with Smith and Mee (2017) that there is a substandard level of advocacy practice amongst nurses, and both authors agree that the reasons for this are multifactorial and include lack of confidence, concerns about hierarchical structures within the workplace and organisational culture challenges.

Choi (2015) identifies the need to conceptualise advocacy to comprehend its relevance in nursing. She describes different forms of advocacy. *Proactive advocacy* is explained as protecting patient rights whilst facilitating patients to make an enlightened choice about their care. *Reactive advocacy* refers to required

interventions when patient safety and self-determination are compromised. The nurse advocate therefore provides a powerful link between vulnerable patients and the local healthcare organisation. There are, however, a number of factors that can affect the ability to advocate effectively. These factors range from capacity issues, patient frailty and vulnerability, which may promote a more paternalistic approach to healthcare, and individual nurse knowledge and skills in advocacy (Smith & Mee, 2017).

Choi (2015) proposes there are four stages that need to be considered when developing advocacy practice. These are consideration of the need for advocacy, stipulating the goal of advocacy, planning and implementing advocacy and evaluating advocacy. In developing effective advocacy practice, Choi (2015) explains that there are individual nurse characteristics that will support effective practice, as detailed previously. Professional competence is a core requirement, and Choi (2015) suggests that identification of a role model and learning from that model are essential, but a team-based approach to the development of these advocacy skills is shown to produce benefit in developing capability. An organisational culture that endorses a whole-team, safe, effective and evidence-based approach to care in a noncritical environment aims to embed advocacy skills. This will safeguard the best outcomes for patients and align with contemporary national healthcare policies.

PROFESSIONALISM, ROLES, RELATIONSHIPS AND POWER

Griffith and Tengnah (2013) offer their definition of *professionalism* as being the knowledge, values, attitudes and behaviours that are required of a registered nurse. The integrity of a registered nurse must be underpinned by professional practice and behaviour (NMC, 2018). Schmidt and McArthur (2018) and Ghadirian et al. (2014) argue that nursing is an evolving profession, and the dynamic nature of it, coupled with rapidly changing societal values, provides regular challenges and ethical dilemmas for nurses. The role evolution is particularly true for GPNs across the UK whose roles are undergoing substantial transformation (NHS England, 2017; PHA/HSCB, 2016; SG, 2018; Welsh Government, 2014).

The NMC is the professional regulator for nurses and midwives registered and practising in the UK and for nursing associates in England (NMC, 2018). The NMC provides comprehensive standards for professional practice and behaviour in the NMC Code (NMC 2018). As the professional regulator, the NMC's role is to protect the public. The NMC professional standards are nonnegotiable, and NMC registrants must commit to upholding them (NMC, 2018). In the current guidance, the NMC state registrants must work within their area of competence and abide by the Code, which provides statements about required behaviour in four key themed areas (NMC, 2018):

- Prioritise people.
- Practise effectively.
- Preserve safety.
- Promote professionalism and trust.

GPNs within the UK must therefore ensure they continually reflect professionalism through their professional attitudes and behaviours, which are aligned to the NMC Code (NMC, 2018).

Explicit within the Code (NMC, 2018) is the requirement to practise effectively, which takes into account the need to 'work co-operatively' (NMC, 2018, p. 10). This requires the registrant to work with colleagues to share information and expertise and to defer appropriately for advice and guidance. Previously, we discussed potential professional conflicts that may challenge effective ethical decision-making (Barlow et al., 2018). GPNs, as NMC registrants, must ensure strong working relationships with GP colleagues. There are arguably barriers within these relationships that may cause challenge.

The introduction of nonmedical prescribing roles in the UK in 1992 (Cope et al., 2016) has facilitated an advanced role for the GPN, who is now be more likely to be managing long-term condition clinics independently. The GPN is likely to be employed by the GP, and as a result of the current role transformations, GPNs will find that they are increasingly involved in complex decision-making and managing the complete care of individual patients (NHS Education for Scotland (NES), 2018).

The concept of power is not widely reported or clarified in nursing literature (Sepasi et al., 2016), with authors articulating that the meaning varies from empowering patients to make their own decisions (Sepasi et al., 2016) to the ability to impose power over someone (Peltomaa et al., 2012), which tends to suggest a paternalistic approach. Peltomaa et al. (2012) state that this imposition of power is likely to be associated with increased knowledge. GPNs will find both interpretations resonant with them, and empowering patients certainly will align with current guidance around ensuring person-centred practice.

As NMC registrants, GPNs are required to ensure they practise in line with the professional behaviours indicated within the NMC Code (NMC, 2018). Clearly, a paternalistic approach to care does not align with either the Code (NMC, 2018) or current national healthcare policies, which aim to ensure care that is person centred. However, as the evidence suggests, although power is a complex concept, it can be used to create positive change and should not be associated with historical interpretations, which indicate it is a negative concept. Moreover, as Sepasi et al. (2016) and Peltomaa et al. (2012) state, empowered nurses can promote quality care, good team relationships and patient advocacy skills, and these researchers concur that self-development is key to promoting an increased sense of power in nurses.

Currently, national healthcare policies (NHS England, 2017; PHA/HSCB, 2016; SG, 2018; Welsh Government, 2014) promote the professional development of GPNs, and if this aligns with the research discussed previously, it should aim to ensure quality care within a strong team of powerful patient advocates.

AUTONOMY AND COMPETENCIES

As discussed previously, Beauchamp and Childress (2013) detail autonomy as the right of an individual to make their own choice without fear of prejudice or penalty. In their 2019 qualitative study, Oshodi et al. attempted to comprehend the meaning of autonomy in nursing for 48 nurses working in hospital settings in England (Oshodi et al., 2019). Whilst not directly relevant to the discipline of general practice nursing, this study provides some insights into UK nurses' comprehension of autonomy. Interestingly, Oshodi et al. (2019) found that there is a lack of agreement about what autonomous practice means, with some nurses feeling it means acting independently to manage practice and others believing that autonomous practice requires interdisciplinary effort to elucidate and corroborate decisions. The authors found, though, that overall, nurses believed that autonomy related to the clinical setting and clinical work and that the ability to make decisions may relate to individual nurses' proficiency and scope of practice. However, they reported that the potential for criticism as seen through the blame culture may affect nurses' confidence in making autonomous decisions (Oshodi et al., 2019).

The RCGP and RCN have developed a framework for GPNs' competence for nurses new to general practice (RCGP/RCN, 2015). This framework aims to standardise GPNs' roles and promote the provision of high-quality care. It also places a requirement on primary care organisations and individual practices to ensure robust workforce planning, recruitment and employment practices are addressed (RCGP/RCN, 2015). In 2017 the QNI/QNIS collaborated to develop voluntary standards to support senior GPNs in their effort to develop the requisite knowledge and skills for their role in general practice (QNI/QNIS, 2017). These competencies and standards, whilst supportive, will possibly place constraints on the degree of autonomy available to a GPN.

Desborough et al. (2016) indicate from their mixed-method study of 21 general practices in Australia that the GPN role is evolving, and there is an increasing demand on primary care that is evident at an international level. Enabling nurses to work within their scope of practice autonomously would provide improvements in interdisciplinary communication and patient care. The authors found that in general practices where nurses had a high level of autonomy and a broad scope of practice, patients were more empowered and satisfied (Desborough et al., 2016). Nurses working in general practice in the UK are required to work as part of interdisciplinary collaborative teams. The GPN role is evolving nationally, and the development and provision of competencies can support the GPN to be clear about the level of knowledge and skill required to work proficiently. The competencies provided by both the RCGP/RCN (2015) and the QNI/QNIS (2017) will support GPNs who are either new to general practice or who are established GPNs to develop the requisite knowledge and skill and be confident that these meet national agreements on the role of the GPN.

The RCGP/RCN (2015) competencies, whilst specific to new GPNs in the UK, have been informed by the World Organization of National Colleges, Academies and Academic Associations of General Practitioners/Family Physicians (WONCA) characteristics of general practice. The competencies aim to ensure new GPNs develop the competencies and skills required for the role, ideally within 18 months of employment. The competencies range from communication skills, leadership, health and safety, personal development, health screening and health promotion to more specific areas of management of long-term conditions and women's and men's health.

As previously indicated, the QNI/QNIS (2017) voluntary standards for general practice are relevant to senior general practice nurses in the UK. They are identified as voluntary to distinguish between mandatory requirements. The authors argue that there are many variables and inconsistencies within general practice across the UK and indicate this has affected GPN role development. The development of these standards was supported by an advisory group from across the four countries, and the standards incorporate four essential domains: clinical practice, leadership and management, facilitation of learning and evidence and research and development (QNI/QNIS, 2017).

SUMMARY

The complex demands and challenges of providing care within the general practice setting mean that the GPN needs to be cognisant of the legal, ethical and professional dimensions that inform care delivery. Additionally, strong interdisciplinary working relationships, knowledge and skills will enable and support GPNs to develop their autonomous role.

RESOURCES

QNI/QNIS (2017) – Voluntary Standards for General Practice:
https://www.qni.org.uk/wp-content/uploads/2016/09/GPN-Voluntary-Standards-for-Web.pdf
RCGP/RCN (2015) – General Practice Nurse Competencies:
https://www.rcgp.org.uk/policy/rcgp-policy-areas/nursing.aspx

REFERENCES

Barlow, N. A., Hargreaves, J., & Gillibrand, W. P. (2018). Nurses' contributions to the resolution of ethical dilemmas in practice. *Nursing Ethics, 25*(2), 230–242.

Beauchamp, T. L., & Childress, J. F. (2013). *Principles of biomedical ethics* (6th ed.). Oxford University Press.

Bolam v. Friern Hospital Management Committee, 1 WLR 583 (1957).

Butts, J. B., & Rich, K. L. (2020). *Nursing ethics across the curriculum and into practice* (5th ed.). Jones and Bartlett Learning.

Choi, P. P. (2015). Patient advocacy: The role of the nurse. *Nursing Standard, 29*(41), 52–58.

Cope, L. C., Abuzour, A. S., & Tully, M. P. (2016). Nonmedical prescribing: Where are we now? *Therapeutic Advances in Drug Safety, 7*(4), 165–172.

Coulter, A., & Collins, A. (2011). *Making shared decision making a reality*. King's Fund.

Department of Health. (2012). *Health and Social Care Act*. http://www.legislation.gov.uk/ukpga/2012/7/contents/enacted

Department of Health. (2014). *The Care Act*. http://www.legislation.gov.uk/ukpga/2014/23/contents/enacted/data.htm

Department of Health and Social Care. (2015). *2010 to 2015 government policy: Health and social care integration*. https://www.gov.uk/government/publications/2010-to-2015-government-policy-health-and-social-care-integration/2010-to-2015-government-policy-health-and-social-care-integration

Desborough, J., Bagheria, N., Banfield, M., Mills, J., Phillips, C., & Korda, R. (2016). The impact of general practice nursing care on patient satisfaction and enablement in Australia: A mixed methods study. *International Journal of Nursing Studies, 64*, 108–119.

Dimond, B. (2015). *Legal aspects of nursing* (7th ed.). Pearson.

Dowie, I. (2017). Legal, ethical and professional aspects of duty of care for nurses. *Nursing Standard, 32*, 16–19, 47–52.

Ghadirian, F., Salsali, M., & Cheraghi, M. A. (2014). Nursing professionalism: An evolutionary concept analysis. *Iranian Journal of Nursing and Midwifery Research, 19*(1), 1–10.

Griffith, R., & Tengnah, C. (2013). *Law and professional issues in nursing* (3rd ed.). Learning Matters.

Health and Social Care (Reform) (Northern Ireland) Act (2009). https://www.legislation.gov.uk/nia/2009/1/pdfs/nia_20090001_en.pdf

Health Education England. (2017). *The general practice nursing workforce development plan*. https://www.hee.nhs.uk/sites/default/files/documents/The%20general%20practice%20nursing%20workforce%20development%20plan.pdf

Hunter v. Hanley, S.C. 200 (1955).

Milliken, A., & Grace, P. (2017). Nurse ethical awareness: Understanding the nature of everyday practice. *Nursing Ethics, 27*(5), 517–524.

NHS Education for Scotland. (2018). *Advanced practice toolkit*. http://www.advancedpractice.scot.nhs.uk/

NHS England. (2017). *General practice – Developing confidence, capability and capacity*. https://www.england.nhs.uk/wp-content/uploads/2018/01/general-practice-nursing-ten-point-plan-v17.pdf

Nursing and Midwifery Council. (2018). *The code: Professional standards of practice and behaviour for nurses, midwives and nursing associates*. https://www.nmc.org.uk/globalassets/sitedocuments/nmc-publications/nmc-code.pdf

Oshodi, T. O., Bruneau, B., Crockett, R., Kinchington, F., Nayar, S., & West, E. (2019). Registered nurses' perceptions and experiences of autonomy: A descriptive phenomenological study. *BMC Nursing, 18*, 51.

Paulsen, J. E. (2011). Ethics of caring and professional roles. *Nursing Ethics, 18*(2), 201–208.

Peltomaa, K., Viinikainen, S., Rantanen, A., Sieloff, C., Asikainen, P., & Suominen, T. (2012). Nursing power as viewed by nursing professionals. *Scandinavian Journal of Caring Sciences, 27*, 580–588.

Polit, D. F., & Beck, C. T. (2017). *Nursing research: Generating and assessing evidence for nursing practice* (10th ed.). Wolters Kluwer.

Public Bodies (Joint Working) (Scotland) Act (2014). http://www.legislation.gov.uk/asp/2014/9/contents/enacted

Public Health Agency & Health and Social Care Board. (2016). *General practice nursing: 'Now and the future'*. https://www.publichealth.hscni.net/sites/default/files/General%20Practice%20Nursing%20Framework_0.pdf

Queen's Nursing Institute/Queen's Nursing Institute Scotland. (2017). *Voluntary standards for general practice*. https://www.qni.org.uk/wp-content/uploads/2016/09/GPN-Voluntary-Standards-for-Web.pdf

Royal College of General Practitioners & Royal College of Nursing. (2015). *General practice nurse competencies*. https://www.rcgp.org.uk/policy/rcgp-policy-areas/nursing.aspx

Schmidt, B. J., & McArthur, E. C. (2018). Professional nursing values: A concept analysis. *Nursing Forum, 53*(1), 69–75.

Scottish Government. (2010). *The healthcare quality strategy for NHSScotland*. https://www.gov.scot/publications/healthcare-quality-strategy-nhsscotland/

Scottish Government. (2015). *Transforming roles: Paper 1: Introduction*. https://www.nes.scot.nhs.uk/media/4031447/cno_paper_1_transforming_nmahp_roles.pdf

Scottish Government. (2018). *Developing the general practice nursing role in integrated community nursing teams*. https://www.gov.scot/publications/developing-general-practice-nursing-role-integrated-community-nursing-teams/

Scottish Government. (2019). *Health and social care integration: Progress review*. https://www.gov.scot/publications/ministerial-strategic-group-health-community-care-review-progress-integration-health-social-care-final-report/

Sepasi, R. R., Abbaszadeh, A., Borhani, F., & Rafiei, H. (2016). Nurses' perceptions of the concept of power in nursing: A qualitative research. *Journal of Clinical and Diagnostic Research, 10*(12), 10–15.

Smith, L., & Mee, S. (2017). Patient advocacy: Breaking down barriers and challenging decisions. *Nursing Times, 113*(1), 54–56.

The Health and Social Care (Quality and Engagement) (Wales) Bill (2019). http://www.assembly.wales/laid%20documents/pri-ld12572-em/pri-ld12572-em-e.pdf

Thompson, J. (2016). *Transforming health and social care in Northern Ireland – Services and governance*. http://www.niassembly.gov.uk/globalassets/documents/raise/publications/2016-2021/2016/health/4016.pdf

Welsh Government. (2014). *Our plan for a primary care service for Wales up to March 2018*. http://www.wales.nhs.uk/sitesplus/documents/986/our%20plan%20for%20primary%20care%20in%20wales%20up%20to%20march%202018.pdf

6

THE CONSULTATION

EVELYN MCELHINNEY

INTRODUCTION

Consultations in primary care are often carried out in an environment where time constraints (10–15 minutes) require the clinician to navigate the reason for attendance whilst trying to reach a working or definitive diagnosis. Patients can present with a differential diagnosis of mental or physical health origin across the life span and/or with exacerbations/complications of long-term conditions (LTCs). Therefore healthcare practitioners require communication, consultation and diagnostic skills for safe and effective practice.

Updates to UK general practitioner (GP) contracts propose a widened, multiprofessional approach to primary care networks, suggesting an increase in the knowledge and skill of existing staff, including general practice nurses (GPNs), and the introduction of other professionals (National Health Service (NHS) England, 2020; Scottish Government (SG), 2017a). In a modern primary care environment, GPNs must be able to consult with patients over the life span and increase their autonomy to enable consultation, clinical decision-making (CDM) and decisions of treatment, management, and discharge in a wider patient group without referral to a doctor. This chapter aims to discuss triage, consultation models and modalities, CDM, health literacy strategies, safety netting and referral required for GPNs in this area of practice.

TRIAGE AND CONSULTATION

A number of modalities can be used to triage patients in primary care. Triage requires decisions with regard to the seriousness of presenting signs and symptoms and the urgency of attendance, as well as directing the patient to the most appropriate place and clinician (Holt et al., 2016). This can be done via telephone, digital methods (virtual waiting rooms) and automated systems.

Once the patient is triaged and attends, consultation is the first step used to explore the reason for attendance and create a plan with the patient for further management, referral or discharge. This can also be completed via telephone and digital methods. The traditional medical model is still taught to healthcare professional students to obtain a medical history, and although this is practitioner centred, it is important to understand when it is useful and when to adapt it. Diagnostic history taking is this model's main task, and it has several steps (Table 6.1). Elements of this model are still adopted in varying degrees in primary care (PC) consultations.

Although, as discussed, this model is seen as practitioner centred, where the patient is passively told what to do, the overall aims of diagnosis and planning treatment and management are incorporated in other models of consultation that take a more shared decision-making approach.

Multiple consultation models have been developed since the 1970s (Byrne & Long, 1976; Kurtz et al., 1998; Neighbour, 1987; Pendleton et al., 1984). Although focussed and written by doctors and arguably adapted by current practitioners and reflecting current thinking, they are still important to review and are relevant to any healthcare practitioner, including GPNs.

Often models build on previous models and include language or strategies that, at the time of writing, reflect the current political, societal, and healthcare practitioner

TABLE 6.1	
Traditional Medical Model	
Task Step	**What Is Included**
Presenting complaint	What the patient sees as the problem or what you have been told by those who have triaged the patient
History of presenting complaint (HPC)	The trajectory of the disease over time; use of a mnemonic such as SOCRATES to quantify a symptom (best used with pain but can be adapted for other symptoms): **S**ite – Where on the body? **O**nset – When did it start? **C**haracter – What does it feel like? **R**adiation – Does it go anywhere else? **A**lleviating factors – What makes it better? **T**iming – How long does it last? Is it constant or intermittent or changed with a certain movement or task (e.g., eating, position, exercise)? **E**xacerbating factors – What makes it worse? **S**everity – Using a scoring tool and checking intervention outcome
Systemic enquiry	Of the organ or system you think the issue is related to (Bickley, 2016; Innes et al., 2018)
Echoing of HPC	Checking your understanding, showing respect to the patient that you have listened to their story and ensuring no misunderstanding or misconception from you or the patient using teach-back
Past medical history: Surgical, medical and investigations	Checking overall health status, relation to presenting complaint and ability to cope with symptoms Ensuring past investigations are noted and not repeated unnecessarily Use of a mnemonic (e.g., THREAD – **t**hyroid issues, **h**eart problems, **r**heumatic fever (possibly related to heart valve issues), **e**pilepsy, **a**sthma, **d**iabetes and tuberculosis, jaundice.
Medication history	Medication(s), dose, timing, ability to still take as prescribed, thinking de-prescribing, combining to reduce polypharmacy
Allergies	What happens?
Family history	What condition, when died – remember genetic conditions
Social history	Employment (past and present), exercise, smoking, alcohol, travel if appropriate, social services use, caring responsibilities

(HCP) approach to healthcare. Similar features or steps are incorporated, including exploring the reason for attendance, determining what is wrong with the patient, finding or not finding a working diagnosis, making supportive shared decisions with the patient, and deciding on a management plan. The following section highlights this in the description of the steps of three influential models.

The Pendleton et al. (1984) model includes a series of tasks: *defining the reason for attendance,* including patients' ideas, concerns and expectations (ICE); *considering the problem;* working with the patient to explore an action for each problem; *shared understanding;* involving the patient in the management plan; *using time effectively and building a relationship* with the patient. Neighbour's (1987) influential model discusses *connecting* (building rapport); *summarising,* or echoing back to the patient their ICE; *handing over,* where the patient is given control of the next steps; *safety netting,* which is different from previous models and deals with the advice given to the patient and considered by the practitioner to ensure the patient knows what to do if things change; and the final step of *housekeeping,* which is a more self-reflective step where the practitioner appraises their own stress levels and ability to perform to their best before the subsequent patient arrives. The Calgary–Cambridge model (Kurtz et al., 1998) has similar steps. These include *initiating the session,* which includes building rapport and finding the reason for the consultation; *gathering information,* where the problem is explored with the patient to understand their perspective; *building the relationship,* including ensuring empathy, support and sensitivity are shown to the patient and respecting the patient's views and feelings; *explanation and planning* using strategies to promote health literacy, such as using small chunks of information and checking for understanding before moving to the next piece of information, echoing back and supportive shared decision-making; and *closing the session,* where an agreed plan is made with the patient.

There is scope to merge the steps of consultation, and GPNs, as with other clinicians, tend to use a structure that is consistent or may be adapted for individuals. Therefore there is no absolutely correct way to consult, although models give a structure and framework that can guide clinicians.

Although the majority of consultations are conducted face to face, they can and have been undertaken via telephone for several years. However, new methods via video conference are increasing, which will require embracing new ways of working. As well as cost and time savings, these systems are arguably more environmentally friendly. Video-conferencing consultations are accessed via platforms such as Attend Anywhere (http://www.attendanywhere.com/) used in NHS Scotland and across other regions of the UK. This browser-based video-conferencing platform has been found to be safe and easy to use for patients and providers and saves on travel, time away from work, carer issues and personal and system financial costs, as well as saving time for secondary and primary care practitioners. However, there were some issues with dropped calls, use of the wrong browser or computer settings and bandwidth, which could lead to inequity of access (Technology Enabled Care, 2019). However, continuous review of the system is mitigating these.

NHS England (2019a) conducted a mixed-method review using surveys and interviews of the use of online systems by practitioners ($n = 1529$) and found that the highest users were GPs (1060; 69.3%), followed by nurses and healthcare assistants (61; 4%). However, only 85 practices offered online consultations. Interestingly, in the same survey, out of a sample of 3066 patients using the online systems, 72% identified as female, and 60% had an LTC, which is a considerable demographic of PC attenders. However, of the 3066, only 85 had used the system to consult with GPs and 14 with nurses. Therefore, despite willingness to use an online system for other tasks, such as ordering repeat prescriptions, checking availability or booking of appointments and checking results, consultation was one of the least frequently used tools. Interestingly, when patients were asked about future consultation methods online, chat via a smartphone was seen as more popular than video chat. However, video conferencing is consistently mooted as an alternative and aim of digital strategies in the UK (NHS England, 2019b; SG, 2018). However, there needs to be careful planning by PC networks on the advantages and disadvantages of online methods, particularly video consultations as opposed to traditional face-to-face and telephone consultations. For further information about setting up online consultations, NHS England's (2019c) toolkit Using Online Consultations in Primary Care is a useful resource for practices that outlines advice on how to initiate online consultations and what to consider before setting up online consultations.

More recent PC models, such as the House of Care based on Wagner's (1998) seminal work, enable care and support planning for self-management and recognise the complex 'work' of living with LTC and multimorbidity (Coulter et al., 2013, 2016). This is an important model increasingly used across the UK. It has been shown to enable supported shared decisions, improved health literacy and increased access to social and supportive resources within communities, as well as enabling the building of relationships with people, a key component of PC (Coulter et al., 2016).

Regardless of which model is used, GPNs need to make clinical decisions during and after consultations on working diagnoses and differentials if possible at this stage, the necessity for further physical examination or investigations and a treatment/management plan with the patient.

ACTIVITY

1. Think about your own consultations. Do you use any of the models in this chapter?
2. Have you adapted or combined models?
3. Discuss with your PC network the possibility of video consultation in your PC network.
4. Consider videoing your consultations and reviewing these with members of your team.

CLINICAL DECISION-MAKING

CDM includes the complex processes of cognition that lead to decisions and judgement in a clinical context. Multiple models and theories have been influential in the areas of medicine and nursing, such as the information-processing–humanistic–deductive (Elstein et al., 1978) and the humanistic–intuitive–novice to expert (Benner, 1984; Benner & Tanner, 1987). However, the current understanding of how humans think and make decisions has shifted the focus to models that include a system 1 intuitive, heuristic (fast) process of thinking and a system 2 analytical (slow, systematic) process (Kahneman, 2013). Croskerry (2009) has integrated this dual approach into his clinical dual-processing model. Intuitive thinking includes heuristics (rules of thumb or cognitive shortcuts). In a clinical context, experienced clinicians often use these when they recognise patterns of disease from the patient's story or nonverbal indicators of distress or function (Benner, 1984; Benner & Tanner, 1987; Croskerry, 2009; Hammond, 1980). Although this can be useful and almost inevitable when an obvious or recognisable patient presentation is seen (Melin-Johansson et al., 2017; Stolper et al., 2009; Van den Brink et al., 2019), this is the phase where the most errors are made (Croskerry et al., 2013; Kahneman, 2013; Van den Brink et al., 2019). Cognitive and affective (emotions) biases are also important to consider when in the intuitive phase, such as 'anchoring' to a specific set of signs or symptoms and using questions that lead to 'confirmation' of a diagnosis that the clinician feels is recognisable without fully exploring alternatives, leading to 'premature closure'. These can also happen in the analytical phase but tend to be higher in the intuitive phase. Several studies have shown that these biases can influence decision-making, leading to errors in diagnosis (Melin-Johansson et al., 2017; Stolper et al., 2009; Van den Brink et al., 2019).

There are over a hundred cognitive biases (Jenicek, 2010), and it is almost impossible for them not to influence judgement; however, being aware of these and how they can influence decisions can help practitioners to mitigate them. Reflection at the time of the decision and/or discussion with patients or colleagues during or after the consultation can help to move into the slower system 2 analytical phase, thus challenging affective or cognitive bias and reassessing decisions. Although more time consuming and mentally taxing, the use of both systems can lead to more thorough diagnostic, treatment or management decisions and reduce errors (Croskerry et al., 2013; Smyth & McCabe, 2017; Van den Brink et al., 2019). Additionally, GPNs should be aware of how factors such as personal fatigue, high stress, negative team dynamics, patient factors, interruptions and constraints of time affect their decisions.

HEALTH LITERACY

Health literacy has been defined as 'the personal characteristics and social resources needed for individuals and communities to access, understand, appraise and use information and services to make decisions about health or that have implications for health. Health literacy includes the capacity to communicate, assert and enact these decisions' (Dodson et al., 2014, p. 1). Globally, low health literacy is considered a critical determinant of health that affects people's ability to be involved in, and make decisions to, self-manage and maintain health. Hence, improving populations' health literacy is crucial to attaining the Sustainable Development Goals (SDGs) (WHO, 2016, 2019). GPNs can promote health literacy by understanding the concept and using strategies to ensure people are able to access, appraise, understand, and use information communicated or required to make health decisions before, during, or after consultations. The following strategies are suggested, which can be used in all areas of healthcare by all practitioners, including PC practitioners.

Plain Language

The use of jargon and acronyms by HCPs and within healthcare systems can cause confusion to the public, especially when individuals are vulnerable, unwell or distressed. Therefore a conscious effort to use plain language in signage, in patient letters and during consultations should be made to reduce this confusion and make healthcare easier to navigate (Pitt & Hendrickson, 2020; SG, 2014, 2017b). When discussing concepts of health with people, replacing jargon with plain, simple language can be achieved by thinking of alternatives, such as those presented in Table 6.2. Other important factors are culture, English as a second language, visual or hearing issues and intellectual or physical disabilities. These may also affect a person's ability to access, appraise or act on information.

ACTIVITY

1. Think of other words that you could replace in your signage, patient correspondence or consultations.
2. Discuss with your PC team and patients how you could improve patient understanding of letters, signage and language to increase health literacy.

Chunk and Check

Many concepts are discussed during clinical consultations, which can become overwhelming to patients, impairing their ability to understand what has been discussed. This can lead to misunderstandings of how to self-manage or carry out next steps or confusion regarding medication regimes (Brega et al., 2015; Rowlands et al., 2015; SG, 2017b). Questions by patients or checking of understanding are often left to the end of consultations, meaning people forget what they wished to ask or leave confused and forgetful of

TABLE 6.2

Replacing Jargon With Plain Language

Jargon	Plain-Language Alternative
Hypertension	High blood pressure
Echocardiogram	Scan of the heart, similar to a baby scan
Palpitations	Racing heart
Cellulitis	Skin infection
Ankle oedema	Swollen ankles

what was discussed. The inclusion of strategies such as chunk and check (Kurtz et al., 1998), where shorter pieces of information are discussed and then checked for understanding using techniques such as teach-back (Schillinger et al., 2003), discussed later in the chapter, with opportunities for patient questions can help check practitioner communication and patient understanding, improve health literacy and aid shared decision-making (WHO, 2018).

Multimodalities

Different methods for the presentation of health information can be used to supplement verbal and text-only information. The following subsections discuss some of the modalities that could be used by GPNs to improve patients' health literacy.

Pictures

The use of pictures during consultations or within printed materials can improve the attractiveness of information, recall and comprehension, leading to improved understanding of health information. This is particularly important for those who have low health literacy or issues with text-only information (Park & Zuniga, 2016). However, the use of pictures should be carefully mapped to the text, culturally sensitive and tested with the target audience to ensure their meaning is relevant and does not add to confusion (Lühnen et al., 2018).

Digital Strategies

The use of digital strategies to improve health literacy, empower people to access and navigate health systems and self-manage and maintain health is the aim of governments throughout the world (WHO, 2018, 2019). Digital political strategies discuss the use of electronic health records, virtual consultations, websites, health wearables, apps, games, online video and emerging technology such as augmented and virtual reality as modalities that can help improve patients' access, understanding and use of health information to enable them to make positive changes in health behaviour (European Commission, 2018; NHS England, 2019b; SG, 2018). GPNs should be aware of these policies and the availability of different modalities that can be used to supplement, improve and empower people's ability to understand

and manage their health. Mobile apps that allow patients to access information, book appointments or offer information or reminders regarding medications have been shown to be useful tools with positive health outcomes (Ernsting et al., 2017; Whittaker et al., 2019).

Games for health have also been shown to lead to positive health outcomes for people across the life span (Egras et al., 2019; Wang et al., 2020). Emerging technologies such as augmented and virtual reality are becoming more accessible to people and are increasingly being used for health research to increase health literacy (Saab et al., 2018) or reduce pain (Mallari et al., 2019). Several UK and international research studies are in progress investigating the use of augmented and virtual reality for promoting health literacy and navigation of health systems (Ahmadvand et al., 2018; Corporation Pop Ltd, 2018; Queensland University of Technology, 2017). These are worth following up to ensure they can positively affect future practice. However, it is also important to be mindful of the practitioner's and the public's ability to use and access digital technologies, ensuring adoption does not increase health inequity and inequalities (United Nations, 2019).

Written Information and Patient Paperwork

Text-based information and forms are consistently used in healthcare. However, across the UK, people still have considerable difficulty with literacy levels and more so for those living in socially deprived communities (Simpson et al., 2020). This means people often have difficulties with completing forms and understanding text-based health information (Morony et al., 2017a; Rowlands et al., 2015; SG, 2017b). Therefore assumptions of people's ability to understand written health information and the ability to complete health forms should be avoided. Where forms do need to be completed, help should always be offered, and written information should always be supplemented with verbal or audio, through recording of consultations for later review. These strategies remove stigma and break down barriers and can help people make sense of information, prepare questions and aid discussion with healthcare practitioners, promoting shared decision-making and improving health outcomes.

Teach-Back

Teach-back (Schillinger et al., 2003) is a simple and quick strategy that can be used in face-to-face and online patient interactions. It allows practitioners to test their communication of information to patients by asking patients to repeat in their own words what has been discussed. Alone or in conjunction with chunk and check, it can improve practitioners' communication and increase patient understanding and recall of information, leading to improved health literacy (Centrella-Niagro & Alexander, 2017; Morony et al., 2017b; Yen & Leasure, 2019). Global health literacy strategies encourage the use of teach-back by all practitioners to improve health literacy across the life span.

ACTIVITY

1. Find out more about teach-back at the Scottish Health Council website (http://scottishhealthcouncil.org/patient__public_participation/participation_toolkit/teach-back.aspx#.XlE8u2j7TlU) and start to introduce it to your practice with the other tools discussed in this chapter.
2. Keep a note of the responses from patients, and reflect on the changes you have made to the language and tools used within your consultations

SAFETY NETTING

As the consultation ends, there needs to be a plan in place for the next steps. This is where safety netting takes place. Introduced over 30 years ago by Neighbour (1987) and also seen in the Calgary–Cambridge model of consultation (Kurtz et al., 1998), safety netting is now seen as fundamental to patient interactions. A recent narrative synthesis of 47 studies by Jones et al. (2019, p. 74), proposed a definition of safety netting as follows:

Safety netting is an essential process to help manage uncertainty in the diagnosis and management of patients by providing information for patients and organising follow-up after contact with a health professional. This aims to empower patients and protect healthcare professionals. Safety netting may be performed at the time of the contact between health professional and patient or may happen after the contact through active monitoring and administrative systems to manage results and referrals.

	TABLE 6.3	
	Components of Safety Netting	
Component of Safety Netting	**Applying Component**	
Communication of uncertainty	Ensuring patients understand there is some uncertainty of diagnosis at this stage of presentation	
Advice on worrying symptoms and 'red flags'	Ensuring patients understand worsening signs and symptoms that would indicate deterioration or require re-attendance or seeking further medical care	
The likely time course of the illness	This would include how long the disease is expected to last and what to do if there is no improvement or the patient becomes worried about worsening symptoms	
How and where to seek further medical care	Ensuring the patient knows when and where to present if there are worsening symptoms or red flags, including how to access and what type of facility should be attended – for example, emergency services, out of hours, telephone advice or re-attendance at general practitioner practice	
Arrange planned follow-up	Ensuring the patient understands when to re-attend for follow-up. This may include making an appointment for the person as opposed to asking them to make an appointment. This can be particularly useful when uncertainty of diagnosis or time constraints warrant a longer consultation or when there is concern with regard to continued engagement.	
Primary care investigations and safety netting	Ensuring investigations are explained and results are followed up with appointments made to discuss results where appropriate, via telephone or face to face	
Organisational components	Good record keeping of the safety netting advice, systems to ensure investigations and results are followed up and given to patients	

The main components of safety netting found by Jones et al.'s (2019) review are shown in Table 6.3. Each component is equally important, and they are interlinked. Chunk and check, teach-back and written information and/or other digital methods or signposting to trustworthy support or informational resources should be used at this stage to ensure the patient understands the material before leaving the consultation.

REFERRAL

Many minor, self-limiting or long-term conditions can be safely managed in PC settings. However, referral to a specialist or secondary care services may be required for acute presentations, investigations or longer-term treatment and management. When this is required, GPNs must be familiar with the systems and processes and urgency of referral (through an understanding of evidence-based guidelines) and the correct practitioner or specialty to refer to. This is often achieved via electronic methods; however, telephone or follow-up letters may be required. Regardless of the method of referral, key components should be included to ensure

the urgency, current health status, investigation results (where available) and reason for referral are clear.

The following resources can assist in writing referrals and ensuring the key components are included:

Allan, A. N. (1997). Effective communication from general practice: The referral letter. *Health Informatics Journal, 3*(1), 37–40. https://doi.org/10.1093%2Finnovait%2Fins036
Wagman, L. (n.d.). *How to write GP referral letters.* https://www.gponline.com/write-gp-referral-letters/article/655978

SUMMARY

This chapter has discussed and described the process, strategies and models of triage, consultation, health literacy strategies, safety netting and referral that GPNs should find useful to consider, particularly to underpin their practice. Consideration and use of contemporary models to structure the person-centred consultation provides the GPN with the basis to support decision-making in the delivery of quality, evidence-based care.

REFERENCES

Ahmadvand, A., Drennan, J., Burgess J., Clark, C., Kavanagh, D., Burns, K., Howard, S., Kelly, F., Campbell, C., & Nissen, L. (2018). Novel augmented reality solution for improving health literacy around antihypertensives in people living with type 2 diabetes mellitus: Protocol of a technology evaluation study. *BMJ Open, 8*(4), Article e019422. https://doi.org/10.1136/bmjopen-2017-019422

Benner, P. (1984). *From expert to novice: Excellence and power in clinical nursing practice.* Addison-Wesley.

Benner, P., & Tanner, C. (1987). Clinical judgment: How expert nurses use intuition. *American Journal of Nursing, 87,* 206–212.

Bickley, L. (2016). *Bates' guide to physical examination and history taking* (12th international ed.). Lippincott Williams and Wilkins.

Brega, A. G., Barnard, J., Mabachi, N. M., Weiss, B. D., DeWalt, D. A., Brach, C., Cifuentes, M., Albright, K., & West, D. R. (2015). *AHRQ health literacy universal precautions toolkit* (2nd ed.) (AHRQ Publication No. 15-0023-EF). Colorado Health Outcomes Program, University of Colorado Anschutz Medical Campus.

Byrne, P. S., & Long, B. E. L. (1976). *Doctors talking to patients.* HMSO.

Centrella-Niagro, A. M., & Alexander, C. (2017). Using the teach-back method in patient education to improve patient satisfaction. *Journal of Continuing Education in Nursing, 48*(1), 47–52.

Corporation Pop Ltd. (2018). *Patient's virtual guide: A healthcare app using augmented reality, gamification and AI to improve a child's knowledge of health interventions.* https://gtr.ukri.org/projects?ref=104123

Coulter, A., Kramer, G., Warren, T., & Salisbury, C. (2016). Building the House of Care for people with long-term conditions: The foundation of the House of Care framework. *British Journal of General Practice, 66*(645), e288–290. https://doi.org/10.3399/bjgp16X684745

Coulter, A., Roberts, S., & Dixon, A. (2013). *Delivering better services for people with long-term conditions: Building the House of Care.* King's Fund. https://www.kingsfund.org.uk/sites/default/files/field/field_publication_file/delivering-better-services-for-people-with-long-term-conditions.pdf

Croskerry, P. (2009). A universal model of diagnostic reasoning. *Academic Medicine: Journal of the Association of American Medical Colleges, 84*(8), 1022–1028. https://doi.org/10.1097/ACM.0b013e3181ace703

Croskerry, P., Singhal, G., & Mamede, S. (2013). Cognitive debiasing 1: Origins of bias and theory of debiasing. *British Medical Journal Quality & Safety, 22,* ii58–ii64. http://dx.doi.org/10.1136/bmjqs-2012-001712

Dodson, S., Beauchamp, A., Batterham, R. W., & Osborne, R. H. (2014). Information sheet 1: What is health literacy? In *Ophelia toolkit: A step-by-step guide for identifying and responding to health literacy needs within local communities. Part A: Introduction to health literacy.* https://www.ophelia.net.au/bundles/opheliapublic/ pdf/Info-Sheet-1-What-is-Health-Literacy.pdf

Egras, A. M., White, N., & Holsinger, K. (2019). Games as a unique teaching strategy used in diabetes shared medical appointments. *AADE in Practice, 7*(2), 12–17. https://doi.org/10.1177/2325160319826960

Elstein, A. S., Shulman, L. S., & Sprafka, S. A. (1978). *Medical problem solving: An analysis of clinical reasoning.* Harvard University Press.

Ernsting, C., Dombrowski, S. U., Oedekoven, M., O'Sullivan, J. L., Kanzler, M., Kuhlmey, A., & Gellert, P. (2017). Using smartphones and health apps to change and manage health behaviors: A population-based survey. *Journal of Medical Internet Research, 19*(4), e101. https://doi.org/10.2196/jmir.6838

European Commission. (2018). *Communication from the Commission to the European Parliament, the Council, the European Economic and Social Committee and the Committee of the Regions on enabling the digital transformation of health and care in the Digital Single Market; empowering citizens and building a healthier society.*

Hammond, K. (1980). *The integration of research in judgment and decision theory.* Colorado University at Boulder Center for Research on Judgment and Policy. https://apps.dtic.mil/dtic/tr/fulltext/u2/a088471.pdf

Holt, T. A., Fletcher, E., Warren, F., Richards, S., Salisbury, C., Calitri, R., Green, C., Taylor, R., Richards, D. A., Varley, A., & Campbell, J. (2016). Telephone triage systems in UK general practice: Analysis of consultation duration during the index day in a pragmatic randomised controlled trial. *British Journal of General Practice, 66*(644), e214–e218. https://doi.org/10.3399/bjgp16X684001

Innes, J. A., Dover, A. R., & Fairhurst, K. (2018). *Macleod's clinical examination* (14th ed.). Elsevier.

Jenicek, M. (2010). *Medical error and harm: Understanding, prevention and control.* Productivity Press.

Jones, D., Dunn, L., Watt, I., & Macleod, U. (2019). Safety netting for primary care: Evidence from a literature review. *British Journal of General Practice, 69*(678), e70–e79. https://doi.org/10.3399/bjgp18X700193

Kahneman, D. (2013). *Thinking, fast and slow.* Farrar, Straus and Giroux.

Kurtz, S. M., Draper, J., & Silverman, J. D. (1998). *Teaching and learning communication skills in medicine.* CRC Press.

Lühnen, J., Steckelberg, A., & Buhse, S. (2018). Pictures in health information and their pitfalls: Focus group study and systematic review. *Zeitschrift für, 77,* 89. https://doi.org/10.1016/j.zefq.2018.08.002

Mallari, B., Spaeth, E. K., Goh, H., & Boyd, B. S. (2019). Virtual reality as an analgesic for acute and chronic pain in adults: A systematic review and meta-analysis. *Journal of Pain Research, 12,* 2053–2085.

Melin-Johansson, C., Palmqvist, R., & Rönnberg, L. (2017). Clinical intuition in the nursing process and decision-making – A mixed-studies review. *Journal of Clinical Nursing, 26,* 3936–3949.

Morony, S., McCaffery, K. J., Kirkendal, S., Jansen, J., & Webster, A. C. (2017a). Health literacy demand of printed lifestyle patient information materials aimed at people with chronic kidney disease: Are materials easy to understand and act on and do they use meaningful visual aids? *Journal of Health Communication, 22*(2), 163–170.

Morony, S., Weir, K., Duncan, G., Biggs, J., Nutbeam, D., & McCaffery, K. (2017b). Experiences of teach-back in a telephone health service. *HLRP: Health Literacy Research and Practice, 1*(4), e173–e181.

Neighbour, R. (1987). *The inner consultation.* Radcliffe Publishing Ltd.

NHS England. (2019a). *Online consultations research: Summary research findings.*

NHS England. (2019b). *Long term plan.* https://www.longtermplan. nhs.uk/publication/nhs-long-term-plan/

NHS England. (2019c). *Using online consultations in primary care: Implementation toolkit.* https://www.england.nhs.uk/wp-content/ uploads/2020/01/online-consultations-implementation-toolkit-v1.1-updated.pdf

NHS England. (2020). *Update to the GP contract agreement 2020/21–2023/24.* https://www.england.nhs.uk/publication/ investment-and-evolution-update-to-the-gp-contract-agreement-20-21-23-24/

Park, J., & Zuniga, J. (2016). Effectiveness of using picture-based health education for people with low health literacy: An integrative review. *Cogent Medicine, 3*(1), Article 1264679. https://doi.or g/10.1080/2331205X.2016.1264679

Pendleton, D., Schofield, T., Tate, P., & Havelock, P. (1984). *The consultation: An approach to learning and teaching.* Oxford University Press.

Pitt, M. B., & Hendrickson, M. A. (2020). Eradicating jargon-oblivion – A proposed classification system of medical jargon. *Journal of General Internal Medicine, 35,* 1861–1864. https://doi. org/10.1007/s11606-019-05526-1

Queensland University of Technology. (2017). *VALiD: The value of augmented reality for improving medicine literacy in diabetes and hypertension.* https://research.qut.edu.au/dmrc/projects/valid-the-value-of-augmented-reality-for-improving-medicine-literacy-in-diabetes-and-hypertension/

Rowlands, G., Protheroe, J., Winkley, J., Richardson, M., Seed, P. T., & Rudd, R. (2015). A mismatch between population health literacy and the complexity of health information: An observational study. *British Journal of General Practice, 65*(635), e379–e386. https://doi.org/10.3399/bjgp15X685285

Saab, M. M., Landers, M., Cooke, E., Murphy, D., & Hegarty, J. (2018). Feasibility and usability of a virtual reality intervention to enhance men's awareness of testicular disorders (E-MAT). *Virtual Reality, 23,* 169–178. https://doi.org/10.1007/s10055-018-0368-x

Schillinger, D., Piette, J., Grumbach, K., Wang, F., Wilson, C., Daher, C., Leong-Grotz, K., Castro, C., & Bindman, A. B. (2003). Closing the loop: Physician communication with diabetic patients who have low health literacy. *Archives of Internal Medicine, 163*(1), 83–90. https://10.1001/archinte.163.1.83

Scottish Government. (2014). *Making it easy: A health literacy action plan for Scotland.*

Scottish Government. (2017a). *The 2018 General Medical Services contract in Scotland.* https://www.gov.scot/publications/gms-contract-scotland/

Scottish Government. (2017b). *Making it easier.*

Scottish Government. (2018). *Scotland's digital health & care strategy: Enabling, connecting & empowering.* https://www.gov. scot/publications/scotlands-digital-health-care-strategy-enabling-connecting-empowering/

Simpson, R. M., Knowles, E., O'Cathian, A. (2020). Health literacy levels of British adults: A cross-sectional survey using two domains of Health Literacy Questionnaire (HLQ). *BMC Public Health, 20,* 1819. https://bmcpublichealth.biomedcentral.com/ track/pdf/10.1186/s12889-020-09727-w.pdf

Smyth, O., & McCabe, C. (2017). Think and think again! Clinical decision making by advanced nurse practitioners in the emergency department. *International Emergency Nursing, 31,* 72–74. https://doi.org/10.1016/j.ienj.2016.08.001

Stolper, E, van Bokhoven, M, Houben P, Van Royen, P., van de Wiel, M., van der Weijden, T., Dinant, G. J. (2009). The diagnostic role of gut feelings in general practice. A focus group study of the concept and its determinants. *BMC Family Practice, 10,* 17.

Technology Enabled Care. (2019). *Attend Anywhere progress report.* NHS Scotland.

United Nations. (2019). *Extreme poverty and human rights. Seventy-Fourth Session Agenda Item 70(b).* https://documents-dds-ny.un.org/doc/UNDOC/GEN/N19/312/13/PDF/N1931213. pdf?OpenElement

Van den Brink, N., Holbrechts, B., Brand, P., Stolper, E., & Van Royen, P. (2019). Role of intuitive knowledge in the diagnostic reasoning of hospital specialists: A focus group study. *BMJ Open, 9*(1), Article e022724. https://doi.org/10.1136/ bmjopen-2018-022724

Wagner, E. H. (1998). Chronic disease management: What will it take to improve care for chronic illness? *Effective Clinical Practice, 1*(1), 2–4.

Wang, Y.-L., Hou, H-T., & Tsai, C. C. (2020). A systematic literature review of the impacts of digital games designed for older adults. *Educational Gerontology, 46*(1), 1–17. https://doi.org/10.1080/03 601277.2019.1694448

Whittaker, R., McRobbie, H., Bullen, C., Rodgers, A., Gu, Y., & Dobson, R. (2019). Mobile phone text messaging and app-based interventions for smoking cessation. *Cochrane Database of Systematic Reviews, 2019*(10).

World Health Organization. (2016). *Shanghai Declaration on promoting health in the 2030 Agenda for Sustainable Development.* https://www.who.int/healthpromotion/conferences/9gchp/ shanghai-declaration/en/

World Health Organization. (2018). *Digital technologies: Shaping the future of primary health care.*

World Health Organization. (2019). *Draft WHO European roadmap for implementation of health available from literacy initiatives through the life course.* http://www.euro.who.int/__data/assets/pdf_file/0003/ 409125/69wd14e_Rev1_RoadmapOnHealthLiteracy_190323. pdf?ua=1

Yen, P. H., & Leasure, A. R. (2019). Use and effectiveness of the teach-back method in patient education and health outcomes. *Federal Practitioner, 36*(6), 284.

7

MANAGING CHRONIC OBSTRUCTIVE PULMONARY DISEASE IN PRIMARY CARE

JACQUELINE ANN DALE

INTRODUCTION

Chronic obstructive pulmonary disease (COPD) is not a disease but an umbrella term that captures the physiological description of a number of functional lung diseases, which specifically causes irreversible obstruction of airflow, depending on the underlying pathophysiology (Global Initiative for Obstructive Lung Disease (GOLD), 2019). Globally, COPD carries a heavy burden, in being one of the top three leading causes of death (GOLD, 2021). The personal cost in individuals is high in living with a disease that is unpredictably variable and distressingly presents as acute breathlessness, resulting in significant morbidity and early mortality. The costs to healthcare providers and the wider society are also high as part of providing care and the number of working days lost. COPD also has the unenviable position of being singled out as the only major cause of death that is on the increase (World Health Organisation 2017), a prevalence rate that is higher within older and deprived populations (CMO, 2020) and lacks prominence as a clinical priority. Underreporting of exacerbations compounds this scenario and, with it, unmet health needs (GOLD, 2021). To understand the diagnosis, treatment and management of COPD, there must be an appreciation of the underlying pathology, which includes chronic asthma, chronic bronchitis and chronic emphysema.

WHO IS AT RISK?

People who smoke and those who engage in occupations that involve exposure to noxious fumes, dust, chemicals and gases (e.g., agricultural, mining, motor and construction careers) are at increased risk of developing COPD. Although COPD can be clinically slow in terms of its progression, it results in considerable morbidity and disability, and work life can be disrupted by breathlessness, frequent chest infections, productive cough and fatigue due to muscle dysfunction.

Lung function in infants and older children born to mothers who smoke shows decreased airway patency (Stocks & Sonnappa, 2013). Lung function that is reduced at birth will further be affected by lower respiratory tract infections in infancy and early childhood, which is an independent risk factor for reduced lung function and developing lung disease in adulthood, a situation that is exacerbated if individuals become smokers or have occupational exposure to noxious fumes. Environmental exposure to air pollutants in childhood and the associated reduction in lung growth is a risk factor for adult-onset respiratory disease and may increase susceptibility to infection in patients with COPD (Grigg, 2009).

From a gender perspective, men are 15% more likely to be diagnosed with COPD, and more men die from COPD. This may reflect historical differences in smoking and occupational choices. However, women are more likely to be underdiagnosed (especially younger women) and are more susceptible to the harmful effects of cigarette smoking, experiencing more severe disease (DeMeo et al., 2018). There is some evidence that oestrogen deficiency may have an important part to play in lung function decline after menopause and is responsible for disease progression in lung disease.

The emergence of COPD is rare under the age of 40, and although the incidence increases with age, other underlying conditions indicate significant risk within the younger age group. Alpha 1 antitrypsin deficiency (AATD) is a rare genetic disorder resulting in the mutation of the protease inhibitor alpha 1 antitrypsin and results in a variation of alpha 1 antitrypsin level in the blood (Soriano et al., 2018). Alpha 1 antitrypsin is a protective enzyme designed to resist damage to the lung tissue from the immune system, when white blood cells are recruited to the lung in the event of an attack by harmful substances, such as cigarette smoke. A reduction in alpha 1 antitrypsin level means that the lung may be more prone to tissue destruction. AATD is rare and affects approximately 1 in every 3,000–5,000 of the UK population. Soriano et al.'s research suggests that AATD is underdiagnosed in the UK. Around 1% of 41- to 50-year-olds have diagnosed COPD compared with 9% of those aged 71 or above.

AETIOLOGY OF COPD

COPD is a complex, heterogeneous syndrome that has both pulmonary and extrapulmonary clinical features. The recent advances in defining phenotypes (or clinical traits) have led to the proposal of several subtypes of COPD, which has implications for prognosis and targeting treatment to optimise the clinical outcome for patients. The predominant but nonspecific symptoms associated with COPD are breathlessness, cough and sputum production.

The respiratory drive (physiological mechanisms that control breathing) probably has a familial or genetic predisposition, giving rise to individual responses to levels of carbon dioxide (CO_2). A normal response to hypoxaemia is to increase the respiratory rate to correct the pH of the blood. Those with a more responsive respiratory drive breathe harder to keep their oxygen levels up (chronic emphysema). But the effort of breathing harder means an increase in energy expenditure as accessory muscles, including the diaphragm, are employed, which in turn disrupts muscle function and muscle mass, leading to weight loss. Patients with a less responsive respiratory drive tolerate a degree of hypoxemia and are less breathless (chronic bronchitis). However, the consequences of chronic hypoxaemia result in reduced life expectancy through the development of pulmonary hypertension (cor pulmonale) and its associated complications.

Patients with COPD are at risk of other comorbidities associated with declining lung function, including pulmonary embolism, pneumonia and cardiorespiratory illnesses.

ASTHMA

Asthma is a complex variable obstructive airway disease typically linked to an allergic response and is usually reversible in nature (Global Initiative for Asthma (GINA), 2019). Chronic asthma is defined as requiring maintenance treatment and may become irreversible over the time course of the disease. Patients with chronic asthma have a higher likelihood of developing bronchiectasis, especially if they are or have also been smokers. There is much debate in the medical domain about defining asthma and COPD and whether there is an 'overlap', and there continues to be no consensus towards an accepted definition. GOLD (2019) suggests that there is a difference in the inflammatory response in asthma leading to obstructive disease and that it differs from the other obstructive-causing pathologies and should remain defined as a separate disease.

BRONCHITIS

Chronic bronchitis is usually characterized by the excess production of sputum through enlarged submucosal glands and inflammation of the bronchial tissues, which narrow and clog the bronchial tubes, causing an obstructive disease process. These patients often develop chronic hypoxaemia (abnormal gas exchange and reduced oxygen levels), predisposing them to the development of pulmonary hypertension, commonly known as *right-sided heart failure* (cor pulmonale), which is characterised by peripheral cyanosis, dependant oedema, pulmonary oedema, abdominal ascites and elevated jugular venous pressure. These patients will typically have a reduced life span.

Patients with chronic bronchitis often have a less responsive respiratory drive, meaning they can tolerate higher levels of CO_2 (hypercapnia) and their breathing (respiratory drive) responds to these higher levels. Hypercapnia develops slowly over time and is a result of chronic shallow breathing and preservation of energy to prevent muscle fatigue. Signs and symptoms of hypercapnia will include memory loss, sleep disturbance, excessive daytime sleepiness, personality changes and gait disturbances. The long-term consequences of hypercapnia and resulting hypoxaemia eventually take their toll on the body. Patients with dominant chronic bronchitis will have oxygen saturations under 92% and are dependent on CO_2 for their respiratory drive. Great caution is needed in patients with low oxygen saturations (under 92%) when receiving oxygen therapy, and they will need to have oxygen saturations maintained between 88% and 92% (British Thoracic Society (BTS), 2015). Uncontrolled oxygen therapy can lead to a reduction in the rate and frequency of breathing, increasing levels of CO_2 and falling pH levels, leading to respiratory acidosis, which is a medical emergency. *Acute-on-chronic respiratory failure* is the term used to describe an acute exacerbation in someone with chronic severe COPD and is deemed *type II respiratory failure*. Signs of acute-on-chronic respiratory failure include hypoventilation and acidosis; symptoms include headache, confusion, anxiety, drowsiness and stupor.

EMPHYSEMA

Emphysema is primarily a pathological diagnosis that affects the air spaces (alveoli) distal to the terminal bronchiole. It is characterized by abnormal permanent enlargement of lung air spaces, with the destruction of their walls but without any fibrosis, and destruction of lung tissue with loss of elasticity (Pahal et al., 2019). This loss of elasticity prevents air from being forced out of the alveoli, and air trapping ensues. Elastic recoil helps prevent dynamic small-airway collapse, which is why patients will often be observed breathing through pursed lips. Pursed-lip breathing helps create resistance in the airways, helping them stay open during expiration and keeping the alveoli ventilated. Pursed-lip breathing also

has the benefit of slowing down and controlling breathing rates. The loss of alveolar walls and destruction of the alveolar capillaries result in a reduction of the surface area available for the transport of oxygen and CO_2 between inhaled air and blood flowing through the lungs.

The predominant symptom of emphysema is breathlessness, largely associated with cigarette smoking. Patients are breathless on exertion; maintain a normal oxygen saturation with mild hypoxaemia; have a mild, nonproductive cough; have a barrel chest; and become cachexic.

Whilst it is important to recognise that chronic asthma, chronic bronchitis and chronic emphysema represent discrete clinical conditions, they exhibit similar pathology, and patients can present with mixed patterns of respiratory diseases. This type of occurrence introduces further complexity in managing and treating patients with COPD.

BRONCHIECTASIS

Bronchiectasis is usually characterised by excessive and chronic production of sputum (as a result of widening of the bronchial tubes), bacterial colonisation of the lower respiratory tract and frequent exacerbations (≥ 2 annually), which can all occur in COPD. Bronchiectasis can be idiopathic or associated with various risk factors, such as childhood infection, measles, tuberculosis (TB), whooping cough and severe pneumonia, and other inflammatory immune conditions, such as rheumatoid arthritis, inflammatory bowel disease, chronic asthma and severe allergic response to fungal and mould spores (e.g., *Aspergillus*). Bronchiectasis should be suspected if the patient has productive, purulent sputum with two or more exacerbations annually and previous identification of positive sputum culture with *Pseudomonas aeruginosa* whilst stable (BTS, 2019). A high-resolution computed tomography (HRCT) scan will be required to confirm the diagnosis. Spirometry testing may show a reduction in the vital capacity (VC), causing a restrictive defect, and any identified airflow obstruction in bronchiectasis is characteristically irreversible to bronchodilator therapy.

COPD ASSESSMENT AND DIAGNOSIS

Any patient presenting with a significant history of smoking (15 pack-years), dyspnoea, cough or productive cough should undergo investigation for COPD. A useful aide-mémoire of clinical signs and investigations is listed in Box 7.1.

A systematic scoping review by Hangaard et al. (2017) found that there were five main themes around the misdiagnosis of COPD (Box 7.2). Within primary care, these errors continue to dominate and perpetuate the missed diagnosis and misdiagnosis of COPD. One of the most challenging aspects of managing COPD in primary care is time. Currently, nurses working in primary care are given as little as 10 to 20 minutes to conduct a COPD review. COPD is complex and requires time to take a thorough history,

review past medical history and results, perform and review appropriate investigations and decide on a systematic, pragmatic approach to diagnosis (if the general practice nurse (GPN) has a respiratory qualification), management and treatment. Education of patients is time consuming because drug regimens are often complex, with a mixture of inhaled therapy devices and oral medication, and the fact that COPD is rarely the only single long-term condition. Patients with COPD frequently have coexisting comorbidities, such as heart disease, diabetes and other autoimmune disease, such as rheumatoid arthritis. An excellent document to help practice nurses assess whether they have the knowledge, skills and training to undertake a COPD review is *Fit to Care: Key Knowledge, Skills and Training for Clinicians Providing Respiratory Care* (Primary Care Respiratory Society (PCRS), 2017).

BOX 7.1
COMMON CLINICAL SIGNS AND INVESTIGATIONS IN COPD

SOFTMASH

Symptoms

To include current symptoms, breathlessness and exercise tolerance, sputum production, cough and frequency of exacerbations. Always consider other diagnoses, such as pneumonia, heart failure, pulmonary embolism and acute coronary syndrome.

Occupation

Consider all occupations that involve exposure to noxious fumes, dust, chemicals and gases.

Family History

Consider heart conditions and immediate relatives who have died under age 50 years, asthma, chronic obstructive pulmonary disease (COPD), lung cancer and any other chest or cardiac diseases.

Triggers

Consider what makes symptoms worse (e.g., allergen exposure, positional, humidity, exercise)

Medication (Current and Past)

Include cardiac and antihypertensives that may cause side effects, such as Atenolol, angiotensin-converting enzyme (ACE) inhibitors and beta blockers, and drugs that interfere with the lungs, such as Methotrexate, Amlodipine, Nitrofurantoin and nonsteroidal anti-inflammatory drugs

(NSAIDs). Detail current inhalers and ensure prescribed by brand and in accordance with local (check clinical commissioning group (CCG) pharmacy prescribing protocol) and national guidance (NICE, 2019).

Check inhaler technique and adherence and concordance with medication before changing prescription (e.g., https://www.rightbreathe.com/).

Alcohol

Use recommended alcohol screening tool.

Smoking History

Ensure pack-year history is documented (see https://www.smokingpackyears.com/) and age commenced smoking; give very brief advice (see http://www.ncsct.co.uk).

History (Medical and Health Beliefs)

Document other relevant medical history affecting chest/shoulder area (e.g., kyphosis, scoliosis, sternotomy) and any comorbidities (e.g., chronic heart disease, chronic kidney disease, diabetes, ventricular assist device).

Consider any personality traits, health beliefs or mental illness that affects their approach to illness, along with adherence and concordance.

PITT

Physical Examination

Note any physical anomalies, such as kyphoscoliosis, pectus carinatum, pectus excavatum, surgical scars, posture,

BOX 7.1—cont'd

COMMON CLINICAL SIGNS AND INVESTIGATIONS IN COPD

chest expansion, finger clubbing and skin colour. Does the patient show use of accessory muscles, pursed-lip breathing, or the ability to talk in full sentences? Also include the following:

Respiratory rate (RR) and depth of breathing pattern (e.g., pursed-lip breathing)

Pulse (May be normal up to 125 bpm – check previous records.)

Chest noise (e.g., wheeze, stridor) – Auscultate the chest if appropriate and trained to do so.

Cyanosis (e.g., blue extremities)

Cough – Productive (amount, consistency, colour, able to expectorate)? Consider bronchiectasis.

Peripheral oedema – Consider heart failure, cor pulmonale.

Height (no shoes), weight

Calculated body mass index (BMI) – If BMI below 19, use Malnutrition Universal Screening Test (MUST) score; use in conjunction with clinical judgement.

INVESTIGATIONS

Blood pressure (BP; a low BP, reduced O_2 saturations, and increased RR >130 may indicate sepsis.)

Oxygen saturation on air (If <90%, refer to long-term oxygen therapy (LTOT) for assessment.)

Quality-assured spirometry – Check contraindications. Presenting history and confirmation of obstructive pattern to confirm diagnosis.

Chest x-ray (CXR) – CXR is a poor predictor of COPD but is useful to exclude other causes of lung disease, such as pneumonia and lung cancer, and cardiac causes, such as heart failure (30% are normal in patients with lung cancer).

Full blood count – To exclude anaemias as a cause of breathlessness and observation of eosinophils because eosinophil recognition may help steer the use of inhaled corticosteroids (ICSs), prevent overuse or help patients to step down ICS therapy.

Liver and renal function, bone profile and thyroid test

Alpha 1 antitrypsin blood test after counselling

Electrocardiogram (ECG) –

Sputum sample – If initial visit, productive cough or frequent exacerbations.

TOOLS

COPD Assessment Test (CAT): https://www.catestonline.org/hcp-homepage.html

Modified Medical Research Council (mMRC) Dyspnea Scale: https://www.mdcalc.com/mmrc-modified-medical-research-council-dyspnea-scale#evidence

Nijmegen Questionnaire to help detect hypersensitivity: https://hgs.uhb.nhs.uk/wp-content/uploads/Nijmegen_Questionnaire.pdf

Hull Cough Questionnaire http://www.issc.info/HullCoughHypersensitivityQuestionnaire.html

Epworth Sleepiness Score: https://epworthsleepinessscale.com/about-the-ess/

TREATMENT

Check current treatment, adherence and concordance.

Self-management plan (see https://shop.blf.org.uk/collections/self-management-hcp)

Vaccinations: Annual flu, PCV23, shingles vaccine (age appropriate)

Pulmonary rehabilitation

Referrals:

Physiology for chest clearance advice and devices to aid mucus excretion (e.g., Acapella, RC Connect, Aerobika (FP10))

Consultant respiratory physician, dietitian, occupational therapist, social services, charities such as the British Lung Foundation and local self-help groups (e.g., https//www.asthmauk.org.uk, http://www.blf.org)

From original SOFTMASH developed by nurses on a COPD diploma course in the South Yorkshire area in the 1990s for COPD review. Extended and revised by J. Dale. Dale, J. (2019). Nurse develops aide memoire for structured respiratory review. *Primary Care Respiratory Update, 18*, 52–54.

BOX 7.2
MISDIAGNOSIS OF COPD IN PRIMARY CARE

1. Thresholds used for defining COPD errors in spirometry (LLN, FEV_1/FVC 0.70)
2. Primary care setting – diagnostic confusion, mislabelled, mistreated, spirometry showing no signs of COPD but diagnosed as COPD
3. Errors linked to performance and interpretation of spirometry
4. Difficulty in distinguishing COPD from other diseases such as heart disease, lung cancer, and asthma
5. Patient related factors: drug use, obesity, ethnicity, lack of symptoms

COPD, Chronic obstructive pulmonary disease; *FEV_1/FVC*, forced expired volume in 1 second divided by the forced vital capacity; *LLN*, lower limit of normal.

Spirometry

Spirometry is considered the main investigation in determining lung function for several respiratory conditions (Pinnock, 2020). Spirometry enables the measurement of dynamic lung function volumes to assess the effects of diseases on the airway that affect the diameter of the bronchioles and the elastic recoil. GPNs are becoming more frequently involved in performing and interpreting spirometry within the surgery setting, which demands being educationally prepared to undertake clinically complex roles.

The use of spirometry in contributing to a diagnosis COPD requires the GPN to recognise and correct poor technique by the patient and the ability to accurately interpret the results. COPD is a clinical diagnosis supported by spirometry and should be interpreted according to the historical context of presenting signs and symptoms.

Spirometry is never an urgent procedure, and therefore careful assessment is required *before* committing the patient for spirometry because they may have contraindication risks.

Lung function naturally declines with age, and spirometry traces produce a range of values based on age, gender, height (without shoes) and ethnicity (termed *patient factors*), which include the lower limit of normal (LLN), predicted values and upper limits of normal, which are based on large cohort studies using patient factors (Global Lung Index (GLI); Quanjar et al., 2012). Results consider the following values:

FEV_1 – Forced expired volume in 1 second (the percentage blown out in 1 second denotes the *severity* of the obstruction). Normal values are $\geq80\%$ and do not improve to over 80% of the predicted value after administration of a bronchodilator or corticosteroids.

FEV_1/FVC – Forced expired volume in 1 second divided by the forced vital capacity. This value relates to *obstruction*. This describes the volume of air blown out in the first second (FEV_1) over the total blown out (FVC). Obstructed values $\leq70\%$ are considered obstructed, but in people over 60 years, LLN values must be considered due to natural lung function decline.

Spirometry forms *part* of lung function assessment, and the results should never be relied on in isolation or labelled as 'COPD'. There are four patterns that can be defined: normal, obstructed, combined, restrictive. Any trace produced should be labelled with one of the four patterns and interpreted in the context of the patient signs and symptoms (Fig. 7.1).

Restrictive spirometry (due to stiff lungs or chest wall abnormalities) is relatively rare and more commonly occurs through poor technique. However, restrictive patterns can be associated with morbid obesity and more serious underlying disease, such as lung cancer and pulmonary fibrosis. It is therefore essential that *all* patients with a restrictive pattern are referred for further investigation of lung function and follow-up by the local respiratory consultant team.

Reversibility testing in COPD helps grade the severity of airflow limitation according to the FEV_1 after bronchodilation. GOLD (2019) advocates post-bronchodilator testing for diagnosis and assessment but states that assessing the degree of reversibility of obstruction is not required. The National Institute for Health and Care Excellence (NICE, 2018) cites that spirometry reversibility testing for most people is not required as part of the diagnostic criteria or to plan initial therapy and can be misleading due to a number of confounding factors, including fluctuations in FEV_1 reversibility, overreliance on a single test and the fact

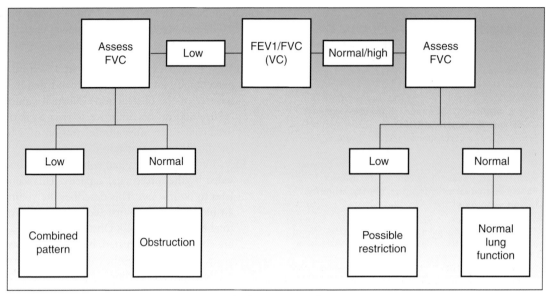

Fig. 7.1 ■ The four patterns of spirometry.

that the response to long-term treatment is not predicted by acute reversibility testing. Unless reversibility exceeds ≥400 ml, any reversibility should not be treated with inhaled corticosteroids (ICSs) on that basis alone. Once a diagnosis of COPD is confirmed by spirometry, as of April 2019, the Quality Outcomes Framework no longer requires annual spirometry at patient review. Full spirometry should be performed in the presence of worsening symptoms or when there has been a sudden worsening from a stable state. A step-by-step, downloadable document was produced to assist health professionals in improving the quality of spirometry undertaken in general practice (Primary Care Commissioning, 2013).

COPD REVIEW

An essential role of the GPN in practice is to provide a review of the treatment and management of COPD and advise in the prevention and immediate management of exacerbations of the disease. The failure to adequately treat and prevent exacerbations has serious consequences for the patient in terms of both morbidity and mortality. The goals of treating exacerbations are to minimise the negative impact of the current exacerbation

and to prevent further exacerbations (GOLD, 2019). Exacerbations of COPD are frequently caused by viral and bacterial pathogens. However, they can also result from other physiological causes (e.g., pulmonary embolism, pneumonia, chronic heart failure, acute coronary syndrome and anaemia) and be triggered by pollution, temperature changes and emotional stress.

Respiratory pathogens increase airway inflammation, mucus production and gas trapping, which drive the exacerbation. Three important factors to consider in exacerbation are as follows:

1. Previous history of exacerbation (≥2 within 12 months)
2. Previous hospital admission (≥1 within 12 months)
3. Purulent sputum

In a seminal paper, Anthonisen et al. (1987) described exacerbations that were defined in terms of increased dyspnoea, sputum production and sputum purulence. During an exacerbation, one of the most important aspects of treatment will be increasing and maintaining maximum bronchodilation.

Exacerbations can be classed as follows (GOLD, 2019, p. 41):

Mild: Increasing use of short-acting beta-agonist (SABA; e.g., Salbutamol)

Moderate: Increasing SABA use and introducing antibiotics and/or oral corticosteroids

Severe: Requiring hospital admission (may precipitate acute respiratory failure)

GPNs can assess the impact of COPD on patients by using the COPD Assessment Test (CAT; https://www.catestonline.org), which was introduced in 2009 as a suitable tool to use in primary care to assess patients' overall wellbeing and quality of life during follow-up review and the modified Medical Research Council (mMRC) scale, which is useful for assessing baseline functional breathlessness impairment in respiratory disease (Fig. 7.2).

Common symptoms of an exacerbation and potential red-flag symptoms are listed in Box 7.3.

Drug Therapy

Inhaled bronchodilators are the preferred treatment for COPD and can help to reduce lung hyperinflation, meaning the patient becomes less breathless, has increased exercise tolerance, has improved wellbeing and

---

BOX 7.3
COMMON SIGNS AND SYMPTOMS OF EXACERBATION

Increase in breathlessness (emphysema – increased risk of lung cancer)
Increase in sputum
Wheeze
Cough, tight chest
Fatigue
Reduced appetite
Reduced exercise capacity
Consider urgent referral (red flags):
Extreme or worsening breathlessness
Peripheral cyanosis
New or worsening oedema
Chest pain
Drowsiness
Confusion
New arrhythmias

---

enjoys an improved quality of life. In stable COPD, longer-acting bronchodilators are given regularly and are the mainstay of treatment. They can be used as a single bronchodilator (long-acting antimuscarinic agonists (LAMAs), which act via the parasympathetic nervous system, blocking M3 receptors to stimulate smooth muscle bronchodilation) or in combination with a long-acting beta$_2$ agonist (LABA), which improves airway patency by stimulating bronchiole smooth muscle.

In acute exacerbations, increased and more frequent doses of short-acting inhaled beta$_2$ agonists are recommended as the initial bronchodilators (GOLD, 2019).

Recent advances in understanding underlying pathology have meant therapy has changed, requiring a more specific reason for ICS use and lower dosages. Triple therapy (LAMA/LABA/ICS) is now only selected for patients with COPD who either have chronic asthma, raised eosinophils above the normal threshold or frequent exacerbators.

Suissa et al. (2013) found that inhalers that contain the corticosteroid Fluticasone increased the risk of serious pneumonia. See Box 7.4 for other factors to consider when using ICSs, which may increase the risk of serious pneumonia.

Modified Medical Research Council (mMRC) Dyspnea Scale	
	mMRC Grade
I only get breathless with strenuous exercise	0
I get short of breath when hurrying on the level or walking up a slight hill	1
I walk slower than people of the same age on the level because of breathlessness, or I have to stop for breath when walking on my own pace on the level	2
I stop for breath after walking about 100 meters or after a few minutes on the level	3
I am too breathless to leave the house or I am breathless when dressing or undressing	4

Stenton C. *Occup Med (Lond)*. 2008;58:226-227.

Fig. 7.2 ■ Modified Medical Research Council (mMRC) Dyspnea Scale. (From Stenton, C. (2008). The MRC Breathlessness Scale. Occupational Medicine, 58, 226–227.)

BOX 7.4

FACTORS THAT INCREASE THE RISK OF PNEUMONIA WITH INHALED CORTICOSTEROIDS

Age >55 years
Previous history of pneumonia
Low body mass index (BMI)
Poor modified Medical Research Council (mMRC) score
Severe airflow limitation
Blood eosinophils <2%

From Suissa, S., Patenaude, V., Lapi, F., & Ernst, P. (2013). Inhaled cortico-steroids in COPD and the risk of serious pneumonia. *Thorax, 68*, 1029–1036.

Inhaler Technique

The least cost-effective and effective inhaler device is the one stockpiled in the patient's cupboard because they cannot use it.

Inhaler technique is pivotal in the treatment and management of COPD, yet nurses' knowledge about how inhalers work, inspiratory flow rates for pressured metered-dose inhalers (pMDIs) and dry-powder inhalers (DPIs) for correct deposition of the drugs in the lung and demonstration of devices continue to be poorly understood (Baverstock et al., 2010; DeTratto et al., 2014). There is a high instance of misuse of inhaler devices among patients, and this lack of knowledge can lead to increased risks for patients, such as increases in exacerbations, hospital admissions and morbidity and mortality and increased costs in healthcare provision. Scullion (2017) provides some insight into the standards and competencies developed to improve inhaler technique through a framework to assess and support the standards of those initiating and checking inhaler therapies. GPNs are ideally placed to ensure adherence to and concordance with inhaler technique at the review appointment, and there are several innovative ways of checking patient inhaler technique. Bryant (2016) discusses the basis of getting inhaler technique right. All registered healthcare professionals have a duty to ensure they are trained in initiating inhaler therapy and reviewing inhaler technique at *every* patient visit.

There are several training aids to assist with coaching patients in correct inhaler technique. They include the In-Check dial (Fig. 7.3a), which enables healthcare providers (HCPs) to coach the patient to use an inhaler device correctly by assessing peak flow inspiratory rate, using various resistance settings that reflect the current pMDI and DPI devices on the market, and training aids that produce a 'tone' when the correct technique is performed (see Fig. 7.3b). GPNs can build a supply of placebos so that demonstration of proficiency and confidence in handling can be gained with each inhaler device. Asthma UK (http://www.asthma.org.uk) and Right Breathe (http://www.rightbreathe.com) both have excellent videos for HCPs to use with patients in the clinic to demonstrate correct inhaler technique.

The use of spacer devices should be encouraged with all pMDI medications. Spacer devices compatible with the pMDI are particularly useful for those with poor inhalation technique, for children, for patients requiring high doses of inhaled corticosteroids, for those prone to oral candidiasis and for treating nocturnal asthma (Joint Formulary Committee, 2021)

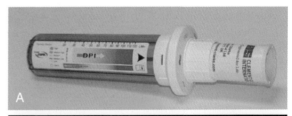

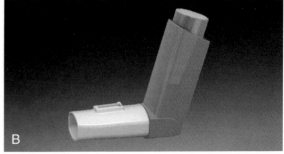

Fig. 7.3 ■ (A) In-Check DIAL G16 (Clement Clarke International Limited). (B) Flo Tone (Clement Clarke International Limited).

Chronic nebuliser use is controversial and is discouraged for most patients and reserved for very severe COPD. Evidence exists that microbial contamination of nebulisers may pose a significant risk for elderly frail patients with COPD, who may not be able to perform recommended cleaning methods, increasing their risk of exacerbation and exposure to serious lung pathogens. A full assessment should be carried out before providing nebulised therapy to ensure that there is objective evidence of either improvement in lung function, a reduction in symptoms or an increase in exercise capacity (NICE, 2018).

Mucolytics

Patients with excessive mucus production may benefit from oral mucolytics, which can improve sputum expectoration by thinning the mucus, making it easier to expectorate. However, caution is advised in elderly patients because gastrointestinal side effects can occur, and patients should be assessed before commencing treatment. There are two mucolytic products: Carbocysteine (consisting of two large capsules three times daily, reducing to one capsule four times daily) or Acetylcysteine, a much-preferred once-daily soluble preparation (BNF Joint Formulary Committee, 2021). The BTS (2019) bronchiectasis guidance recommends that mucolytics should not be used routinely, and if there is no benefit after a 3- to 6-month trial period, treatment should be stopped. Pragmatic use should be considered in exacerbations, where mucolytics can be used for shorter periods.

Rescue Packs and Antibiotics

Patients have traditionally been issued with repeat prescriptions (rescue packs) containing antibiotic and oral corticosteroid drug therapy to self-manage exacerbations. Hurst and Robinson (2020) highlight the challenges for people living with COPD in recognising when they need to commence steroids, antibiotics or both and how clinicians should select the people most likely to benefit from using such 'rescue packs'. NICE (2019) guidance details the need for education in self-management and an action plan for each person so they can respond to significant changes in their symptoms and optimize steroid and antibiotic usage. The importance of shared decision making and liaising with the community respiratory team or GP is emphasised by Hurst and Robinson (2020) with safety of the patient as the key focus alongside evidence-based prescribing. Following the PACE study by Butler et al. (2019), C-reactive protein testing is recommended in acute exacerbations, and general practice has seen an increase in point-of-care (POC) testing. GPNs may encounter POC testing and should encourage its use to help reduce the burden of antimicrobial prescribing in acute exacerbation.

Recurrent oral candidiasis (thrush) through use of high doses of ICS/oral corticosteroids can be difficult to eradicate. Ensure any pharmacological treatment includes the care of dentures (Joint Formulary Committee, 2021).

SMOKING

Smoking is the biggest preventable cause of COPD, with at least 20% of smokers going on to develop the irreversible airflow obstruction that is a primary feature of COPD (Terzikhan et al., 2016).

Peak lung function is achieved by the age of 25 years and declines steadily in the 30- to 40-year age range, but the decline is considerably accelerated in smokers. Taking an accurate smoking history is a vital part of understanding the insult that has occurred to the lung through the specific smoking product and length of time smoked. The use of a smoking pack-years calculator (available online) can help to give an accurate smoking history. Pack-years are calculated as follows: 1 pack-year is equivalent to 20 cigarettes smoked daily for 1 year. A history of 15 pack-years is considered significant.

Increasingly, vaping has become fashionable and popular as a method for helping smokers to quit tobacco smoking, and the UK government has stated that vaping is 95% safer than tobacco smoking. However, because vaping is such a new phenomenon, there are concerns about the long-term unknown effects, which may give rise to similar current lung diseases. The UK government continues to endorse the use of e-cigarettes as an effective method to assist smokers in quitting. A study published in 2019 showed that the most common reason for using e-cigarettes was to quit smoking, that there had been an increase in adults using e-cigarettes from 3.7% in 2014 to 6.7% and that the trend was increasing. However, people over 60 were least likely to take up vaping, and yet these are the patients who may benefit the most (NHS Digital

2019). Brief interventions have been shown to increase the likelihood of quit attempts, and the very brief advice (VBA) technique is recommended for all HCPs. Short, effective online training for VBA is available from the National Centre for Smoking Cessation and Training (NCSCT).

Healthcare professionals should continue to make quitting smoking a top priority for patients with COPD.

NONPHARMACOLOGICAL MANAGEMENT

Lifestyle changes can make a significant difference in the quality of life, and every effort should be made to encourage patients to make healthy changes. This will include stopping smoking advice and smoking cessation referral, nutrition advice in line with current recommendations and encouraging activity and social interaction. To prevent exacerbation through the prevention of lower respiratory tract infection, up-to-date vaccination is recommended. Currently, the annual flu vaccination and pneumococcal vaccination are recommended for all patients with COPD. However, it is prudent to ensure all adult vaccinations are up to date, including measles, mumps, and rubella (MMR) and shingles status (age dependent).

Pulmonary Rehabilitation

Pulmonary rehabilitation (PR) has long been the cornerstone of managing COPD. PR is a structured, supervised programme that is offered to patients with moderate through to very severe COPD. The aim of PR is to provide an individually tailored program to promote self-care and promote long-term commitment to exercise and activity. Programmes often include education about COPD, including both pharmacological and nonpharmacological management; symptom control of breathlessness and anxiety; increasing exercise tolerance, stamina and muscle strength; as well as improving independent living, self-confidence and quality of life.

To encourage management of breathlessness in the community, the Breathing, Thinking, Functioning Model was proposed by Spathis et al. (2017) as a way of managing breathlessness in chronic COPD (Fig 7.4).

COPD Action Plans

Self-management plans have long been indicated in the management of asthma but are relatively new in COPD management. Taylor and Pinnock (2017) discuss some of the frequently asked questions and evidence surrounding supported self-management for respiratory conditions in primary care and conclude that supporting self-management is a shared responsibility but one that puts the patient at the centre of holistic care and results in improved outcomes for the majority of patients.

LONG-TERM OXYGEN THERAPY

Patients with chronic hypoxemia and a resting oxygen saturation rate of ≤92% should be assessed for long-term oxygen therapy (LTOT). Treatment with LTOT is evidenced to improve survival rates and pulmonary hemodynamics, including polycythemia. Assessment should be carried out by the LTOT specialist team and will include the measurement of arterial blood gases (BTS, 2015). LTOT needs to be given for a minimum of 15 hours a day to improve life expectancy, and there are many factors to be considered before LTOT can be prescribed. Patients who continue to smoke are not usually considered for LTOT, for as well as providing little clinical benefit, they remain an explosion and fire risk, not only to themselves but also to the people who care for them.

THE ROLE OF CARERS IN COPD

The carers of patients with COPD often suffer poorer physical health and emotional, social, financial and relational stresses when caring for their loved ones. The role of carers is well recognised and one that has been extensively researched. A literature research–base narrative review by Cruz et al. (2017) found that there were unique challenges to family carers related to the specificities of the disease. It also found that interventions to support them were lacking. It is important to involve carers, with the consent of patients, when discussing diagnosis, management and treatment to ensure that appropriate and timely support can be offered in terms of emotional, financial and relationship help. Charities such as the British Lung Foundation (BLF) offer practical support for carers in supporting

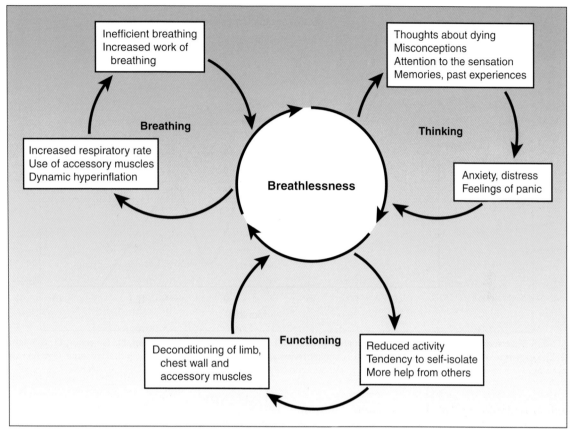

Fig. 7.4 ■ Breathing, Thinking, Functioning Model. (From Spathis, A., Booth, S., Moffat, Hurst, R., Ryan, R., Chin, C., & Burkin, J. (2017). The Breathing, Thinking, Functioning clinical model: A proposal to facilitate evidence-based breathlessness management in chronic respiratory disease. NPJ: Primary Care Respiratory Medicine, 27, Article 27. https://www.nature.com/articles/s41533-017-0024-z)

their relative with COPD, but they offer little in the way of interventions to improve carers' own lives. Probably the two most important interventions for carers are psychological support and, for relatives with severe COPD, respite services.

END-OF-LIFE CARE

Patients with COPD and their families are often ill prepared for the possibility of death and have often had near-death experiences, only to recover, to the surprise of clinician, family and friends. The course of events can be unpredictable in end-stage COPD, creating difficulties for HCPs as to when to discuss end-of-life care.

Landers et al. (2017) describe patients with severe COPD as having a chaotic trajectory towards death, with numerous difficulties in trying to decide the transition from continuing care to a 'palliative approach' (Fig. 7.5).

Palliative care has traditionally been the domain of cancer but has begun expanding the management of advanced but chronic long-term conditions, rather than palliative care adopting a palliative approach in the uncertainty of the condition. The Supportive and Palliative Care Tool (SPICT; University of Edinburgh, 2019) guides the identification of patients at risk of deteriorating and dying with one or more progressive conditions. The key indicators for

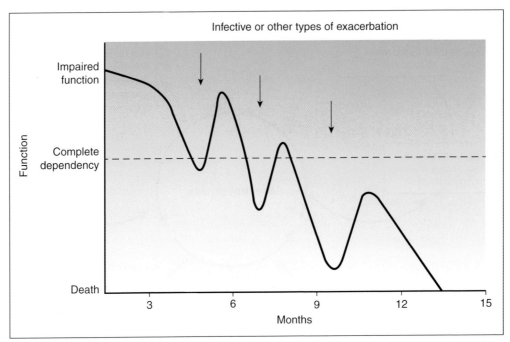

Fig. 7.5 ■ Trajectory of chronic obstructive pulmonary disease (COPD). (From Giacomini, M., DeJean, D., Simeonov, D., & Smith, A. (2012). Experiences of living and dying with COPD: A systematic review and synthesis of the qualitative empirical literature. Ontario Health Technology Assessment Series, 12(13), 1–47. http://www.hqontario.ca/en/mas/tech/pdfs/2012/rev_COPD_Qualitative_March.pdf)

respiratory decline include breathlessness at rest or minimal effort, long-term oxygen use associated with chronic persistent hypoxia and previous ventilation or ventilation contradicted (University of Edinburgh, 2019).

The palliative approach is aimed at reducing anxiety, treating persistent breathlessness through opiates and nonpharmacological treatments such as fan therapy, specialist pain management and access to psychologists for cognitive–behavioural therapy (e.g., Cambridge Breathlessness Intervention Service). Landers et al.'s (2017, p. 312) research acknowledges that 'the palliative approach is the responsibility of all; conversations about the illness and what to expect is everybody's business' and that collaboration across specialist services should be integrated to provide holistic, patient-centred care.

Hospitalisation for acute exacerbation may provide the trigger for a discussion about advanced care planning, resuscitation orders and place of death to enable patient wishes to be discussed and acted upon.

SUMMARY

COPD is a multifaceted disease. It therefore requires a multidisciplinary collaborative approach with the overarching principle of preventing and managing exacerbations. The GPN is in a prime position to co-ordinate and optimise holistic, patient-centred care. The importance of preventing and reducing exacerbations in patients with COPD cannot be overemphasised. A thorough history of symptoms, including breathlessness and exercise tolerance, sputum production, frequency of exacerbations and lifestyle modifications (e.g., smoking cessation, optimising inhaler treatment, technique and concordance, pulmonary rehabilitation, nutrition, vaccination), and a review of assessment using CAT and the mMRC, as well as self-management plans to assist in detecting functional deterioration, anxiety and depression, will enable prevention, treatment and management of acute exacerbations, which can have a devastating impact on patient morbidity and mortality.

REFERENCES

Anthonisen, N. R., Manfreda, J., Warren, C. P., Hershfield, E. S., Harding, G. K., & Nelson, N. A. (1987). Antibiotic therapy in exacerbations of chronic obstructive pulmonary disease. *Annals of Internal Medicine, 106*(2), 196–204.

Baverstock, M., Woodhall, N., & Maarman, V. (2010). P94: Do healthcare professionals have sufficient knowledge of inhaler techniques in order to educate their patients effectively in their use? *Thorax, 65,* A117–A118.

BNF Joint Formulary Committee. (2019). *British national formulary* (78th ed.). BMJ Group and Pharmaceutical Press.

British Thoracic Society. (2015). *Guidelines for home oxygen use in adults.* https://www.brit-thoracic.org.uk/quality-improvement/guidelines/home-oxygen/

British Thoracic Society. (2019). *Guideline for bronchiectasis in adults.* https://www.brit-thoracic.org.uk/quality-improvement/guidelines/bronchiectasis-in-adults/

Bryant, T. (2016) Getting the basics right. *Primary Care Respiratory Update, 3*(1).

Butler, C. C., Gillespie, D., White, P., Bates, J., Lowe, R., Thomas-Jones, E., Wootton, M., Hood, K., Phillips, R., Melbye, H., Llor, C., Cals, J. W. L., Naik, G., Kirby, N., Gal, M., Riga, E., and Francis, N. A. (2019). C-reactive protein testing to guide antibiotic prescribing for COPD exacerbations. *New England Journal of Medicine, 381,* 111–120.

Chief Medical Officer's Annual Report. (2020). *Health trends and variation in England.* https://assets.publishing.service.gov.uk/government/uploads/system/uploads/attachment_data/file/945929/Chief_Medical_Officer_s_annual_report_2020_-_health_trends_and_variation_in_England.pdf

Cruz, J., Marques, A., & Figueiredo, D. (2017). Impacts of COPD on family carers and supportive interventions: A narrative review. *Health and Social Care in the Community, 25*(1), 11–25.

DeMeo, D., Ramagopalan, S., Abishek, K., Vegesna, A., Han, M. K., Yadao, A., Wilcox, T. K., & Make, B. J. (2018). Women manifest more severe COPD symptoms across the life course. *International Journal of Chronic Obstructive Pulmonary Disease, 13,* 3021–3029. https://www.ncbi.nlm.nih.gov/pmc/articles/PMC6171761/

Department of Health. (2010). *Consultation on a strategy for services for chronic obstructive pulmonary disease (COPD) in England.* https://assets.publishing.service.gov.uk/government/uploads/system/uploads/attachment_data/file/213840/dh_113279.pdf

DeTratto, K., Gomez, C., Ryan C., Bracken, N., Steffen, A., & Corbridge, S. J. (2014). Nurses' knowledge of inhaler technique in the inpatient hospital setting. *Clinical Nurse Specialist, 28*(3), 156–160.

Global Initiative for Asthma. (2019). *Pocket guide for asthma management and prevention.* https://ginasthma.org/wp-content/uploads/2019/04/GINA-2019-main-Pocket-Guide-wms.pdf

Global Initiative for Chronic Obstructive Lung Disease. (2019). *Pocket guide to management diagnosis, management and prevention.* https://goldcopd.org/wp-content/uploads/2018/11/GOLD-2019-POCKET-GUIDE-FINAL_WMS.pdf

Global Initiative for Obstructive Lung Disease. (2021). *Global strategy for the diagnosis, management and prevention of COPD.*

https://goldcopd.org/wp-content/uploads/2020/11/GOLD-REPORT-2021-v1.1-25Nov20_WMV.pdf

Grigg, J. (2009). Particulate matter exposure in children. Relevance to chronic obstructive pulmonary disease. *Proceedings of the American Thoracic Society, 6,* 564–569.

Hangaard, S., Helle, T., Nielsen, C., & Hejlesen, O. K. (2017). Causes of misdiagnosis of chronic obstructive pulmonary disease: A systematic scoping review. *Respiratory Medicine, 129,* 63–84.

Hurst, Robinson (2020). The appropriate use of rescue packs. Primary care respiratory update. *Primary Care Respiratory Society* https://www.pcrs-uk.org/sites/pcrs-uk.org/files/pcru/articles/2020-Winter-Issue-21-Appropriate-Use-of-Rescue-Packs.pdf

Joint Formulary Committee. (2021). *British National Formulary.* www.medicinescomplete.com

Landers, A., Wiseman, R., Pitama, S., & Beckert, L. (2017). Severe COPD and the transition to a palliative approach. *Breathe, 13*(4), 310–316.

National Institute for Health and Care Excellence. (2018). *Chronic obstructive pulmonary disease in over 16s: Diagnosis and management (NG115).* https://www.nice.org.uk/guidance/NG115

National Institute for Health and Care Excellence. (2019). *Pneumonia (community-acquired): Antimicrobial prescribing (NG138).* https://www.nice.org.uk/guidance/ng138

NHS Digital. (2019). *Statistics on smoking – England 2019.* https://digital.nhs.uk/data-and-information/publications/statistical/statistics-on-smoking/statistics-on-smoking-england-2019

Pahal, P., Avula, A., & Sharma, S. (2019). Emphysema. In *StatPearls* [Internet]. https://www.ncbi.nlm.nih.gov/books/NBK482217/

Pinnock, H. (2020). Respiratory problems. In A. Staten & P. Staten (Eds.), *Practical general practice guidelines for effective clinical management* (7th ed., pp. 93–108). Elsevier.

Primary Care Respiratory Society. (2017). *Fit to care: Key knowledge, skills and training for clinicians providing respiratory care.* https://www.pcrs-uk.org/resource/fit-care

Quanjer, P. H., Stanojevic, S., Cole, T. J., Baur, X., Hall, G. L., Culver, B. H., Enright, P. L., Hankinson, J. L., Ip, M. S. M., Zheng, J., Stocks, J., & the ERS Global Lung Function Initiative. (2012). Multi-ethnic reference values for spirometry for the 3-95-yr age range: The global lung function 2012 equations. *European Respiratory Journal, 40,* 1324–1343.

Robinson, F. (2018). The appropriate use of rescue packs. *Primary Care Update, 5*(1).

Scullion, J. (2017). *Standards and competencies to improve inhaler technique.* http://www.independentnurse.co.uk/clinical-article/standards-and-competencies-to-improve-inhaler-technique/151138/

Soriano, J., Jones, R., Lucas, S., Mahadeva, M., & Miravitlles, J. (2018). Modern epidemiology of alpha(1)-antitrypsin deficiency (AATD) in the UK. *American Journal of Respiratory and Critical Care Medicine, 197,* Article A1955.

Spathis, A., Booth, S., Moffat, Hurst, R., Ryan, R., Chin, C., & Burkin, J. (2017). The Breathing, Thinking, Functioning clinical model: A proposal to facilitate evidence-based breathlessness management in chronic respiratory disease. *NPJ: Primary Care Respiratory Medicine, 27,* Article 27. https://www.nature.com/articles/s41533-017-0024-z

Stocks, J., & Sonnappa, S. (2013). Early influences on the development of chronic obstructive pulmonary disease. *Therapeutic Advances in Respiratory Disease, 7*(3), 161–73.

Suissa, S., Patenaude, V., Lapi, F., & Ernst, P. (2013). Inhaled cortico-steroids in COPD and the risk of serious pneumonia. *Thorax, 68,* 1029–1036.

Taylor, S., & Pinnock, H. (2017). Supported self-management for respiratory conditions in primary care. *Primary Care Update, 4*(3).

Terzikhan, N., Verhamme, K. M., Hofman, A., Stricker, B. H., Brusselle, G. G., & Lahousse, L. (2016). Prevalence and incidence of COPD in smokers and non-smokers: The Rotterdam Study. *European Journal of Epidemiology, 31*(8), 785–792.

University of Edinburgh. (2019). *SPICT*. http://www.spict.org.uk/the-spict/

World Health Organization. (2017). Chronic obstructive pulmonary disease (COPD). Key facts. https://www.who.int/news-room/fact-sheets/detail/chronic-obstructive-pulmonary-disease-(copd)

8

MANAGING ASTHMA IN PRIMARY CARE

COLETTE HENDERSON

INTRODUCTION

Asthma is a common long-term respiratory condition that causes significant morbidity and mortality, with UK mortality being amongst the highest in Europe (Asthma UK, 2019d). The annual cost of asthma to the National Health Service (NHS) is in excess of £1.1 billion; the vast majority of this total relates to prescription costs and the estimated 6.4 million consultations in UK primary care settings (Mukherjee et al., 2016). Because the bulk of asthma care is undertaken in the community setting, general practice nurses (GPNs) who have been suitably educated are ideally placed to provide person-centred asthma care for individuals and their families. This chapter will discuss the definition and aetiology of asthma, presenting symptoms, assessment and diagnosis and management of asthma, with a focus on the role of the GPN.

Asthma is a common long-term respiratory condition that affects approximately 5.4 million people in the UK; 4.3 million adults and 1.1 million children currently receive treatment for asthma (Asthma UK, 2019a). The World Health Organisation (WHO, 2019) reports that asthma is the most common noncommunicable disease in children. Mukherjee et al. (2016) state that the UK has one of the highest incidences of allergies and asthma in the world.

Asthma can occur at any point throughout the life span and causes significant morbidity and mortality; in 2016/2017 the UK had 77,124 hospital admissions and 1484 deaths (Asthma UK, 2019a). The Royal College of Physicians (2014) testifies that many of these deaths could be prevented with improvements in asthma care. Asthma UK specialists attribute the UK's high asthma mortality rate to lack of knowledge about the severity of the disease and poor basic care, such as lack of asthma action plans, inhaler technique reviews or annual reviews (Asthma UK, 2019d). Because most asthma care is undertaken in the community setting (Asthma UK, 2019a; Mukherjee et al., 2016), GPNs who have been suitably educated are ideally placed to provide person-centred asthma care for individuals and their families. Good asthma control will reduce the risk of asthma attacks, which are known to be associated with poor outcomes (Mukherjee et al., 2016).

Traditionally, UK asthma guidance has come from British Thoracic Society/Scottish Intercollegiate Guidelines Network (BTS/SIGN) collaborations. Although guidelines exist to promote best practice, both BTS/SIGN (2019) and the Global Initiative for Asthma (GINA, 2019) stress the importance of making clinical decisions in consultation with the patient and based on all available clinical data.

DEFINITION, AETIOLOGY AND PRESENTING SYMPTOMS

BTS/SIGN (2019) and GINA (2019) report that the definition of asthma is inclusive of the existence of more than one of the symptoms of cough, wheeze, shortness of breath or tight chest and variable airflow obstruction, airway hyperresponsiveness and airway inflammation. Whilst the exact cause of asthma remains unclear, there are factors that increase the risk of developing asthma, such as genetics and environmental pollutants (WHO, 2019). A familial predisposition for asthma, eczema and allergies increases the risk of developing asthma, as do tobacco smoking or exposure to tobacco smoke, premature birth, low birth weight and bronchiolitis. Exposure to air pollutants and certain chemicals is also thought to increase the risk of developing asthma (Asthma UK, 2019a; WHO, 2019).

Having a clear understanding of the pathophysiology of asthma will support the GPN in comprehending the diagnosis and assisting patients in managing their disease. Asthma is characterised by airway inflammation, which is associated with variable airflow obstruction and airway hypersensitivity to various stimuli (GINA, 2019). Stimuli such as air temperature, pollen, foods, exercise or emotional upset, for example, can cause airway hypersensitivity. Narrowing or obstruction of the airways may be caused by smooth muscle inflammation, which leads to an increase in mucus production that will obstruct the airways, but in addition, an immune response causes oedema, further narrowing inflamed airways (Tortora & Derrickson, 2015). Poor asthma control can lead to cell and tissue changes within the airways that cause permanent damage and result in remodelling of the airways. The subsequent commonly reported symptoms of cough, wheeze, shortness of breath and tight chest are a result of the disease, although these symptoms are not mutually exclusive for asthma. BTS/SIGN (2019) guidance cautions that solitary symptoms alone are not unique or specific for asthma.

The WHO (2019) indicates that persistent asthma symptoms can result in additional challenges for individuals, such as lethargy or a decline in activity, and may ultimately affect attendance at school or work. A comprehensive clinical review by a suitably educated health professional is therefore indicated to ensure optimum assessment and appropriate asthma management (BTS/SIGN, 2019; White et al., 2018) and to avoid overtreatment or misdiagnosis (GINA, 2019).

ASSESSMENT AND DIAGNOSIS

BTS/SIGN (2019) and GINA (2019) highlight the challenge of diagnosing asthma and indicate that there is no single diagnostic test that will be conclusive for an asthma diagnosis, but a comprehensive assessment should be inclusive of signs, symptoms and diagnostic evidence. A thorough history should ensure detail is provided regarding any symptoms of cough, wheeze, shortness of breath or tight chest; variation in time and intensity of symptoms; and variation in airflow obstruction, airway hyperresponsiveness to stimuli and exposure to triggers (BTS/SIGN, 2019). It is vital that the history incorporates detail regarding risk factors for asthma (GINA, 2019). Questions about past medical history should provide key data about birth history and childhood infections. Information about current medications should be ascertained; this will include prescribed, over-the-counter, herbal or illicit drugs and any association between taking these medications or drugs and the development of asthma symptoms. This level of detail will enable the GPN to consider potential causes and differential diagnoses (BTS/SIGN, 2019; GINA, 2019). Family history is relevant to provide evidence about familial predisposition to asthma, eczema or allergies and exposure to tobacco smoke. A thorough social history will supply information about personal smoking and alcohol history, pets and hobbies and any link between the development of symptoms after exposure to pets or with new hobbies. Smoking and alcohol history provide detail about potential challenges in the management of asthma and are implicated in associated morbidity and mortality.

Occupational information linked with symptom development or resolution will support considerations of whether there is an occupational element to the development of asthma symptoms (BTS/SIGN, 2019).

Physical examination should be integral to a holistic assessment. GINA (2019) suggests that whilst this may often be normal, expiratory wheeze can be identified during chest auscultation, and a nasal examination may reveal allergic rhinitis. Expiratory wheeze and allergic rhinitis will support a diagnosis of asthma, whereas repeated normal chest auscultation will aid in discounting an asthma diagnosis (GINA, 2019).

In assessing a child presenting with symptoms suggestive of asthma, the history detail, as identified previously, can be provided by parents. This should include a discussion about lethargy and a reduction in or lack of activity (WHO, 2019). Bhatt and Parker (2019) counsel the practitioner to ensure that an exact understanding of wheeze is obtained, and they suggest that this diagnosis of wheeze must be confirmed by a doctor. BTS/SIGN (2019) guidance indicates, however, that a trained healthcare professional could reliably identify wheeze. Bhatt and Parker (2019) confirm that infants and small children make asthma diagnosis more challenging due to the difficulty in obtaining objective test data, and GINA (2019) concurs with this view. Bhatt and Parker (2019) suggest assessment of children should consist of history, physical examination and, in children over 5 years of age, variation in peak expiratory flow rates and a trial of treatment. GINA (2019) agrees and advises that in under 5s, consideration of symptoms, patterns of symptoms, risk factors and response to treatment trials will support the clinician to make a diagnosis. Bhatt and Parker (2019) and GINA (2019) highlight that these data are useful, but for all children, alternate diagnoses should be considered and excluded. BTS/SIGN (2019) guidance indicates that for adults, obesity, dysfunctional breathing, anxiety and comorbidities such as chronic obstructive pulmonary disease (COPD) and other explanations for symptoms that may imitate asthma must be contemplated.

Objective tests such as spirometry, bronchodilator reversibility, peak expiratory flow variability and fractional exhaled nitric oxide can all provide relevant indicative detail to support or refute an asthma diagnosis. A key concern is that diagnostic tests should demonstrate the variation in airflow obstruction or airway inflammation (BTS/SIGN, 2019; GINA, 2019). BTS/SIGN (2019) guidance highlights that one of the significant challenges to diagnosing asthma is that of false positives and false negatives in relation to both assessment data and objective testing; additionally, the variable nature of asthma can cause challenges with undertaking objective tests because the patient may not be symptomatic at the time of testing, and therefore the result may signify a false negative. The BTS/SIGN (2019) guidance reinforces the need to ensure all clinical assessment data are utilised alongside test results when assessing for asthma. The GPN should be cognisant of this during any patient assessment.

Spirometry

GINA (2019) and BTS/SIGN (2019) agree that spirometry is the preferred diagnostic test to demonstrate airflow obstruction for adults, adolescents and children over the age of 5. Spirometry testing and interpretation of results should be undertaken by trained practitioners, and it is vital that equipment is maintained and calibrated. Whilst spirometry testing in under 5s requires specialist referral, trained GPNs can undertake spirometry in general practice settings for children over 5 years of age.

The British Lung Foundation (BLF, 2019) advises that the test itself involves information about the patient's age, sex, height and ethnicity being entered into the spirometer. This enables a prediction to be made about what result would be expected based on the details provided. The patient is asked to perform a prolonged forced exhalation after maximum inspiration into a mouthpiece that is attached to a spirometer. They are given the opportunity to provide at least three breaths to attempt to ensure reliability, and the highest of these three measurements will be used. The test measures the forced expiratory volume in the first second (FEV_1) and the forced vital capacity (FVC), which is the amount of air that is blown out in each forced breath (BLF, 2019). The ratio of FEV_1 to FVC provides the measure of airway obstruction. The actual result is then compared with the predicted result. An FEV_1/FVC ratio value that is 75% to 80% of that predicted for adults and 90% of that predicted for children (GINA, 2019) is considered normal. BTS/SIGN (2019) guidance, however, indicates the challenge with the interpretation of this FEV_1/FVC ratio because it changes with age; BTS/SIGN guidance therefore directs the practitioner to the European Respiratory Society Global (2019) Lung Function Initiative to review normal results for adults and children.

If spirometry demonstrates obstruction, bronchodilator reversibility testing is indicated. An inhaled short-acting beta-agonist is given, and spirometry is repeated after 15 to 20 minutes. An improvement in FEV_1 of 12% or more in children is seen to be a positive test; for adults, an improvement in FEV_1 of 12% or more and an increased volume of 200 ml or more is seen to be a positive test. If the improvement in FEV_1 is more than 400 ml, this is suggestive of asthma (BTS/SIGN, 2019). In children, adolescents and adults, a normal result for someone who is asymptomatic at the time of testing does not preclude asthma (BTS/SIGN, 2019).

Peak Expiratory Flow Variation

Peak expiratory flow (PEF) measurement can be useful to assess airflow variability. BTS/SIGN (2019) guidance advises that the patient can be sitting or standing and should record the best of three forced expiratory breaths. The measurements should be recorded multiple times over at least 2 weeks. Twice-daily readings, morning and evening, provide detail of some variation, but BTS/SIGN (2019) guidance advises that more frequent readings will produce a better assessment of variation. Variation in readings of 20% or more is indicative of asthma.

BTS/SIGN (2019) and GINA (2019) indicate there are additional objective tests that can be utilised for adults when airway obstruction is not evident but for whom a diagnosis of asthma is still being considered, such as challenge tests or bronchiole provocation tests. If these are indicated, the patient will require specialist referral.

Fractional Exhaled Nitric Oxide

Fractional exhaled nitric oxide (FeNO) measurement will provide detail about the level of eosinophilic inflammation in the lungs and complements an asthma assessment but is not conclusive for asthma. BTS/SIGN (2019) guidance recommends its use if available and advises that a positive test will increase the likelihood of asthma, but asthma is not rejected if the test is negative.

Atopy Tests

GINA (2019) and BTS/SIGN (2019) advise that atopy can be assessed through skin-prick or allergen-specific immunoglobulin E (sIgE) testing and will increase the likelihood of asthma, but it is not specific for asthma, and these tests should not be routinely used.

BTS/SIGN (2019) guidance suggests that the likelihood of asthma is based on the following:

- Knowledge of recurrent symptoms supported by objective tests detailing variation in peak flows when symptomatic and asymptomatic
- Symptoms of shortness of breath, cough, tight chest and wheeze

- Healthcare professional identification of wheeze
- Familial predisposition for asthma, eczema and allergies or personal history of eczema or allergies
- No evidence or symptoms suggesting other diagnoses

If diagnostic doubt remains, alternate diagnoses and referral for further testing should be considered.

MANAGEMENT OF ASTHMA

GINA (2019) advises that the main objectives of asthma management are to ensure symptoms are well controlled and that the risks of asthma morbidity and mortality and treatment side effects are reduced. It is vital that the patient is an equal partner in managing their care. BTS/SIGN (2019) guidance indicates that if there is a high likelihood of asthma, this should be documented, and a 6-week trial of inhaled corticosteroids should begin. A review appointment in 6 to 8 weeks' time should seek to ascertain any improvement through the use of a validated symptom questionnaire, such as the Asthma Control Questionnaire, and objective lung function tests, either FEV_1 or PEF measured when the patient is symptomatic and asymptomatic. If symptoms and objective tests indicate a good response the diagnosis can be confirmed. Pharmacological treatment can then be reviewed and adjusted if required. BTS/SIGN (2019) guidance advises that patients should be on the lowest possible dose of medication with their symptoms controlled. The GPN should ensure the patient is given self-management advice and instruction, and a personal asthma action plan should be agreed upon, which will provide detail about how asthma should be managed.

If diagnostic doubt remains based on the review assessment, initial consideration should include a review of adherence with prescribed medication and a check of their inhaler technique. If this does not provide an answer, alternate diagnoses and referral for further testing should be considered (BTS/SIGN, 2019). GINA (2019) concurs with this and suggests it is also important to review comorbidities that may be affecting the quality of life and consider repeated allergen exposure to agents such as tobacco smoke. BTS/SIGN (2019) and GINA (2019) indicate that these areas should be reviewed at regular opportunities, such as annual review.

Pharmacological Management

BTS/SIGN (2019) guidance advises that short-acting bronchodilators should be prescribed for adults and children who have been diagnosed with asthma. They propose that short-acting inhaled beta$_2$ agonists (SABAs), known as 'relievers', should be prescribed because of their speed of action and side-effect profile. These medicines should be used infrequently for symptom relief, but if one inhaler is being used monthly, then an urgent asthma assessment should be undertaken. SABAs act on the β2-adrenoceptors of bronchial muscle, producing bronchodilatation and relieving symptoms (Billington et al., 2017).

GINA (2019) confirms that it does not advise SABA use alone for the treatment of asthma, instead advocating the use of inhaled corticosteroids (ICSs) as required or to be taken daily to control symptoms and decrease the chance of asthma exacerbation. BTS/SIGN (2019) guidance proposes that for some individuals who have sporadic or short-term wheeze, a SABA may be the only medication needed.

ICSs reduce inflammation and decrease bronchial hyperresponsiveness and are the recommended treatment for adults and children to achieve control of asthma. BTS/SIGN (2019) guidance advises that ICSs should be considered in patients who use a SABA three times a week or more, have symptoms three times a week or more, wake with asthma symptoms 1 night weekly or have had an asthma attack in the preceding 2 years. Both BTS/SIGN (2019) and GINA (2019) indicate it is too challenging to provide the full details of all available doses but prefer to express the dose as very low for paediatrics, low as a starting dose for adults and medium and high. They further advise that there is evidence available that demonstrates safety and efficacy in children under 5 if taken at recommended doses. The recommended doses are detailed in the BTS/SIGN (2019) guidance.

BTS/SIGN (2019) guidance offers counsel in considering the safety of prescribed ICSs. For adults, the guidance advises that side effects of oral candidiasis and dysphonia have been reported, and concerns about bone density have been raised. For this reason, the guidance recommends ensuring the patient is taking the lowest possible dose of ICS whilst maintaining symptom control.

Children taking ICSs might be at risk of systemic side effects, such as failure to grow and adrenal insufficiency. BTS/SIGN (2019) guidance instructs that children's height and weight should be measured annually but also advises ensuring the child is taking the lowest possible dose of ICS with symptoms controlled. Additionally, children who are taking either medium- or high-dose ICSs should have specialist care and written guidance about steroid replacement.

Asthma control may not be achieved with ICSs alone, and add-on therapy may have to be considered. However, BTS/SIGN (2019) guidance states that before initiating any additional therapy, a thorough review is indicated. This provides an opportunity to reconsider adherence, inhaler technique and triggers.

BTS/SIGN (2019) guidance advocates the use of a long-acting inhaled beta$_2$ agonist (LABA) as an appropriate next step for adults, but this should not be prescribed without ICS treatment. LABAs also produce a bronchodilatory effect but have a longer duration of action, lasting for 12 hours or longer (Billington et al., 2017). A combination ICS/LABA inhaler might encourage compliance and should be considered when initiating add-on therapy (BTS/SIGN, 2019).

For children, BTS/SIGN (2019) guidance recommends either LABAs or leukotriene receptor antagonists (LTRAs) as initial add-on therapy. The guidance advises that LABAs are not licensed for children under 4, and there is limited evidence for LTRA use in children under 4. LTRAs block leukotrienes, which cause airway inflammation, thereby reducing airway inflammation and narrowing (Asthma UK, 2019c).

BTS/SIGN (2019) guidance advises that if asthma control has not been achieved after introducing a LABA, the dose of ICS should be titrated from low to medium in adults and from very low to low in children age 5 to 12, or the addition of an LTRA could be contemplated.

If these steps fail to control asthma, a referral to specialist services is indicated (BTS/SIGN, 2019). GINA (2019) highlights that a stepwise approach to asthma management will ensure treatment is increased as required, but if symptoms have been controlled for

3 months, a step-down of treatment should be considered to ensure the lowest possible dose of medication is being taken whilst symptoms remain controlled.

GINA (2019) recommends that when managing asthma, consideration should be given to cost-effectiveness. GPNs should ensure their prescribing aligns with local formularies and evidence-based guidance.

Influenza is implicated in exacerbations of asthma, and GINA (2019) advocates for the promotion of this vaccination to patients with an asthma diagnosis in an effort to reduce the risk of asthma exacerbation.

Comorbidities

GINA (2019) advises that several comorbidities are present in patients with difficult-to-treat asthma and proposes that this may affect asthma control. Managing these comorbidities is endorsed because of the potential influence on asthma symptoms and medication interactions.

The Royal College of General Practitioners (RCGP, 2015) indicates that approximately 60% of the UK population is classed as overweight or obese. Obesity has the potential to adversely affect health, may cause breathing difficulties and could obscure an asthma diagnosis. GINA (2019) and BTS/SIGN (2019) agree that weight-reduction or weight-loss programmes should be offered to obese adults and children with asthma to ameliorate symptoms and promote an appropriate diagnosis and general good health. Ensuring a healthy diet, they argue, is linked with a reduced decline in lung function.

Smoking cessation should be encouraged, and parents of children with asthma should be advised appropriately about the danger of passive smoking (BTS/SIGN, 2019; GINA, 2019). Patients with asthma who continue to smoke may require an increased dose of ICS to control their asthma symptoms, and as discussed earlier, ICSs have the potential to cause side effects, which may affect adherence. Additionally, consideration should be given as to whether symptoms are attributable to asthma or asthma/COPD overlap, which will require further investigation.

GINA (2019) stresses the importance of considering whether a mental health assessment is required, indicating that this may help to distinguish between anxiety-related disorders and an asthma diagnosis, but the GINA guidance also notes that for patients with

asthma and increasing stress, a reduction in adherence might occur, increasing the risk of exacerbations. The GPN who is providing an asthma clinic should be cognisant of this and provide appropriate advice, self-help literature or referral if necessary.

ASTHMA EDUCATION

There is convincing evidence to support a reduction in morbidity and mortality when regular reviews and supported self-management are available (Asthma UK, 2019d; Royal College of Physicians, 2014; Pinnock et al., 2015). Knowledge of asthma and lack of asthma action plans, inhaler technique reviews and annual reviews are areas that have been identified as being suboptimal (Asthma UK, 2019d; Royal College of Physicians, 2014). GINA (2019) advises that those with low health literacy will find education more challenging and suggests methods of ameliorating the impact of low health literacy, which are detailed in the GINA (2019) asthma strategy. The GPN should take the opportunity to review this information.

BTS/SIGN (2019) and GINA (2019) provide guidance regarding the requisite patient education required to promote self-management. They suggest that key components are education and written, personalised asthma action plans.

Education should include detail about asthma aetiology and management. Prescribed medications and the difference between 'relievers' for symptomatic control and 'preventers', which act to reduce inflammation and decrease bronchial hyperresponsiveness, are key topics. Patients may avoid taking ICSs because of concerns about the side-effect profile or perceived lack of benefit, which may increase their risk of an exacerbation of asthma. Advice can be given about common side effects, such as oral candidiasis, and about rinsing the mouth after taking the ICS if this is identified as a problem (BTS/SIGN, 2019). If the GPN understands the patient view about prescribed medication, they can work to provide detailed explanations, which may ameliorate concerns and promote medication adherence. Monitoring prescription rates will support the GPN in understanding if asthma is controlled.

Inhaler technique has been identified as a concerning area (Asthma UK, 2019d; Royal College of

Physicians, 2014). GINA (2019) advises that 70% to 80% of patients have a poor inhaler technique, and this will affect asthma management. An additional challenge is the selection of an appropriate device, according to the patient's wishes and ability, because comorbidities, such as arthritis, may affect inhaler ability (GINA, 2019). There are many devices available, and GPNs should have expertise in the commonly used devices because they will be required to check the patient's technique. There are instructional inhaler technique videos available, and it would be appropriate to direct patients to these resources, for example, https://www.asthma.org.uk/advice/inhaler-videos/ (Asthma UK, 2019b).

Asthma UK (2019d) identified a lack of knowledge about the severity of asthma as an area of concern. The GPN should therefore ensure that patients' knowledge of signs and symptoms of deterioration is discussed, and written detail should be provided in a personalised asthma action plan detailing what they should do if deterioration is identified. This asthma action plan will also detail the indicators that asthma control is deteriorating. BTS/SIGN (2019) guidance advises that any discussion should include trigger recognition and avoidance of triggers where possible to reduce the risk of exacerbations.

ASTHMA REVIEW

Key components of an asthma review include revisiting the patient's knowledge of asthma; their assessment of asthma control, inhaler technique, adherence to medication and personalised asthma action plan; and for children, growth must be checked and documented (BTS/SIGN, 2019). Patients should be invited to an annual review; this is in addition to any acute review and follow-up that may have been required. At the annual review, the GPN can revisit asthma knowledge and provide or update the patient about any variation, check inhaler technique and advise appropriately, or discuss if change is required. The review also provides an opportunity for the GPN to monitor and review prescribed asthma medication. This may highlight overuse of SABAs or adherence being an issue and will enable a discussion about any concerns about medication side effects or

safety. Comorbidities can also be discussed, and the GPN will have an opportunity to advise appropriately regarding healthy diet, weight loss and smoking cessation. Personal asthma action plans should be revisited at this point, and any updates to the plan should be made. Children who attend for review should have growth measured and charted, and a discussion should be held if there are any parental concerns (BTS/SIGN, 2019).

The asthma review provides an opportunity to assess asthma control. Asthma control can vary over time and in response to exposure to triggers or deterioration in physical or mental health (GINA, 2019). Because the patient is a partner in their care, assessment of their view of asthma control is vital and may identify relevant areas for discussion, such as level of control or severity. BTS/SIGN (2019) guidance provides recommendations about several tools that may be utilised to garner information about asthma control. A validated questionnaire, such as the Asthma Control Questionnaire or the Asthma Control Test (BTS/SIGN, 2019), which contains five questions, including symptoms and reliever use, provides detail about asthma control and enables a frank discussion about limitations as a result of symptoms and risk of exacerbations. The GPN can therefore utilise this opportunity to promote asthma symptom control.

ACUTE EXACERBATIONS OF ASTHMA

Asthma UK (2019d) indicates that the UK has one of the highest mortality rates in Europe. BTS/SIGN (2019) guidance advises that most deaths from asthma occur outside hospital settings and in patients whose asthma treatment or monitoring was suboptimal. The patients most at risk are those with learning difficulties, mental ill health, social problems, chaotic or unhealthy lifestyles, previous life-threatening asthma, more severe disease or repeated nonattenders (BTS/SIGN, 2019). Moderate exacerbations of asthma can be treated in the community, but BTS/SIGN (2019) guidance advises that patients who present with acute/severe or life-threatening asthma should be immediately referred to the hospital. Levels of severity of asthma exacerbations for adults are

TABLE 8.1	
Levels of Severity of Asthma Attacks in Adults	
Moderate acute asthma	Increasing symptoms
	PEF >50–75% best or predicted
	No features of acute severe asthma
Acute severe asthma	Any one of:
	■ PEF 33–50% best or predicted
	■ Respiratory rate ≥25/min
	■ Heart rate ≥110/min
	■ Inability to complete sentences in one breath
Life-threatening asthma	Any one of the following in a child with severe asthma:

Clinical signs	Measurements
Exhaustion	PEF <33% best or predicted
Hypotension	
Cyanosis	SpO$_2$ <92%
Silent chest	
Poor respiratory effort	
Confusion	

Near-fatal asthma	Raised PaCO$_2$ and/or requiring mechanical ventilation with raised inflation pressures

PEF, Peak expiratory flow.
Scottish Intercollegiate Guidelines Network (SIGN). British guideline on the management of asthma. Edinburgh: SIGN; 2019. (SIGN publication no. 158). [cited July 2019]. Available from URL: http://www.sign.ac.uk

TABLE 8.2	
Levels of Severity of Asthma Attacks in Children	
Moderate acute asthma	Able to talk in sentences
	SpO$_2$ ≥92%
	PEF ≥50% best or predicted
	Heart rate ≤140/min in children aged 1–5 years, ≤125/min in children >5 years
	Respiratory rate ≤40/min in children aged 1–5 years, ≤30/min in children >5 years
Acute severe asthma	Can't complete sentences in one breath or too breathless to talk or feed
	SpO$_2$ <92%
	PEF 33–50% best or predicted
	Heart rate >140/min in children aged 1–5 years, >125/min in children >5 years
	Respiratory rate >40/min in children aged 1–5 years, >30/min in children >5 years
Life-threatening asthma	Any one of the following in a child with severe asthma:

Clinical signs	Measurements
Exhaustion	PEF <33% best or predicted
Hypotension	
Cyanosis	SpO$_3$ <92%
Silent chest	
Poor respiratory effort	
Confusion	

PEF, Peak expiratory flow.
Scottish Intercollegiate Guidelines Network (SIGN). British guideline on the management of asthma. Edinburgh: SIGN; 2019. (SIGN publication no. 158). [cited July 2019]. Available from URL: http://www.sign.ac.uk

detailed in Table 8.1. Levels of severity of asthma exacerbations in children are detailed in Table 8.2. Figs. 8.1 and 8.2 detail the treatment advocated by BTS/SIGN (2019) for adult and child patients who present to general practice.

SUMMARY

The UK has one of the highest incidences of asthma in the world (Mukherjee et al., 2016), and asthma mortality is amongst the highest in Europe (Asthma UK, 2019d). The Royal College of Physicians (2014)

argues that many of these deaths could be prevented with improvements in asthma care. The vast majority of asthma care is undertaken in community settings, and the GPN is ideally placed to provide a pivotal role in the assessment and management of asthma. GPNs require appropriate education to undertake this role, and knowledge and use of evidence-based guidance will support the GPN to improve the management of asthma and reduce associated morbidity and mortality.

Management of acute asthma in adults in general practice

Many deaths from asthma are preventable. Delay can be fatal. Factors leading to poor outcome include:

- Clinical staff failing to assess severity by objective measurement
- Patients or relatives failing to appreciate severity
- Under use of corticosteroids

Regard each emergency asthma consultation as for acute severe asthma until shown otherwise.

Assess and record:

- Peak expiratory flow (PEF)
- Symptoms and response to self treatment
- Heart and respiratory rates
- Oxygen saturation (by pulse oximetry)

Caution: Patients with severe or life-threatening attacks may not be distressed and may not have all the abnormalities listed below.
The presence of any should alert the doctor.

Moderate asthma	Acute severe asthma	Life-threatening asthma

INITIAL ASSESSMENT

PEF>50–75% best or predicted	PEF 33–50% best or predicted	PEF<33% best or predicted

FURTHER ASSESSMENT

• SpO_2 ≥92% • Speech normal • Respiration <25 breaths/min • Pulse <110 beats/min	• SpO_2 ≥92% • Can't complete sentences • Respiration ≥25 breaths/min • Pulse ≥110 beats/min	• SpO_2 <92% • Silent chest, cyanosis or poor respiratory effort • Arrhythmia or hypotension • Exhaustion, altered consciousness

MANAGEMENT

Treat at home or in surgery and **ASSESS RESPONSE TO TREATMENT**	**Consider admission**	**Arrange immediate ADMISSION**

TREATMENT

• β_2 bronchodilator: – via spacer* If no improvement: – via nebuliser (preferably oxygen-driven), salbutamol 5 mg • Give prednisolone 40–50 mg • Continue or increase usual treatment If good response to first treatment (symptoms improved, respiration and pulse settling and PEF >50%) continue or increase usual treatment and continue prednisolone	• Oxygen to maintain SpO_2 94–98% if available • β_2 bronchodilator: – via nebuliser (preferably oxygen-driven), salbutamol 5 mg – or if nebuliser not available, via spacer* • Prednisolone 40–50 mg or IV hydrocortisone 100 mg • **If no response in acute severe asthma: ADMIT**	• Oxygen to maintain SpO_2 94–98% • β_2 bronchodilator with ipratropium: – via nebuliser (preferably oxygen-driven), salbutamol 5 mg and ipratropium 0.5 mg – or if nebuliser and ipratropium not available, β_2 bronchodilator via spacer* • Prednisolone 40–50 mg or IV hydrocortisone 100 mg immediately

Admit to hospital if any: • Life-threatening features • Features of acute severe asthma present after initial treatment • Previous near-fatal asthma Lower threshold for admission if afternoon or evening attack, recent nocturnal symptoms or hospital admission, previous severe attacks, patient unable to assess own condition, or concern over social circumstances	**If admitting the patient to hospital:** • Stay with patient until ambulance arrives • Send written assessment and referral details to hospital • β_2 bronchodilator via oxygen-driven **nebuliser in ambulance**	**Follow up after treatment or discharge from hospital:** • Continue prednisolone until recovery (minimum 5 days) • **GP review within 2 working days** • Monitor symptoms and PEF • Check inhaler technique • **Written asthma action plan** • Modify treatment according to guidelines for chronic persistent asthma • Address potentially preventable contributors to admission

*β_2 bronchodilator via spacer given one puff at a time, inhaled separately using tidal breathing; according to response, give another puff every 60 seconds up to a maximum of 10 puffs

Fig. 8.1 ■ Management of acute asthma in adults in general practice. *GP*, General Practitioner. (Scottish Intercollegiate Guidelines Network (SIGN). British guideline on the management of asthma. Edinburgh: SIGN; 2019. (SIGN publication no. 158). [cited July 2019]. Available from URL: http://www.sign.ac.uk)

Management of acute asthma in children in general practice

Age 2–5 years

ASSESS AND RECORD ASTHMA SEVERITY

Moderate asthma
- SpO$_2$ ≥92%
- Able to talk
- Heart rate ≤140/min
- Respiratory rate ≤40/min

Acute severe asthma
- SpO$_2$ <92%
- Too breathless to talk
- Heart rate >140/min
- Respiratory rate >40/min
- Use of accessory neck muscles

Life-threatening asthma
SpO$_2$ <92% plus any of:
- Silent chest
- Poor respiratory effort
- Agitation
- Confusion
- Cyanosis

- Oxygen via facemask to maintain SpO$_2$ 94–98% if available

Moderate:
- β$_2$ bronchodilator:
  – via spacer ± facemask*
- Consider oral prednisolone 20 mg

Acute severe:
- β$_2$ bronchodilator
  – via nebuliser (preferably oxygen driven), salbutamol 2.5 mg
  – or, if nebuliser not available, via spacer*
- Oral prednisolone 20 mg

Assess response to treatment 15 mins after β$_2$ bronchodilator

Life-threatening:
- β$_2$ bronchodilator with ipratropium:
  – via nebuliser (preferably oxygen-driven), salbutamol 2.5 mg and ipratropium 0.25 mg every 20 minutes
  – or, if nebuliser and ipratropium not available, β$_2$ bronchodilator via spacer*
- Oral prednisolone 20 mg or IV hydrocortisone 50 mg if vomiting

IF POOR RESPONSE ARRANGE ADMISSION

IF POOR RESPONSE REPEAT β$_2$ BRONCHODILATOR AND ARRANGE ADMISSION

REPEAT β$_2$ BRONCHODILATOR VIA OXYGEN-DRIVEN NEBULISER WHILST ARRANGING IMMEDIATE HOSPITAL ADMISSION

GOOD RESPONSE
- Continue β$_2$ bronchodilator via spacer or nebuliser, as needed but not exceeding 4 hourly
- If symptoms are not controlled repeat β$_2$ bronchodilator and refer to hospital
- Continue prednisolone until recovery (minimum 3–5 days)
- Arrange follow-up clinic visit within 48 hours
- Consider referral to secondary care asthma clinic if 2nd attack within 12 months

POOR RESPONSE
- Stay with patient until ambulance arrives
- Send written assessment and referral details
- Repeat β$_2$ bronchodilator via oxygen-driven nebuliser in ambulance

LOWER THRESHOLD FOR ADMISSION IF:
- Attack in late afternoon or at night
- Recent hospital admission or previous severe attack
- Concern over social circumstances or ability to cope at home

NB: If a patient has signs and symptoms across categories, always treat according to their most severe features

Age >5 years

ASSESS AND RECORD ASTHMA SEVERITY

Moderate asthma
- SpO$_2$ ≥92%
- Able to talk
- Heart rate ≤125/min
- Respiratory rate ≤30/min
- PEF ≥50% best or predicted

Acute severe asthma
- SpO$_2$ <92%
- Too breathless to talk
- Heart rate >125/min
- Respiratory rate >30/min
- Use of accessory neck muscles
- PEF 33–50% best or predicted

Life-threatening asthma
SpO$_2$ <92% plus any of:
- Silent chest
- Poor respiratory effort
- Agitation
- Confusion
- Cyanosis
- PEF <33% best or predicted

- Oxygen via facemask to maintain SpO$_2$ 94–98% if available

Moderate:
- β$_2$ bronchodilator:
  – via spacer*
- Consider oral prednisolone 30–40 mg

Acute severe:
- β$_2$ bronchodilator
  – via nebuliser (preferably oxygen-driven), salbutamol 5 mg
  – or, if nebuliser not available, via spacer*
- Oral prednisolone 30–40 mg

Assess response to treatment 15 mins after β$_2$ bronchodilator

Life-threatening:
- β$_2$ bronchodilator with ipratropium:
  – via nebuliser (preferably oxygen-driven), salbutamol 5 mg and ipratropium 0.25 mg every 20 minutes
  – or, if nebuliser and ipratropium not available, β$_2$ bronchodilator via spacer*
- Oral prednisolone 30–40 mg or IV hydrocortisone 100 mg if vomiting

IF POOR RESPONSE ARRANGE ADMISSION

IF POOR RESPONSE REPEAT β$_2$ BRONCHODILATOR AND ARRANGE ADMISSION

REPEAT β$_2$ BRONCHODILATOR VIA OXYGEN-DRIVEN NEBULISER WHILST ARRANGING IMMEDIATE HOSPITAL ADMISSION

GOOD RESPONSE
- Continue β$_2$ bronchodilator via spacer or nebuliser, as needed but not exceeding 4 hourly
- If symptoms are not controlled repeat β$_2$ bronchodilator and refer to hospital
- Continue prednisolone until recovery (minimum 3–5 days)
- Arrange follow-up clinic visit within 48 hours
- Consider referral to secondary care asthma clinic if 2nd attack within 12 months

POOR RESPONSE
- Stay with patient until ambulance arrives
- Send written assessment and referral details
- Repeat β$_2$ bronchodilator via oxygen-driven nebuliser in ambulance

LOWER THRESHOLD FOR ADMISSION IF:
- Attack in late afternoon or at night
- Recent hospital admission or previous severe attack
- Concern over social circumstances or ability to cope at home

NB: If a patient has signs and symptoms across categories, always treat according to their most severe features

*β$_2$ bronchodilator via spacer given one puff at a time, inhaled separately using tidal breathing; according to response, give another puff every 60 seconds up to a maximum of 10 puffs

Fig. 8.2 ■ Management of acute asthma in children in general practice. (Scottish Intercollegiate Guidelines Network (SIGN). British guideline on the management of asthma. Edinburgh: SIGN; 2019. (SIGN publication no. 158). [cited July 2019]. Available from URL: http://www.sign.ac.uk)

REFERENCES

Asthma UK. (2019a). *Asthma facts and statistics.* https://www.asthma.org.uk/about/media/facts-and-statistics/

Asthma UK. (2019b). *How to use your inhaler.* https://www.asthma.org.uk/advice/inhaler-videos/

Asthma UK. (2019c). *Leukotriene receptor antagonists (LTRAs).* https://www.asthma.org.uk/advice/inhalers-medicines-treatments/add-on-treatments/ltra/

Asthma UK. (2019d). *UK asthma death rates amongst worst in Europe.* https://www.asthma.org.uk/about/media/news/press-release-uk-asthma-death-rates-among-worst-in-europe

Bhatt, J. M., & Parker, G. (2019). The diagnosis of asthma in children. *British Journal of Family Medicine, 3,* 12.

Billington, C. K., Penn, R. B., & Hall, I. P. (2017). β2 agonist. In C. P. Page & P. J. Barnes (Eds.), *Pharmacology and therapeutics of asthma and COPD* (pp. 23–40). Springer.

British Lung Foundation. (2019). *Spirometry and bronchodilator responsiveness testing.* https://www.blf.org.uk/support-for-you/breathing-tests/spirometry-and-reversibility?cmp_id51519530222&adg_id562024389801&kwd5spirometry&device5c&gclid5EAIaIQobChMIp6quxK6H5gIVCbLtCh2PxQRtEAAYASAAEgKMYPD_BwE

British Thoracic Society/Scottish Intercollegiate Guidelines Network. (2019). *BTS/SIGN guideline for the management of asthma 2019.* https://www.brit-thoracic.org.uk/quality-improvement/guidelines/asthma/

European Respiratory Society. (2019). *Global Lung Function Initiative.* https://www.ers-education.org/guidelines/global-lung-function-initiative.aspx

Global Initiative for Asthma. (2019). *Global strategy for asthma management and prevention.* https://ginasthma.org/wp-content/uploads/2019/06/GINA-2019-main-report-June-2019-wms.pdf

Mukherjee, M., Stoddart, A., Gupta, R. P., Nwaru, B. I., Farr, A., Heaven, M., Fitzsimmons, D., Bandyopadhyay, A., Aftab, C., Simpson, C. R., Lyons, R. A., Fischbacher, C., Dibben, C., Shields, M. D., Phillips, C. J., Strachan, D. P., Davies, G. A., McKinstry, B., & Sheikh, A. (2016). The epidemiology, healthcare and societal burden and costs of asthma in the UK and its member nations: Analyses of standalone and linked national databases. *BMC Medicine, 14,* Article 113.

Pinnock, H., Epiphaniou, E., Pearce, G., Parke, H., Greenhalgh, T., Sheikh, A., Griffiths, C. J., & Taylor, S. J. C. (2015). Implementing supported self-management for asthma: A systematic review and suggested hierarchy of evidence of implementation studies. *BMC Medicine, 13,* Article 127.

Royal College of General Practitioners. (2015). *RCGP position statement on obesity and malnutrition.* https://www.rcgp.org.uk/-/media/Files/CIRC/Nutrition/Nutrition-position-statement-Oct-2015.ashx?la5en

Royal College of Physicians. (2014). *Why asthma still kills: The National Review of Asthma Deaths (NRAD).* https://www.asthma.org.uk/293597ee/globalassets/campaigns/nrad-full-report.pdf

Tortora, G. J., & Derrickson, B. (2015). *Introduction to the human body: The essentials of anatomy and physiology* (10th ed.). Wiley.

White, J., Paton, J. Y., Niven, R., & Pinnock, H. (2018). *Guidelines for the diagnosis and management of asthma: A look at the key differences between BTS/ SIGN and NICE.* https://thorax.bmj.com/content/thoraxjnl/73/3/293.full.pdf

World Health Organisation. (2019). *Asthma.* https://www.who.int/news-room/fact-sheets/detail/asthma

9

MANAGING CARDIOVASCULAR CONDITIONS IN PRIMARY CARE

EVELYN WALTON

INTRODUCTION

As an umbrella term, *cardiovascular disease* (CVD) is an expression for diseases affecting the heart and blood vessels, whose origins are genetic and/or acquired across the life course. CVDs are ranked as the leading cause of mortality globally, representing 31% of all deaths (World Health Organisation (WHO), 2019); however, this is considered to be a conservative estimate. Within the UK, whilst there have been significant improvements in mortality and morbidity rates, these have reached a plateau over the past decade. National Health Service (NHS) England (2019) confirms that CVD affects over 7 million people, resulting in significant disability and death. Public Health England (PHE, 2019a) poignantly comments that CVD is responsible for in 1 in 4 deaths, equating to 1 death every 4 minutes. CVD is also a major cause of health inequalities, with people living in the most deprived communities being 4 times more likely to suffer premature death in comparison to those living in the least deprived communities.

Against this backdrop, general practice plays a crucial and multifaceted role in responding to CVD health needs (NHS England, 2019). Pragmatically, this entails deploying primary prevention strategies to promote healthy lifestyles/behavioural change to prevent the onset of CVD via risk-based assessment and awareness-raising campaigns. For those patients who have developed CVD, secondary prevention strategies support the diagnosis, treatment, management and, where indicated, the onward referral to special services to prevent further risk of morbidity, comorbidity and premature mortality.

The general practice nurse (GPN) plays a major role in contributing to these strategies and thus must acquire and demonstrate the knowledge and skills to promote health and manage care for people presenting with CVD (Queen's Nursing Institute, 2020; Royal College of General Practitioners, 2012). With a focus on secondary prevention, this chapter specifically explores the care required in managing hypertension, coronary heart disease, and chronic kidney disease (CKD), conditions that are commonly managed within primary care and in which the GPN is likely to have a significant role.

HYPERTENSION: ASSESSMENT, DIAGNOSIS AND MANAGEMENT

Hypertension is associated with an increased risk of angina, myocardial infarction (MI), heart failure, stroke, peripheral vascular disease and abdominal aortic aneurysm and is a leading cause of death and disability-adjusted life-years worldwide (Forouzanfar et al., 2017; Rapsomaniki et al., 2014a, 2014b). Nearly 30% of people in the UK have hypertension, with up to half not receiving treatment (British Heart Foundation, 2019); however, the risk of developing concomitant conditions, such as those identified earlier, can be greatly reduced by achieving optimal blood pressure (BP) control.

Prompt assessment, diagnosis and management are crucial in reducing the risk of death and disability due to hypertension, as evidenced within the updated evidence-based guidelines of the National Institute for Health and Care Excellence (NICE, 2019a). These guidelines include clinical guidance in relation to managing hypertension in type 2 diabetes; however, there are separate NICE guidelines for BP targets in relation to type 1 diabetes and CKD.

NICE (2019a) hypertension guidelines stress the importance of obtaining an accurate BP measurement to enable the classification of hypertension to guide the management and, importantly, assess cardiovascular risk. Competency in measuring BP is essential, and this includes the use of validated and calibrated equipment; a relaxed clinical atmosphere with the person seated, arm supported and outstretched; and the use of an appropriate BP cuff size (NICE, 2019a). The cuff should be sized accurately, with 22 to 26 cm for a small adult, 27 to 34 cm for an adult, and 35 to 44 cm for a large adult. The cuff should be positioned at the level of the right atrium or mid-sternum, and two readings should be recorded on two occasions (American College of Cardiology/American Heart Association (ACA/AHA), 2017). A radial pulse must be checked to exclude irregularity before measuring BP. If an irregular pulse is detected, such as in the case of atrial fibrillation, then the BP measurement should be taken manually with direct auscultation of the brachial artery (NICE, 2019a).

If hypertension is suspected, measurements should be taken in both arms. This is essential because a difference of 15 mmHg or more can be an indicator of peripheral arterial disease, increasing the risk of death from stroke (Clarke et al., 2012). Hypertension is diagnosed if the BP is 140/90 mmHg or above or with an ambulatory blood pressure measurement (ABPM) or home BP monitoring (HBPM) of 135/80 mmHg or higher (NICE, 2019a). ABPM or HBPM should be used to diagnose hypertension if the BP in the clinical setting is between 140/80 and 180/110 mmHg. At least two measurements per hour should be taken for ABPM and twice-daily readings for 7 days when using HBPM. ABPM is viewed to be the gold standard in the diagnosis of hypertension (NICE, 2019a).

Classification and Management of Hypertension

The stages of hypertension have been classified by NICE (2019a), and these provide the thresholds for clinical treatment and management. If the BP is above 180/110 mmHg with evidence of retinal haemorrhage, papilledema, new confused mental state, chest pain,

signs of heart failure, renal impairment or suspected pheochromocytoma, the patient should be referred urgently for same-day assessment in secondary care (NICE, 2019a). Immediate referral to the general practitioner (GP) is required should the GPN detect the presence of clinical 'red flags' to ensure swift onward referral and management in secondary care.

Evidence-based guidance recommends a treatment threshold for patients who have a 10% or greater risk of developing CVD, and this includes lipid modification (Cannon, 2017; NICE, 2014). The JBS3 risk calculator offered by the Joint British Society (JBS) is a useful tool that the GPN can use to demonstrate and communicate a person's risk of developing CVD in the next 10 years (JBS, 2014). In utilising this type of tool, the GPN can help patients with hypertension make informed choices about lifestyle changes and treatment to reduce their overall CVD risk. Similarly, the QRISK3 is an evidence-based prediction algorithm that can be used to estimate cardiovascular risk (Hippisley-Cox et al., 2017). This prediction model includes conditions such as severe mental illness and migraine as potential new risk factors, providing an opportunity for discussion around modifiable risks.

THE GPN ROLE IN THE MANAGEMENT OF HYPERTENSION

Helping patients make behaviour changes to optimise health outcomes is a fundamental aspect of nursing practice (Johnson & May, 2015), which the GPN must exploit regarding the nonpharmacological management of hypertension. The GPN has a crucial role in providing a person-centred approach in ensuring that the patient is aware of the potential high-risk complications of poorly controlled hypertension and the necessity to make, where indicated, lifestyle changes. Lifestyle advice should be tailored, and this may include advice on limiting alcohol consumption to 14 units per week (Chief Medical Officer (CMO), 2016). Dietary advice can be personalised with the visual aid of the Eatwell Guide (PHE, 2016). The Dietary Approaches to Stop Hypertension (DASH) diet should be promoted to help improve BP and the lipid profile (National Heart, Lung and Blood Institute (NHLBI), 2010). Where appropriate, smoking cessation advice and assistance should be offered (NICE, 2019a).

Physical activity should be individualised and based on recommended guidelines (PHE, 2019b). Where necessary, the GPN should instigate referral pathways to specialist services to support the modification of lifestyle factors.

Pharmacological therapy is indicated for those aged under 80 with stage 1 hypertension who have one or more of the following: a 10% or greater cardiovascular risk, target-organ damage, established CVD, renal disease or diabetes. NICE guidelines (2019a) do not recommend a reduced target BP for patients with type 2 diabetes. Adults of any age with stage 2 hypertension should be offered pharmacological therapy, but clinical judgement is needed when prescribing for the over-80 age group, who are at increased risk of falls, are frail, have other comorbidities and may live alone. These issues stress the importance of undertaking holistic assessment, which must take account of the social situation in parallel with the biophysical measurements.

Specific cautions exist regarding the prescribing of angiotensin-converting enzyme (ACE) inhibitors and angiotensin-receptor blockers (ARBs); these should be avoided in women of childbearing potential, and specific guidelines should be followed for those who are pregnant or breastfeeding (NICE, 2019b).

The GPN must be aware of the recommended target BP for the person presenting, record BP accurately, initiate nonpharmacological management and trigger referral for pharmacological therapy where indicated. This treatment will be lifelong, so it is crucial that the GPN communicates effectively to ensure that the patient is aware of the benefits of maintaining a target BP.

Clinical examination, such as urinalysis for proteinuria, HbA1c, electrolyte profile, estimated glomerular filtration rate (eGFR), lipid profile, fundoscopy and electrocardiogram are the essential investigations required when a person receives a diagnosis of hypertension (Blane, 2020). If the person is prescribed an ACE or ARB, renal function must be checked before and 1 to 2 weeks after commencing medication or following an increase in the dosage (NICE, 2019a).

BP measurements obtained during clinic attendance should be used when monitoring the response to treatment. HBPM and ABPM can be used, but the target is lower, at 135/85 mmHg. The target for those over 80 years is 150/90 mmHg (NICE, 2019a). Annual review is recommended, in which BP is monitored, and diet, lifestyle and medications are discussed. This is an excellent opportunity to check the person's understanding of their condition, discuss any side effects of medication and provide support to aid concordance with therapy. The GPN should be mindful of person-centred approaches and avoid a communication style based on an outdated, paternalistic model of compliance in supporting patients to make lifestyle changes. The aim is to empower patients to accept responsibility for self-management as part of a collaborative relationship (Phillips, 2017); however, there will be instances where not all patients want to, or are able to, take control of their self-management. Shared decision-making ensures that the different treatment and management options are discussed and explored, including risks and benefits, with the patient and the healthcare professional reaching a decision together (NICE, 2019a).

Hypertension is one of the most important treatable causes of premature morbidity and mortality in the world, and the GPN can demonstrate person-centred management to protect those in this high-risk group. There is an expectation that every nurse should be a health-promoting practitioner (Nursing and Midwifery Council (NMC), 2018), with the GPN ideally placed to use their knowledge and skills to improve the health and wellbeing of those living with hypertension.

CORONARY HEART DISEASE

Coronary heart disease (CHD) is the most prevalent type of CVD, occurring when the coronary arteries become narrowed as a result of a build-up of fatty atheroma (Grossman & Porth, 2014). A serious consequence of CHD is MI, defined pathologically as myocardial cell death resulting from prolonged ischaemia (Grossman & Porth, 2014). In the UK, CVD causes 450 deaths per day, and of these, 170 deaths are directly attributable to CHD (British Heart Foundation, 2021). MI causes most of these deaths, with 1 hospital admission for MI occurring every 5 minutes. In the 1960s more than 7 out of 10 of these people died, whereas today, at least 7 out of

10 survive an MI. This reduction is attributable to a greater use of reperfusion therapy, primary percutaneous coronary intervention (PCI), modern antithrombotic therapy and implementation of secondary prevention (Huber et al., 2019). Nevertheless, all-cause and cardiac death rates remain substantial, with a 5-year mortality risk of greater than 20% (Rapsomaniki et al., 2014a).

Management of Coronary Heart Disease

The GPN role frequently involves caring for the patient who has suffered an MI in the context of secondary prevention to prevent reoccurrence. This entails carrying out a holistic annual review comprising a comprehensive history and assessment of symptoms, notably any new symptoms such as chest pain, shortness of breath, ankle/leg oedema, dizziness, fatigue or leg cramps.

Current guidelines (NICE, 2013) for rehabilitation and secondary prevention following acute MI are based on landmark randomised controlled trials, such as 4S (van Boven et al., 1994), CARE (Sacks et al., 1996) and LIPID (LIPID Study Group, 1998). These trials revealed that a reduction of total serum cholesterol and low-density lipoprotein (LDL) in the region of 25% to 35% using statin therapy led to a reduction in CHD of approximately the same degree. A blood cholesterol level over 5.2 mmol/l contributes to 46% of deaths from CHD (Mozaffarian et al., 2016). NICE (2013) suggests starting people with CHD with Atorvastatin 80 mg. Measure total cholesterol, high-density lipoprotein (HDL) cholesterol and non-HDL cholesterol after 3 months of treatment, with an aim of greater than 40% reduction in non-HDL cholesterol (NICE, 2013).

Further evidence supporting secondary prevention strategies for MI is derived from a large body of evidence showing the beneficial effects of several single-drug therapies, such as dual antiplatelet therapy (DAPT) with aspirin and a P2Y12 inhibitor (prasugrel, ticagrelor or clopidogrel), lipid-lowering drugs, ACE inhibitors or ARBs and beta-blockers (Ibanez et al., 2018; Roffi et al., 2016). Ticagrelor, in combination with aspirin, is recommended as an option for preventing atherothrombotic events in adults who have had an MI and who are at risk of a further event (NICE, 2016). Renal function, serum electrolytes and BP should be measured before starting an ACE

inhibitor or ARB and again within 2 weeks of starting treatment. More frequent monitoring may be required in people who are at risk of deterioration in renal function (NICE, 2013).

The Framingham study (Kannel & Magee, 1979), one of the most prestigious epidemiological studies on CVD, determined that the presence of diabetes doubles the risk for CVD in men and triples it for women. People living with diabetes are 50% more likely to have a fatal MI, indicating that achieving good glycaemic control can positively influence mortality in patients with diabetes (Bergenstal, 2015). Management of glycaemic control is an essential part of secondary prevention in this group of people in reducing their long-term risks. The close association between CVD and diabetes means that the GPN has a key role in the clinical management of patients living with multiple morbidities.

Physical inactivity contributes to 37% of CHD deaths, compared with smoking, which contributes to 19% of CHD deaths (Mozaffarian et al., 2016). The UK CMO recommends at least 150 minutes of moderate-intensity training, 75 minutes of vigorous activity or a mixture of both. This is in combination with strengthening activities on 2 days and reducing periods of extended sitting (PHE, 2019b). Local exercise groups can offer support and tailored activities, and consequently, GPNs should be aware of local initiatives and signpost the appropriate patients to these groups. A Mediterranean-style diet is recommended, but oily fish and omega-2 supplementation is not endorsed. Healthy eating advice should be individually tailored and extended to the whole family (NICE, 2013). The DASH diet may be beneficial, especially if there is a concurrent diagnosis of hypertension (NHLBI, 2010). Smokers should be encouraged to stop at every opportunity, offering behavioural support in a way that is sensitive to their preferences and needs. Pharmacological therapies such as nicotine replacement therapy (NRT), bupropion, or varenicline are recommended, as is referral to a specialist stop smoking service, where expert advice on quitting can be tailored to each individual (NICE, 2018). Advice on e-cigarettes is that they are substantially less harmful to health than smoking, but they are not risk-free (NICE, 2018).

Post-MI, all patients, regardless of their age, should be offered a cardiac rehabilitation programme with an exercise component, and partners or relatives should be involved if the patient wishes (NICE, 2013). GPNs are ideally placed to discuss any factors that may stop patients from attending, such as transport difficulties.

Holistic assessment also involves screening for depression in patients with CHD because these conditions are closely linked; CHD can cause depression, and depression is an independent risk factor for CHD and its complications. Depression may also contribute to sudden cardiac death and increase all causes of mortality. It is crucial to screen for depression annually and initiate treatment plans if the person with CHD is experiencing depression. The PHQ9 tool can be used for initial depression screening (see Chapter 12).

A vital aspect of the GPN's role is helping to increase the quality of life of the person living with CHD. A holistic and compassionate approach will significantly increase their confidence in coping with and managing their condition. Patients who have had an MI are often anxious and fearful and may require support on issues that range from understanding the disease and its pharmacological management to driving, employment and sexual and personal issues that can be adversely affected by this long-term condition. The diagnosis of MI can sometimes come as a surprise, and patients may not associate a PCI with having a 'heart attack'. Providing them with the relevant information and bespoke health promotion can enable them to make positive health decisions and set realistic goals.

CHRONIC KIDNEY DISEASE

CKD has a number of complex causes but is also identified as a comorbidity of hypertension, CHD and diabetes. The prevalence of CKD is estimated to be 13% in adults and up to 35% in those aged 75 years (NICE CKS, 2019), and with the longevity of older populations, the prevalence of CKD is likely to increase (Mendez, 2015).

The pathophysiology of CKD indicates the progressive loss of nephrons, resulting in deterioration in glomerular filtration, tubular reabsorption and the endocrine function of the kidney (Grossman & Porth 2014), which has been present for more than 3 months

(NICE 2015). CKD represents the gradual impairment of kidney function, which, over time, can progress to end-stage renal disease (ESRD). With careful management, it can be slowed or even reversed (Guidelines and Audit Implementation Network (GAIN), 2015).

Screening for CKD

CKD is often asymptomatic, particularly in the early stages, and is usually discovered by chance following a routine blood or urine test. Specific symptoms usually only emerge as the disease progresses and can include nausea, insomnia, anorexia, headache, peripheral oedema (digital/ankle), headache, muscle cramps and polyuria (Lowth, 2013). This is an important consideration in that, beyond hypertension, diabetes and cardiovascular disease, other known risk factors for CKD include acute kidney injury, structural renal tract disease, systemic lupus erythematosus, rheumatoid arthritis, haematuria and obesity. Further, those at risk also include patients taking nephrotoxic drugs such as ACE inhibitors, ARBs, ciclosporin, diuretics, Lithium and nonsteroidal anti-inflammatory drugs (GAIN, 2015).

Within the general practice setting, patients at risk of CKD should be screened serologically by assessing their eGFR and urine albumin:creatinine ratio (ACR) (GAIN, 2015). The diagnosis of CKD is established when tests have persistently (more than 3 months) shown proteinuria or a reduction in kidney function. The diagnosis is confirmed if the eGFR is persistently less than 60 ml/min and/or the urinary ACR is greater than 3 mg/mmol (NICE, 2015). NICE (2015) guidelines for the assessment and management of CKD have adopted the US National Kidney Foundation Kidney Disease Outcomes Quality Initiative (NKF-KDOQI) classification (Inker et al., 2014), which describes five stages of CKD in relation to the progressive loss of renal function (Fig. 9.1).

Fig. 9.1 recognises that an increased ACR and a decreased eGFR are each associated with a higher risk of adverse outcomes and that if both are present, the risk is multiplied (Inker et al., 2014). Consideration should be given to using eGFRcystatin C at initial diagnosis to confirm or rule out CKD in people with an eGFR of 45 to 59 ml/min/1.73 m^2, sustained for at least 90 days and no proteinuria, ACR less than 3 mg/mmol or other marker of kidney disease (NICE, 2015).

Classification of chronic kidney disease using GFR and ACR categories

GFR and ACR categories and risk of adverse outcomes			ACR categories (mg/mmol), description and range		
			<3 Normal to mildly increased	3–30 Moderately increased	>30 Severely increased
			A1	A2	A3
GFR categories (ml/min/1.73 m²), description and range	≥90 Normal and high	G1	No CKD in the absence of markers of kidney damage		
	60–89 Mild reduction related to normal range for a young adult	G2			
	45–59 Mild-moderate reduction	G3a[1]			
	30–44 Moderate-severe reduction	G3b			
	15–29 Severe reduction	G4			
	<15 Kidney failure	G5			

Increasing risk →

Increasing risk (vertical)

[1]Consider using eGFRcystatinC for people with CKD G3aA1 (see recommendations 1.1.14 and 1.1.15)

Abbreviations: ACR, albumin:creatinine ratio; CKD, chronic kidney disease; GFR, glomerular filtration rate

Fig. 9.1 ■ Classification of chronic kidney disease using glomerular filtration rate *(GFR)* and albumin:creatinine ratio *(ACR)* categories. (Adapted with permission from Kidney Disease: Improving Global Outcomes (KDIGO) CKD Work Group. (2013). KDIGO 2012 clinical practice guidelines for the evaluation and management of chronic kidney disease. *Kidney International Supplements, 3*(1), 1–150.)

CKD can progress to ESRD in a very small proportion of people – about 2%. In fact, people with CKD are roughly 20 times more likely to die from CVD than progress to ESRD. The all-cause mortality rate for CKD is up to 60% higher than the rate for the general population (NICE, 2015).

Management of Chronic Kidney Disease

Management and referral of patients to specialist services should follow current evidence-based guidelines (NICE, 2015). The aims for the management of CKD are to prevent disease progression and its associated risks. Treatment can effectively slow the progression of the disease and the associated risk factors, with early diagnosis and intervention producing significant results (Jameson et al., 2014). Assessment and management of risk factors will include identifying underlying causes, nephrotoxic drugs and modification of lifestyle risk factors. A comprehensive blood profile, including lipids, should be obtained and include analysis of serum calcium, phosphate, vitamin D, and parathyroid hormone tests to exclude renal metabolic and bone disorders for people with CKD category stages 4 or 5. The frequency of subsequent monitoring depends on the results and clinical judgement (NICE CKS, 2019). An accelerated progression of CKD is indicated by a sustained decrease in eGFR of 25% or more in 1 year or a sustained decrease in eGFR of 15 ml/min per year (NICE, 2015).

Treatment with statins contributes to lowering mortality and major cardiovascular events by 20% in people with CKD (Palmer et al., 2014). Pharmacological management involves the use of atorvastatin and increasing the dose if they have not had more than a 40% decrease in non-HDL with an eGFR >30 (NICE, 2014). Antiplatelet drugs are beneficial for the prevention of cardiovascular disease, but there is an increased risk of bleeding (NICE, 2015).

BP should be kept below 140/80 mmHg, or under 130/80 mmHg if the person has diabetes or the ACR is greater than 70 mg/mmol (NICE CKS, 2019). An ACE inhibitor should be used if the person has diabetes and the ACR is 3 mg/mmol or more, if there is hypertension with an ACR greater than 30 mg/mmol or if the ACR is greater than 70 mg/mmol. ACE inhibitors and ARBs should not be used in combination (NICE, 2015). Renal function should be checked before starting these drugs and between 1 and 2 weeks of starting or increasing the dose (Lowth, 2013).

Patients with stage 4 or 5 CKD should have their body mass index (BMI) and body weight recorded regularly and receive dietary advice to restrict their sodium intake to <2.4 g/daily. The risk of hyperkalaemia can be reduced by avoiding some fruits, coffee and chocolate (Ramlan, 2015). Lifestyle advice around smoking, alcohol and physical activity is a priority when managing this high-risk group. The links between CKD and hypertension and cardiovascular risk need to be explained. The person with CKD will unquestionably need to consider lifestyle changes, with the practice nurse negotiating change strategies through motivational interviewing (Miller & Rollnick, 2013) (see Chapter 2).

Referral to a nephrology specialist is required if the eGFR is less than 30 or has decreased by 25% or more in 1 year. Refer if the ACR is above 70 mg/mmol (unless the person has diabetes and is being treated) or the ACR is over 30 mg/mmol with persistent haematuria, after infection has been ruled out (NICE CKS, 2019).

CKD is a common presentation in general practice, and support and compassion are paramount in caring for this high-risk group. The challenges for the nurse are early identification of CKD and implementing an appropriate management plan. Patients with CKD need appropriate lifestyle advice and support, combined with pharmacological therapies and monitoring. This will require ongoing effort and engagement from the GPN to help reduce their risk of dying from cardiovascular disease.

SUMMARY

Cardiovascular conditions remain the most prevalent cause of morbidity and premature death in the UK, and as such, they are a priority within the healthcare agenda. The role that general practice plays is evident, hence the professional knowledge and skills needed by the GPN in providing evidence-based care for patients with hypertension, CHD and CKD. Whilst the clinical complexities associated with providing care based on achieving biometric targets, pharmacological treatment and non-pharmacological management are obvious in the context of evidence-based care, also obvious is the GPN's crucial role in coordinating holistic quality care, which also entails being a supportive and informative resource for patients.

REFERENCES

American College of Cardiology/American Heart Association. (2017). Guidelines for the prevention, detection, evaluation and management of high blood pressure in adults – A report of the American College of Cardiology and American Heart Association Task Force on Clinical Practice Guidelines. *Hypertension, 15,* 13–115.

Bergenstal, R. (2015). Glycaemic variability and diabetes complications – Does it matter? *Diabetes Care, 38*(8), 1615–1621.

Blane, D. N. (2020). Cardiovascular problems. In A. Staten & P. Staten (Eds.), *Practical general practice guidelines for effective clinical management* (7th ed., pp. 65–92). Elsevier.

British Heart Foundation. (2021). *British Heart Foundation UK factsheet*. http://www.bhf.org.uk

Cannon, J. (2017). Implications of the joint European cardiovascular disease prevention guidelines. *British Journal of Family Medicine, 4*(5).

Chief Medical Officer. (2016). *Low drinking guidelines*. https://assets.publishing.service.gov.uk/government/uploads/system/uploads/attachment_data/file/489795/summary.pdf

Clarke, C., Taylor, R., Shore, A., Ukkoumunne, O., & Campbell, J. (2012). Association of a difference in systolic blood pressure between arms with vascular disease and mortality: A systemic review and meta-analysis. *The Lancet, 379*(9819), P905–914.

Forouzanfar, M. I., Lui, P., Roth, G. A., Ng, M., Biryukov, S., Marczak, L., Alexander, L., Estep, K., Hassen Abate, K., Akinyemiju, T. F., Ali, R., Alvis-Guzman, N., Azzopardi, P., Banerjee, A., Bärnighausen, T., Basu, A., Bekele, T., Bennett, D. A., Biadgilign, S., . . . Murray, C. J. L. (2017). Global burden of hypertension and systolic blood pressure of at least 110 to 115 mmHg, 1990–2015. *Journal of the American Medical Association, 317*, 165–182.

Grossman, S., & Porth, C. (2014). *Porth's pathophysiology – Concepts and altered health states* (9th ed.). Wolters Kluwer, Lippincott Williams and Wilkins.

Guidelines and Audit Implementation Network. (2015). *Northern Ireland guidelines for management of chronic kidney disease*. https://rqia.org.uk/RQIA/files/7c/7c79b895-22e6-4b6d-95e8-3261f83baa34.pdf

Hippisley-Cox, J., Coupland, C., & Brindle, P. (2017). Development and validation of QRISK3 risk prediction algorithms to estimate future risk of cardiovascular disease: Prospective cohort study. *British Medical Journal, 357*, Article j2099.

Huber, C., Meyer, M., Steffel, J., & Blozik, E. (2019). Post-myocardial infarction (MI) care: Medication adherence for secondary prevention after MI in a large real-world population. *Clinical Therapeutics, 41*(1), 107–117.

Ibanez, B., James, S., & Agewall, S. (2018). ESC guidelines for the management of acute myocardial infarction in patients presenting with ST-elevation. *European Heart Journal, 39*, 119–177.

Inker, L., Astor, B., & Fox, C. (2014). KDOQI US commentary on the 2012 KDIGO clinical practice baseline for the evaluation and management of CKD. *American Journal of Kidney Disease, 36*(5), 713–715.

Jameson, K., Jick, S., & Hagberg, K. (2014). Prevalence and management of chronic kidney disease in primary care patients in the UK. *International Journal of Clinical Practice, 68*(9), 1110–1121.

Johnson, M., & May, C. (2015). Promoting professional behaviour change in healthcare: what interventions work, and why? A theory-led overview of systematic reviews. *British Medical Journal Open, 5*(9), Article e008592. https://doi.org/10.1136/bmjopen-2015-008592

JBS3 Board. (2014). Joint British Societies' consensus recommendations for the prevention of cardiovascular disease (JBS3). *Heart, 100*(2), ii1–ii67.

Kannel, W. B., & McGee, D. L. (1979). Diabetes and cardiovascular disease: The Framingham Study. *Journal of the American Medical Association, 241*(19), 2035–2038. https://doi.org/10.1001/jama.1979.03290450033020

LIPID Study Group. (1998). Prevention of cardiovascular events and death with pravastatin in patients with coronary heart disease and a broad range of initial cholesterol levels. *New England Journal of Medicine, 339*, 1349–1357.

Lowth, M. (2013). Chronic kidney disease. *Practice Nurse, 43*(1), 24–29.

Mendez, A. (2015). Chronic kidney disease: Supporting at risk and diagnosed patients. *British Journal of Community Nursing, 20*(2), 97–99.

Miller, W. R., & Rollnick, S. (2013). *Motivational interviewing. Helping people change* (3rd ed.). Guilford Press.

Mozaffarian, D., Benjamon, E., & Go, A. S. (2016). Heart disease and stroke statistics – 2016 update: A report from the American Heart Association. *Circulation, 133*(4), e338–360.

National Heart, Lung and Blood Institute. (2010). *DASH eating plan*. https://www.nhlbi.nih.gov/health-topics/dash-eating-plan

National Institute for Health and Care Excellence. (2013). *Myocardial infarction: Cardiac rehabilitation and prevention of further cardiovascular disease* (CG172). https://www.nice.org.uk/guidance/cg172

National Institute for Health and Care Excellence. (2014). *Cardiovascular risk assessment and management*. https://www.nice.org.uk/guidance/CG181

National Institute for Health and Care Excellence. (2015). *Chronic kidney disease in adults – Assessment and management*. https://www.nice.org.uk/guidance/cg182/

National Institute for Health and Care Excellence. (2016). *Ticagrelor for preventing atherothrombotic events after myocardial infarction*. https://www.nice.org.uk/ta420

National Institute for Health and Care Excellence. (2018). *Stop smoking interventions and services*. https://www.nice.org.uk/guidance/ng92/resources/stop-smoking-interventions-and-services-pdf-1837751801029

National Institute for Health and Care Excellence. (2019a). *Hypertension in adults, diagnosis and management*. https://www.nice.org.uk/guidance/GID-NG10054/documents/draft-guideline

National Institute for Health and Care Excellence. (2019b). *Hypertension in pregnancy – Diagnosis and management*. https://www.nice.org.uk/guidance/ng133

NHS England. (2019). *Long term plan*. https://www.longtermplan.nhs.uk/publication/nhs-long-term-plan/

NICE CKS. (2019). *NICE clinical knowledge summary: Chronic kidney disease*. https://cks.nice.org.uk/chronic-kidney-disease#!scenario

Nursing and Midwifery Council. (2018). *The code – Professional standards of practice and behaviour for nurses and midwives*.

Palmer, S., Navaneethan, S., & Craig, J. (2014). HMG CoA reductase inhibitors (statins) for people with chronic kidney disease not requiring dialysis. *Cochrane Database of Systematic Reviews, 2014*(5), Article CD00784. https://doi.org/10.1002/14651858.CD007784.pub2

Phillips, E. (2017). Evaluation of a coaching experiential learning project on OT student abilities and perceptions. *The Open Journal of Occupational Therapy, 5*(1), Article 9.

Public Health England. (2016). *The eatwell guide*.

Public Health England. (2019a). *Cardiovascular disease*. https://www.gov.uk/government/publications/health-matters-preventing-cardiovascular-disease/

Public Health England. (2019b). *Physical activity: Applying All Our Health.*

Queen's Nursing Institute. (2020). *Standards for education and practice for nurses new to general practice.* https://www.qni.org.uk/wp-content/uploads/2020/05/Standards-of-Education-and-Practice-for-Nurses-New-to-General-Practice-Nursing.pdf

Ramlan, G. (2015). Dietary challenges in patients with diabetes and CKD. *Journal of Renal Nursing, 7*(2), 58–63.

Rapsomaniki, E., Shah, A., & Perel P. (2014a). Prognostic models for stable coronary artery disease based on electronic record cohort of 102,023 patients. *European Heart Journal, 35,* 844–852.

Rapsomaniki, E., Timmis, A., George, J., Pujades-Rodriguez, M., Shah, A. D., Denaxas, S., White, I. R., Caulfield, M. J., Deanfield, J. E., Smeeth, L., Williams, B., Hingoran, A., & Hemingway, H. (2014b). Blood pressure and incidence of twelve cardiovascular diseases – Lifetime risks, healthy life years lost and age-specific associations in 1.25 million people. *The Lancet, 383,* 1899–1911.

Roffi, M., Patrono, C., & Collet, J. P. (2016). ESC guidelines for the management of acute coronary syndromes in patients presenting without persistent ST-segment elevation. *European Heart Journal, 37,* 267–315.

Royal College of General Practitioners. (2012). *Practice nurse competencies.* https://www.rcgp.org.uk/membership/practice-teams-nurses-and-managers/,/media/Files/Membership/GPF/RCGP-GPF-Nurse-Competencies.ashx

Sacks, M. D., Pfeffer, M. D., & Moye, L. (1996). The effect of pravastatin on coronary events after myocardial infarction in patients with average cholesterol levels. *New England Journal of Medicine, 335,* 1001–1009.

van Boven, J., Brügemann, A., & de Graeff, P. (1994). Randomised controlled trial of cholesterol-lowering in 4444 patients with coronary heart disease – the Scandinavian Simvastatin Survival Study (4S). *The Lancet, 344,* 1383–1389.

World Health Organisation. (2019). *Cardiovascular diseases.* https://www.who.int/news-room/fact-sheets/detail/cardiovascular-diseases-(cvds)

10

MANAGING ENDOCRINE CONDITIONS IN PRIMARY CARE

JOANNE POWELL ■ SUSAN F. BROOKS

INTRODUCTION

This chapter describes the role of the general practice nurse (GPN) in the management of disorders caused by endocrine dysfunction (ED). Most commonly, GPNs will be involved in ED management in relation to disorders affecting the thyroid gland and pancreas. This is the third-largest diagnostic category in primary care (Roberts et al., 2018), indicating how ED presentations are a common occurrence that the GPN needs to be vigilant to identify as part of sustained engagement with the practice population to enable early diagnosis. It is vitally important to establish the diagnosis and initiate management and referral to secondary care where appropriate (National Institute for Health and Clinical Excellence (NICE), 2018). As such, this chapter will discuss the diagnostic criteria to enable GPNs to assess for early recognition and support of people living with these long-term conditions (LTCs), especially because there is an increasing incidence of these diseases nationally and globally.

THE ENDOCRINE SYSTEM

The endocrine system is an extensive system of ductless glands that release hormones from secretory cells, which are diffused into the bloodstream via a network of capillaries (Waugh & Grant, 2014). Hormones are carried in the bloodstream to target organs for cell growth and metabolism. The glands and cells that produce these hormones operate independently of each other and have no physical connections (Waugh & Grant, 2014); however, the system is controlled by homeostasis and feedback mechanisms controlled by the hypothalamus and the autonomic nervous system (Tortora, 2017).

MANAGEMENT OF THYROID DYSFUNCTION

Anatomy and Physiology

The thyroid gland consists of two connected lobes situated on each side of the trachea (Fig. 10.1) and controls the rate at which glucose is oxidised and converted to body heat and energy for tissue growth and development. As a highly vascularised organ, the thyroid extracts iodine from the blood, which is required to produce two principal thyroid hormones, thyroxine (T_4) and triiodothyronine (T_3), with the subscript number relating to the number of iodine atoms. T_4 is an inactive hormone, which is changed into active T_3 by the conversion of iodine. T_3 is five times more active than T_4. Dietary sources of iodine, such as seafood, vegetables grown in iodine-rich soil and iodinated table salt, importantly support this process.

Aetiology

Waugh and Grant (2014), in noting the importance of dietary iodine, indicate thyroid dysfunction can occur as a result of a deficiency of dietary iodine, which in turn can result in increased production of thyroid-stimulating hormone (TSH), causing enlarged thyroid glands and goitre. The release of T_3 and T_4 into the bloodstream is stimulated by TSH from the anterior pituitary gland, and TSH is stimulated by thyrotropin-releasing hormone (TRH) from the hypothalamus. The thyroid hormones affect most organs, and underproduction or

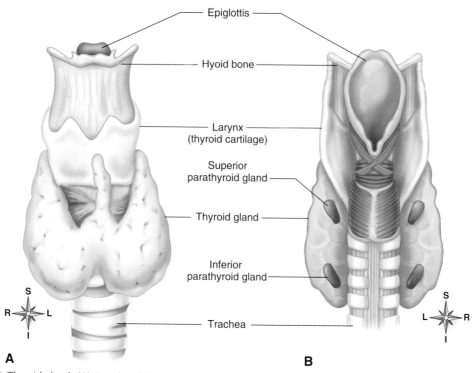

Epiglottis

Hyoid bone

Larynx
(thyroid cartilage)

Superior
parathyroid gland

Thyroid gland

Inferior
parathyroid gland

Trachea

A

B

Fig. 10.1 ■ Thyroid gland. (A) Anterior. (B) Posterior. (From Washington: Washington and Leaver's principles and practice of radiation therapy, 5th edition, 2021, Elsevier.) [[1st from Chabner screen 10 2nd from Washington and Leaver screen 1]]

overproduction of hormone can have physiological effects on the skeletal muscles, skin, reproductive and digestive systems.

Hypothyroidism is the clinical result of underproduction of thyroid hormones. In hyperthyroidism, the thyroid gland is overactive and produces excessive amounts of T_4 (Waugh & Grant, 2014). In addition, autoimmune diseases can cause thyroid dysfunction, such as Graves' disease, in which an antibody mimics the release of T_3 and T_4, leading to an increased amount of these hormones. Conversely, in Hashimoto's disease (autoimmune thyroiditis), the thyroid gland is attacked and destroyed by antibodies, resulting in hypothyroidism (British Thyroid Foundation, 2020).

Presenting Symptoms

To facilitate early identification and management of thyroid dysfunction, it is important for GPNs to be able to identify patients who require screening and management. The main signs and symptoms are related to high or low levels of T_3 and T_4 because of their relationship to the basal metabolic rate (Table 10.1). For instance, in Graves' disease, the presenting symptoms are nervousness and anxiety accompanied by weight loss, despite having a good appetite. Graves' disease is more prevalent in women than men and occurs most commonly between the ages of 30 and 50 years. However, hypothyroidism (again more common in women) presents as feeling 'tired all the time' and weight gain. Hypothyroidism can result from autoimmune thyroiditis (Hashimoto's disease), iodine deficiency, anti-thyroid medications, surgical removal of the thyroid or ionising radiation. A simple goitre can arise from a lack of T_3 and T_4, resulting in stimulation of TSH, causing hyperplasia of the thyroid gland. This can be triggered by persistent iodine deficiency, genetic disorders, anti-thyroid

TABLE 10.1
Signs and Symptoms of Thyroid Dysfunction

Hypothyroidism	Hyperthyroidism
Weight gain	Weight loss
Constipation	Frequent and loose bowel movements
Tiredness	Hyperactivity
Dry skin	Sweating
Hair loss	Agitation
Intolerance to cold	Exophthalmos
Hoarse voice	Tachycardia
Muscle stiffness and pain	Palpitations
Mental slowing and depression	
Nonpitting oedema of face, eyelids, feet and hands	

Adapted from NHS Conditions. (2020). *Symptoms of underactive thyroid (hypothyroidism)*. https://www.nhs.uk/conditions/underactive-thyroid-hypothyroidism/symptoms/and NHS Conditions. (2020). *Symptoms of overactive thyroid (hyperthyroidism)*. https://www.nhs.uk/conditions/overactive-thyroid-hyperthyroidism/symptoms/

medications or surgical removal of the thyroid (Waugh & Grant, 2014).

Assessment and Diagnosis

After the identification of clinical signs and symptoms, assessment of thyroid dysfunction is made through blood tests. According to NICE (2019a), the standard test for thyroid dysfunction is serological analysis of the TSH level; reference ranges are given in Table 10.2.

TABLE 10.2
Reference Ranges for Thyroid Hormones

	Hypothyroidism	Normal	Hyperthyroidism
TSH	> 10 mIU/l	0.4–4.0 mIU/l	TSH <0.1 mIU/l
FT_4	Below reference range	9–25 pmol/l	Above reference range
FT_3	Below reference range	3.5–7.8 pmol/l	Above reference range

TSH, Thyroid-stimulating hormone.
From British Thyroid Foundation. (2019). *Thyroid function tests*. https://www.btf-thyroid.org/thyroid-function-tests

In addition, NICE (2019a) states that for an accurate diagnosis, the test should also include free T_4, free T_3 and thyroid antibodies. Whilst these are relatively cheap tests, approximately 300 million tests are completed annually in the UK at an estimated cost of £30 million (Roberts et al., 2018). A cross-sectional study of 16,000 patients in a UK GP practice identified that the TSH test is overused and under-evidenced because only one-third of patients tested had results suggesting thyroid dysfunction (Werhun & Hamilton, 2015). Additionally, Roberts et al. (2018) found that thyroid function tests are requested for approximately 30% of older people without overt symptoms indicative of thyroid dysfunction. Consequently, clinical judgement is required in determining the appropriateness of initiating testing. Subclinical hypothyroidism may be diagnosed where blood test results are within the reference range, but patients report symptoms and may represent mild thyroid dysfunction.

Prognosis/Comorbidities

Having thyroid dysfunction may predispose individuals to other metabolic and endocrine disorders, so it is important that the GPN is aware of these links and considers screening appropriately for early diagnosis. Thyroid function may alter carbohydrate metabolism and result in type 2 diabetes mellitus (T2DM) (Chen et al., 2019). The risk of T2DM is higher in women with thyroid dysfunction. Thyroid dysfunction is also associated with a higher risk for cardiovascular disease and heart failure (Bano et al., 2019). Hypothyroidism is associated with dyslipidaemia, especially with higher levels of total and low-density lipoprotein (LDL) cholesterol. Thyroid dysfunction can also cause cardiac arrhythmia, where hyperthyroidism can lead to atrial arrhythmia and hypothyroidism to ventricular arrhythmia (Chen et al., 2019). Overt hyperthyroidism is associated with an increased risk of osteoporosis and fracture and is a concern in menopausal women. In addition, people with hyperthyroidism may experience reduced quality of life as a result of palpitations, heat intolerance and anxiety. Maternal hypothyroidism can lead to obstetric complications such as increased risk of miscarriage, placental abruption and preterm delivery, and it is vital that GPNs have an awareness of these rare but important clinical features patients can experience.

Treatment/Medication Options/ Other Contextual Issues

Primary hypothyroidism is a common condition and is generally managed in primary care (Drummond et al., 2020), usually with the replacement of synthetic hormone, levothyroxine. Evidence-based guidance (NICE, 2019a) indicates that the aim of treatment should be to normalise thyroid function and resolve symptoms using levothyroxine. Generally, dosage adjustments are made in incremental amounts and adjusted every 4 weeks, depending on the clinical response. And careful attention is required to the age of the patient requiring treatment for primary hypothyroidism with levothyroxine as this will determine the initial and maintenance dosing. If symptoms continue, further investigation should be made, including referral to an endocrinologist to investigate secondary hypothyroidism or a non-thyroid cause of symptoms. In subclinical hypothyroidism, some patients may benefit from symptom improvement with replacement levothyroxine.

Treatment of hyperthyroidism depends on the cause and is generally managed in secondary care, although general practitioners can initiate beta-blocker therapy to manage symptoms whilst individuals are awaiting referral. Where malignancy is suspected, referral should be made according to the cancer care pathway under the 2-week rule (NICE, 2016). *Primary hyperthyroidism* refers to a condition that arises from the thyroid gland rather than a pituitary or hypothalamic disorder. It is mainly caused by Graves' disease (an autoimmune disorder mediated by antibodies that stimulate the TSH receptor). Other causes include toxic nodular goitre (autonomously functioning thyroid nodules that secrete excess thyroid hormone) and drug-induced thyrotoxicosis. For patients with Graves' disease, treatment involves anti-thyroid medications, and patients generally achieve normal thyroid function within 4 to 6 weeks of commencing treatment (NICE, 2019a). Anti-thyroid drugs can also be used to prepare for thyroidectomy or for long-term management. In the UK, carbimazole is the most commonly used medication, which reduces the amount of circulating thyroid hormones. The GPN may be involved at this juncture because before starting anti-thyroid drugs, blood tests for a full blood count and liver function tests should be taken; GPNs should be aware of potentially serious side effects of carbimazole, such as bone marrow suppression and the associated increased risk of congenital malformations when used during pregnancy, especially in the first trimester and at high doses (daily dose of 15 mg or more). Women of childbearing potential should use effective contraception during treatment with carbimazole, and propylthiouracil may be considered for patients who experience side effects with carbimazole, are pregnant or are trying to conceive within the following 6 months or have a history of pancreatitis (Joint Formulary Committee, 2020). Other treatments include radioactive iodine and surgery through specialist endocrinology services.

ROLE OF GPN

In general practice, it is important that the GPN can recognise the signs and symptoms of thyroid dysfunction within a clinical assessment and make arrangements or referral for appropriate screening and diagnosis. Therefore knowledge of the reference ranges for thyroid tests is important to ensure appropriate onward referral. Often, patients with thyroid dysfunction may have other comorbidities for which they are monitored by the GPN (e.g., diabetes). Because thyroid dysfunction is associated with cardiovascular disease, the GPN will need to assess cardiovascular risk using a validated scoring system such as Q Risk (https://www.qrisk.org/). Where there are associated risk factors, the GPN can use a coaching approach to promote lifestyle modification with the aim of disease prevention. Where there are concordance issues with medication regimes, it is important that the GPN understands treatment regimens for thyroid dysfunction and can advise appropriately. For instance, in most cases, thyroid dysfunction is lifelong, and the resolution of symptoms can take up to 6 months. Generally, patients with thyroid dysfunction will be monitored annually unless the patient becomes symptomatic. The GPN can also advise that in the UK, levothyroxine treatment entitles the patient to medical exemption for prescription charges (FP92). Patients may require significant support from the GPN because of the impact of symptoms on quality of life, often experiencing prolonged delays in diagnosis and effective treatment that affects their ability to function and work (British Thyroid Foundation, 2020).

MANAGEMENT OF PANCREATIC DYSFUNCTION

In the UK, 4.8 million people have diabetes, and of these, 900,000 are undiagnosed (Diabetes UK, 2020). It is anticipated that this figure will rise to greater than 5 million people by 2035, with approximately 90% being diagnosed with T2DM (Diabetes UK, 2020).

Increasing levels of diabetes place an immense burden on the National Health Service (NHS), accounting for 10% of the health budget. This has implications for primary care, where the largest proportion of people diagnosed with diabetes are supported. In addition, those with T2DM are 2.5 times more likely to have a myocardial infarction or heart failure and 2 times more likely to have a stroke (Diabetes UK, 2019).

Anatomy and Physiology

The pancreas has both endocrine and exocrine functions (Fig. 10.2). Most pancreatic cells are arranged in

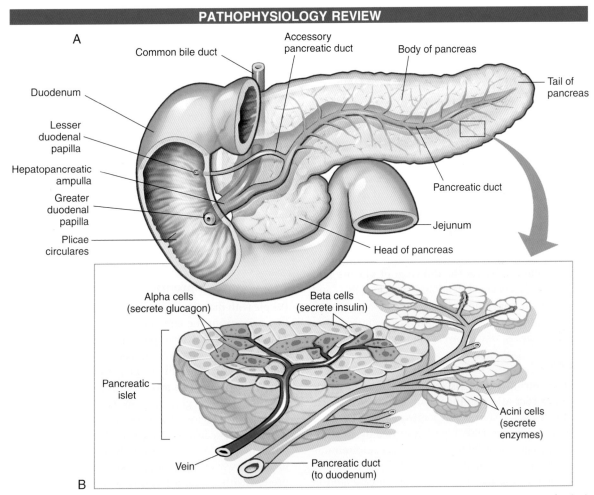

PATHOPHYSIOLOGY REVIEW

Fig. 10.2 ◼ Pancreas. (From Hockenberry MJ: Wong's nursing care of infants and children, 11th edition, 2019, Elsevier.) [[1. Blumgart's video atlas screen 3 2. NCIC screen 1]]

TABLE 10.3

Cells in Pancreatic Islets

Cell	Hormone	Function
Alpha cells (20% of cells)	Glucagon	Raise blood glucose
Beta cells (70% of cells)	Insulin	Lower blood glucose
Delta cells (5% of cells)	Somatostatin	Inhibit glucagon and insulin release

From Da Silva, X. (2018). The cells of the islets of Langerhans. *Journal of Clinical Medicine, 7*(3), 54.

clusters, which produce digestive enzymes through a network of ducts. Within these clusters, pancreatic islets (Table 10.3) are found, which contain hormone-secreting cells releasing hormones directly into the bloodstream.

The level of blood glucose is controlled by the secretion of glucagon and insulin via negative-feedback mechanisms. Normal fasting blood glucose levels are between 3.5 and 6.0 mmol/l (Waugh & Grant, 2014). Hypoglycaemia stimulates the release of glucagon from alpha cells, which acts on liver cells to convert glycogen into glucose (glycogenolysis) and promote the formation of glucose from lactic acid and amino acids (gluconeogenesis). This releases glucose into the bloodstream and raises blood glucose levels. Conversely, hyperglycaemia inhibits the release of glucagon and stimulates the release of insulin from beta cells. Insulin accelerates the diffusion of glucose into the cells – especially skeletal and muscle cells – and speeds up the conversion of glucose to glycogen in the liver (glycogenesis). It also slows glycogenolysis and gluconeogenesis, which lowers blood glucose levels.

Aetiology

Diabetes mellitus (DM) is the most common endocrine disorder affecting the ability to produce or use insulin, which results in hyperglycaemia. There are two major types of DM. Type 1 is caused by an absolute deficiency of insulin caused by an autoimmune disorder. It is known that certain human leukocyte antigens increase susceptibility to the disease, and in susceptible individuals, environmental factors (e.g., vitamin D intake, infections, antibiotic use) may trigger the destruction of the pancreatic beta cells

(Esposito et al., 2019). In contrast, T2DM is caused largely by insulin resistance and beta-cell dysfunction resulting in relative insulin deficiency and may have a background genetic predisposition. Insulin resistance is associated with ageing, physical inactivity and obesity. A further risk factor for T2DM is gestational diabetes mellitus (GDM) occurring in pregnancy and associated with insulin resistance and hyperglycaemia. GDM is associated with a 30% increased risk of developing T2DM (Mengying et al., 2019). Insulin resistance is also associated with metabolic changes at the cellular level resulting in high triglyceride levels, reduced high-density lipoprotein (HDL) cholesterol levels and hypertension – termed *metabolic syndrome* or *syndrome X* (Nolan & Prentki, 2019). This has demonstrable links with an increased risk of cardiovascular disease. In men, Hackett (2019) has presented convincing evidence demonstrating that low levels of testosterone are associated with obesity, T2DM and components of the metabolic syndrome. In addition, a study of people living in London by Pham et al. (2019) concluded that compared with people from a White ethnic group, the likelihood of having a T2DM diagnosis was more than double among those of Asian ethnicity and elevated by 65% among the Black group and by 17% among those from mixed and other ethnic groups. This has implications for health inequalities and how GPNs need to consider the ethnic diversity of their area with their teams in regard to screening, provision of healthcare and education.

Presenting Symptoms

People with diabetes will often present with symptoms that arise from the consequences of hyperglycaemia. These include polyuria, polydipsia, tiredness, weight loss, blurred vision and infections. Polyuria arises when the proximal tubules in the kidney exceed the capacity to pump glucose back into the circulation, resulting in excess glucose being excreted in the urine. Glycosuria increases the osmotic effect and loss of water. This predisposes to dehydration and creates an unquenchable thirst. Osmotic changes can also occur in the lens, causing blurred vision. People may also present with fungal infections, which are accelerated in the presence of glucose (e.g., *Candida albicans* causing balanitis and vulvovaginal candidiasis). People with type 1 diabetes mellitus (T1DM) may also present with weight loss caused by the loss of glucose/calories in the urine and aggravated by insulin deficiency accelerating glucose production by breaking down fat and protein. People with T1DM are at risk of developing ketoacidosis (DKA), where ketones develop from the breakdown of proteins and fat and result in a life-threatening situation if not remedied. It is therefore vital that GPNs have knowledge of this condition and how to recognise and refer anyone showing signs or symptoms of DKA. T1DM often has a rapid onset and usually occurs in childhood, whereas T2DM is usually slow and insidious in onset and occurs in later life. However, T2DM is increasingly being seen globally in adolescents and young adults, with a prevalence of 3.3% to 14.3%, and in their systematic review, Spurr et al. (2020) noted this is commonly associated with obesity, family history and ethnicity.

Assessment and Diagnosis

Given the increasing prevalence of diabetes, it is important that the GPN can recognise the signs and symptoms of pancreatic dysfunction within a clinical assessment and make arrangements for appropriate screening and diagnosis. Since 2011, the UK has been using the World Health Organisation (WHO, 2006) diagnostic criteria for diagnosing diabetes and has accepted the WHO guidelines of using glycated haemoglobin (HbA1c) for diagnosis (John, 2012). Therefore those who present in primary care with a clinical history and symptoms of diabetes should have blood tests for fasting plasma glucose and HbA1c. Previously, people being tested for diabetes were investigated using an oral glucose tolerance test (OGTT). This involved fasting and ingestion of a measured oral carbohydrate load with measurements of blood glucose before and 2 hours after. The HbA1c represents a cheaper and easier alternative for the diagnosis of diabetes, although it is not appropriate for all. In women with suspected GDM, the OGTT remains the gold standard (NICE, 2015). The diagnosis of diabetes should not be made based on a single measurement of plasma glucose or HbA1c.

The recommendations for diagnosis are two readings of fasting plasma glucose of 7.0 mmol/l or more or two readings of HbA1c of 48 mmol/mol. It is not always necessary to use fasting blood glucose levels as measures for diagnosis because these can be

inaccurate as a result of potentially poor fasting practices (John, 2012). However, where a person has a medical condition that would prevent accurate measurement of HbA1c (children or young people, those with suspected T1DM or people with haemoglobinopathies), fasting blood glucose should also be used to confirm the diagnosis. In addition, there also needs to be caution with the HbA1c in conditions where people have been acutely ill or taking medication that may cause a rapid glucose rise, such as corticosteroids or antipsychotic medications. The presence of pancreatic damage, such as acute pancreatitis or haemoglobinopathies, can also give rise to incorrect HbA1c values. The measurement of C-peptide or specific diabetes antibodies is not generally undertaken in primary care and is the responsibility of secondary care delivery (NICE, 2016). In patients with known haemoglobinopathies, serum fructosamine can be used as an alternative to HbA1c.

In addition, the GPN has a key role in the risk assessment for pre-diabetes and diabetes. NICE (2019b) recommends that a validated computer-based risk assessment tool should be used to identify those on the practice register who are at higher risk of T2DM. Alternatively, the validated Diabetes Risk Score Assessment tool from Diabetes UK (2020) can be used. Additionally, this risk assessment can be used for those attending NHS Health Checks aged between 40 and 74 years. Where the risk assessment identifies those at high risk, blood tests should be advised to confirm the diagnosis. The GPN also has a crucial role in health coaching with the aim of disease prevention through lifestyle modification. The role of the GPN will be focussed on encouraging self-management with people living with T2DM because they represent the largest proportion of the diabetes caseload. People with stable T1DM may be discharged to primary care for their support, but GPNs must consider their scope of competence when monitoring people on insulin regimens, and additional study and training in the titration of different insulins and their management is advised for this role.

Prognosis

It is estimated that people living with T2DM are likely to have a lower life expectancy as a result of the condition. Seminal research from the Diabetes

Complications and Control Trial (DCCT) published in 1993 (DCCT Research Group, 1993) and the UK Prospective Diabetes Study (UKPDS) published in 2008 (UKPDS Group, 2008) showed that diabetes increases the risk of microvascular and macrovascular complications. These studies showed that intensive management of glycaemic and blood pressure control is crucial in preventing diabetes-related macrovascular (heart attack and stroke) and microvascular (retinopathy, nephropathy and neuropathy) complications. These issues are still relevant because more recently, a recent systematic review of 10 studies combining the results of 34,385 participants demonstrated that for those living with T2DM, there is a doubled risk of cardiovascular death (Zhang et al., 2019). When consulting with people living with T2DM, GPNs should support and encourage maintenance of optimal weight, avoidance of smoking and heavy drinking, adoption of a healthy diet and increased physical activity levels.

Treatment and Monitoring

The financial cost of treating diabetes is around £8.8 million (Roberts & Greenhalgh, 2018), so lifestyle intervention programmes are increasingly being used as effective prevention methods. Therefore GPNs can play an integral role in identifying and engaging with people at risk of disease to recommend lifestyle interventions aimed at disease prevention. In the UK, GPNs can refer people at risk of diabetes to the NHS Diabetes Prevention Programme (NHSDPP), which is a combination of behavioural interventions enabling weight loss, increased physical activity and improved nutrition through a minimum of 13 face-to-face group-based sessions over 9 months (Barron et al., 2017). This scheme is open to adults who are registered with a general practitioner (GP) who have blood glucose levels putting them at risk of diabetes who can take part in light exercise. Barron et al. (2017) have shown in their evaluation of the NHSDPP that behavioural interventions supporting people to maintain a healthy weight and being more active can reduce the risk of diabetes. A total of 43,603 referrals were received between June 2016 and March 2017, and 49% of those referred attended the first session. In particular, Barron et al. (2017) noted that attendance rates among men and

ethnic groups showed the programme was effective in reaching those at risk of T2DM who typically access healthcare less effectively.

However, if diabetes is diagnosed, as a result of the findings of the studies noted previously, the key priorities of treatment and management are to control blood glucose to as near normal as possible, control blood pressure and reduce the person's cardiovascular risk and risk of microvascular complications (NICE, 2019b). As with diabetes prevention, it is recognised that structured education is a powerful mechanism to achieve this. On average, a person with diabetes will spend approximately 3 hours with a healthcare professional (Diabetes UK, 2016). Therefore strategies to improve self-management and self-empowerment are crucial. A systematic review of 23 studies investigating structured education in 6747 people with T2DM concluded that it significantly improves glycaemic control in terms of HbA1c and also improves self-management skills – in terms of diabetes knowledge, self-efficacy, satisfaction and body weight (McCay et al., 2019). As such, NICE (2019b) recommends that all newly diagnosed people with diabetes should be referred to structured education, of which DESMOND is well recognised (https://www.desmond-project.org.uk/). The aim of management should be to promote individualised care and shared decision-making, largely around lifestyle modification (NICE, 2019b). However, many patients report negative reactions at the time of diagnosis of diabetes (termed 'diabetes distress' by Polonsky et al. (2017)). These feelings can persist over time and are linked to poor glycaemic control. Health coaching has been defined by Wolever et al. (2013) as 'a person-centred process that is based upon behaviour change theory and is delivered by health professionals with diverse backgrounds' and has been shown to reduce diabetes distress across four different dimensions – emotional burden, regimen distress, interpersonal distress and physical distress (Allison et al., 2019). Health coaching, whether in individual or group settings, has been demonstrated to show significant improvements in empowerment and quality of life and reduction in emotional distress (Cheng et al., 2019). In the UK, group consultations are a relatively new strategy being used in general practice to enable adults to take control and actively manage their condition. One group consultation project reported a 70% reduction in HbA1c and 61% improvement in blood pressure (NHS England, 2019). This project was in an area of South West London with acute deprivation and serving a largely Black and minority ethnic (BME) population where there was a large variation in accessing services. In addition, the project reported that 90% of attendees of group consultations reported feeling more listened to and less isolated. The attendees noted that peer learning and support were incredibly powerful. One attendee stated:

> We come together. We can relate to each other. We encourage one another to look after our health. This is important to us as diabetic people… I love it because I am learning a lot about how to manage my diabetes… I feel like crying because it changed my life.

The potential for primary care to lead weight management and lifestyle modification has also been exciting and evaluated in the Diabetes Remission Clinical Trial (DiRECT) (Lean et al., 2019). This randomised controlled trial in primary care practices in the UK (in Tyneside and Scotland) built on the work of Steven and Taylor (2015), who demonstrated remission of diabetes after following a very low-calorie diet. This study has demonstrated that 46% of the intervention structured weight-management group with T2DM of up to 6 years' duration could achieve remission at 12 months and rose to 86% of those in the intervention group who achieved a target weight loss of 15 kg or more. The legacy effect of this intervention has been shown to exist at 2 years, with 35% still in remission in the intervention group, compared with 3% of the control group. The resulting message to new GPNs is that there is exciting partnership work with individuals with diabetes to identify key goals and mechanisms for promoting healthy behaviours, acknowledging that living with this LTC can be a huge challenge and consultations need to be nonjudgemental and empowering rather than conveying blame or shame (Been-Dahmen et al., 2015).

Whilst NICE (2019b) notes that the main aim of diabetes management is lifestyle modification,

medications may be clinically indicated for optimum control. NICE (2019b) offers an algorithm for blood-glucose-lowering therapy in adults with T2DM, which features a step-wise progression for optimising glycaemic control. However, before recommending optimisation of a medication regimen, the GPN should discuss concordance with therapeutic regimens. One approach that could be utilised in general practice is to evaluate medicine usage. The GPN can liaise with the GP and clinical pharmacist to facilitate this. Routine monitoring of diabetes via self-monitoring of blood glucose is not routinely recommended (NICE, 2019b) unless the person is using a glucose-lowering therapy such as a sulfonylurea or insulin. The optimization of blood glucose levels is a complex process of negotiation between the clinician and the person living with diabetes. Knowledge of the newer drugs for diabetes that maximize cardiovascular outcomes may require referral to a diabetes specialist as there are novel and exciting options available (Basu et al, 2021)

ROLE OF GPN

It is apparent that the role of the GPN in the management of pancreatic dysfunction is multifaceted. At one end of the continuum, the role will be with education and coaching regarding diet and lifestyle issues for health promotion and disease prevention. However, at the other end of the continuum, the GPN may initiate and titrate medications to manage disease processes and prevent complications of the condition. The GPN needs to be competent to discuss lifestyle interventions and to be familiar with the signs and symptoms of the disease to facilitate prompt assessment, diagnosis and management. As such, the GPN needs to be able to understand the diagnostic criteria for pancreatic dysfunction. GPNs also need to have excellent communication skills to liaise with and refer to multidisciplinary colleagues (e.g., retinal screening, podiatry) and make referrals for the relevant structured education based on the individual needs of the person. All care must be individualised and recognise the importance of the person's biological and psychosocial needs. As with any role, the GPN needs to work within their scope of competence. An example of this is with the monitoring of foot health as part of the general practice annual health review for people with diabetes. It is crucial that the GPN has the necessary education, training and supervision for the roles undertaken in this field.

SUMMARY

This chapter has described the role of the GPN in the management of disorders caused by ED of the thyroid gland and pancreas. GPNs have great opportunities to be involved in raising awareness of these conditions and supporting people who are living with the challenges of medication and other treatments that are often lifelong. Knowledge of ED can be gained through experiences of meeting people who have become experts in living with their individual condition and through specific study to become a specialist practitioner. Empathetic consulting alongside this knowledge can make a positive contribution to the lives of many people accessing general practice for their main source of healthcare, and GPNs continue to be ideally placed to fulfil this important role.

REFERENCES

Allison, M., Srivastava, S., Burton, S. B., et al. (2019). 51-LB: The impact of digital health coaching on the Diabetes Distress Scale. *Diabetes, 68*(Suppl. 1). https://doi.org/10.2337/db19-51-LB

Bano, A., Chaker, L., Mattace-Raso, F., Terzikhan, N., Kavousi, M., & Arfan Ikram, M., & Peeters, R. P., & Franco, O. H. (2019). Thyroid function and life expectancy with and without noncommunicable diseases: A population-based study. *PLoS Medicine, 16*(10), Article e1002957. https://journals.plos.org/plosmedicine/article?id=10.1371/journal.pmed.1002957

Barron, E., Clark, R., Smith J., & Valbhii, J. (2017). Progress of the Healthier You: NHS Diabetes Prevention Programme: Referrals, uptake and participant characteristics. *Diabetes Medicine, 35*(4), 513–518. https://doi.org/10.1111/dme.13562

Basu, A., Patel, D., Winocour, P. and Ryder, R.J. (2021) Cardiovascular impact of new drugs (GLP-1 and gliflozins): the ABCD position statement *The British Journal of Diabetes* https://bjd-abcd.com/index.php/bjd/article/view/711/909.

Been-Dahmen, J., Dwarswaard, J., Hazes, J., Loes van Staa, A., & Ista E. (2015). Nurses' views on patient self-management: A qualitative study. *Journal of Advanced Nursing, 71*(12), 2834–2845.

British Thyroid Foundation. (2020). *Thyroiditis.* https://www.btf-thyroid.org/thyroiditis

Chen, R. H., Chen, H. Y., Man, K. M., et al. (2019). Thyroid diseases increased the risk of type 2 diabetes mellitus. *Medicine,*

98(20), Article e15631. https://doi.org/10.1097/MD.0000000000015631

Cheng, L., Sit, J. W. H., & Choi, K. C. (2019). The effects of an empowerment-based self-management intervention on empowerment level, psychological distress and quality of life in patients with poorly controlled type 2 diabetes: A randomised controlled trial. *International Journal of Nursing Studies, 3*(21), Article 103407. https://doi.org/10.1016/j.ijnurstu.2019.103407

Diabetes Control and Complications Trial (DCCT) Research Group. (1993). The effect of intensive treatment of diabetes on the development and progression of long-term complications in insulin dependent diabetes mellitus. *New England Journal of Medicine, 329*(14), 977–986.

Diabetes UK. (2016). *Diabetes education and self-management.* https://www.diabetes.org.uk/professionals/resources/shared-practice/diabetes-education

Diabetes UK. (2019). *Know your risk – professionals.* https://www.diabetes.org.uk/professionals/diabetes-risk-score-assessment-tool

Diabetes UK. (2020). *Know diabetes. Fight diabetes.* https://www.diabetes.org.uk/

Drummond, R., McManus, F., Hughes, K., Mackin, S., & Carty, D. (2020). Diabetes and endocrinology. In Staten and Staten *practical general practice guidelines of effective clinical management* (7th Ed., pp. 409–425). Elsevier.

Esposito, S., Giada, T., Santi, E., et al. (2019). Environmental factors associated with type 1 diabetes. *Frontiers in Endocrinology, 10,* Article 592. https://www.ncbi.nlm.nih.gov/pmc/articles/PMC6722188/

Hackett, G. (2019). Type 2 diabetes and testosterone therapy. *World Journal of Men's Health, 37*(1), 31–44. https://doi.org/10.5534/wjmh.180027

John, W. G. (2012). Use of HbA1c in the diagnosis of diabetes mellitus in the UK. The implementation of World Health Organization guidance 2011. *Diabetic Medicine, 29*(11), 1350–1357. https://doi.org/10.1111/j.1464-5491.2012.03762.x

Joint Formulary Committee. (2020). *British national formulary.* http://www.medicinescomplete.com

Lean, M. E. J., Leslie, W. S, Barnes, A. C., et al. (2019). Durability of a primary care led weight management intervention for remission of type 2 diabetes mellitus: 2-year result of the DiRECT open label, cluster randomised trial. *The Lancet, 7*(5), 344–355.

McCay, D., Hill, A., Coates, V., et al. (2019). Structured diabetes education outcomes: looking beyond HbA1C. A systematic review. *Practical Diabetes, 36*(3), 86–90.

Mengying, L., Rahman, M., Jing, W., et al. (2019). 1705-P genetic risk score of type 2 diabetes and progression risk from gestational diabetes mellitus to type 2 diabetes: Results from 2 independent populations. *Diabetes, 68*(Suppl. 1). https://doi.org/10.2337/db19-1705-P

National Health Service England. (2019). *Introducing group consultations for adults living with type 2 diabetes at Brigstock Medical Practice.* https://www.england.nhs.uk/atlas_case_study/introducing-group-consultations-for-adults-living-with-type-2-diabetes-at-brigstock-medical-practice/

National Institute for Health and Care Excellence. (2015). *Diabetes in pregnancy: management from preconception to the postnatal period (NG3)*. https://www.nice.org.uk/Guidance/NG3

National Institute for Health and Care Excellence. (2016). *Head and neck cancers – Recognition and referral*. https://cks.nice.org.uk/topics/head-neck-cancers-recognition-referral/

National Institute for Health and Care Excellence. (2018). *Type 2 diabetes in adults: Management (NICE Guideline NG28)*. https://www.nice.org.uk/guidance/ng28

National Institute for Health and Care Excellence. (2019a). *Guideline for thyroid disease: assessment and management (NICE Guideline NG145)*. https://www.nice.org.uk/guidance/ng145

National Institute for Health and Care Excellence. (2019b). *Type 2 diabetes in adults: Management (NICE Guideline NG28)*. https://www.nice.org.uk/guidance/ng28

Nolan, C. J., & Prentki, M. (2019). Insulin resistance and insulin hypersecretion in the metabolic syndrome and type 2 diabetes: Time for a conceptual framework shift. *Diabetes and Vascular Disease Research, 16*(2), 118–127. https://doi.org/10.1177/1479164119827611

Pham, T., Carpenter, J., Morris, T., Sharma, M., & Peterse, I. (2019). Ethnic differences in the prevalence of type 2 diabetes diagnoses in the UK: Cross-sectional analysis of the Health Improvement Network Primary Care Database. *Clinical Epidemiology, 11*, 1081–1088.

Polonsky, W. H., Capehorn, M., Belton, A., et al. (2017). Physician-patient communication at diagnosis of type 2 diabetes and its links to patient outcomes: New results from the global IntroDia study. *Diabetes Research and Clinical Practice, 237*, 265–274. https://doi.org/10.1016/j.diabres.2017.03.016

Roberts, L., McCahon, D., Johnson, O., et al. (2018). Stability of thyroid function in older adults: The Birmingham Elderly Thyroid Study. *British Journal of General Practice, 68*(675), e718–e726. https://doi.org/10.3399/bjgp18X698861

Roberts, S., & Greenhalgh, T. (2018). *Weighing up the costs of type 2 diabetes prevention programs*. On Medicine [Blog].

https://blogs.biomedcentral.com/on-medicine/2018/01/30/weighing-up-the-costs-of-type-2-diabetes-prevention-programs/

Spurr, S., Bally, J., Hill, P., et al. (2020). Exploring the prevalence of undiagnosed prediabetes, type 2 diabetes mellitus and risk factors in adolescents: A systematic review. *Journal of Pediatric Nursing, 50*, 94–104. https://doi.org/10.1016/j.pedn.2019.09.025

Steven, S., & Taylor, R. (2015). The glycaemic and anti-hypertensive effects of a very low-calorie diet are maintained over 6 months in both short and long duration type 2 diabetes. *Diabetic Medicine, 32*(Suppl. 1), 53.

Tortora, G. J. (2017). *Tortora's principles of anatomy and physiology* (15th ed.). John Wiley and Sons.

United Kingdom Prospective Diabetes Study (UKPDS) Group. (1998). Intensive blood-glucose control with sulphonylureas or insulin compared with conventional treatment and risk of complications in patients with type 2 diabetes (UKPDS 33). *The Lancet, 352*, 837–853.

Waugh, A., & Grant, A. (2014). *Ross and Wilson anatomy and physiology in health and illness* (13th ed.). Elsevier.

Werhun, A., & Hamilton, W. (2015). Thyroid function in primary care: overused and under-evidenced? A study examining which clinical features correspond to an abnormal thyroid function result. *Family Practice, 32*(2), 187–191.

Wolevar, R., et al. (2013). A systematic review of the literature on health and wellness coaching: Defining a key behavioural intervention in healthcare. *Global Advances in Health and Medicine, 2*(4), 38–57.

World Health Organisation. (2006). *Use of glycated haemoglobin (HbA1c) in the diagnosis of diabetes mellitus*. http://www.who.int/diabetes/publications/report-hba1c_2011.pdf

Zhang, Y., et al. (2019). Combined lifestyle factors and risk of incident type 2 diabetes and prognosis among individuals with type 2 diabetes: A systematic review and meta-analysis of prospective cohort studies. *Diabetologia, 63*, 21–33.

11

MANAGING NEUROLOGICAL CONDITIONS IN PRIMARY CARE

DEBORAH LOUISE DUNCAN

INTRODUCTION

Neurological conditions, in terms of their scale, range and clinical complexity, present significant challenges to individuals, families and the health and social care systems. Furthermore, people with neurological conditions often experience the lowest health-related quality of life in relation to other long-term conditions, signalling unmet needs. Consequently, improving the standard of care represents a priority within the UK, where the aim is to support self-management, independence and the delivery of coordinated quality care (Welsh Government, 2017; Scottish Government, 2019; National Institute for Healthcare Excellence (NICE), 2021). Building the capacity within general practice to care for people with neurological conditions is a key facet of action plans and policies.

Specialist clinicians within secondary care normally oversee the diagnosis and management of patients presenting with serious neurological conditions. However, as a front-line service, these patients, for a variety of reasons, may consult with the general practice nurse (GPN), and in some instances, this may entail the ongoing monitoring of their condition. Consequently, the GPN may have a varied and complex role in supporting a patient with a neurological disease and their family (Hickey, 2013). From this perspective, knowledge of neurological diseases the GPN is likely to encounter, their evidence-based management and approaches to ongoing monitoring is imperative.

This chapter critically considers the role of the GPN in relation to three neurological diseases: epilepsy, Parkinson's disease (PD), and multiple sclerosis (MS).

CARING FOR PATIENTS WITH A NEUROLOGICAL DISEASE

The GPN plays a critical role in supporting patients with neurological diseases to optimise their quality of life. This may entail, depending on the stability of the patient's condition, the GPN undertaking annual monitoring for some neurological diseases as part of the evidence-based management (NICE, 2017, 2019, 2020; Scottish Intercollegiate Guidelines Network (SIGN), 2018). Furthermore, under the auspices of the Quality Outcomes Framework for primary care (England, Wales and Northern Ireland) and the Global Sum (Scotland), there is an expectation that general practice will collate registers of patients with neurological diseases (NHS Digital, 2019). This provides the GPN with the opportunity to deliver person-centred care in discussing self-management, engaging in shared decision-making and providing psychological and practical support (Carrier, 2015). The GPN has an important role in initiating discussions with patients on health-related quality of life (HRQoL) issues, such as anxiety and depression, because a third of patients with a neurological disease are predicted to experience depression, and this figure appears to be rising (Fernie et al., 2015). Whilst sensitive inquiry and exploration of mental health issues may be challenging for the GPN (see Chapter 12), early identification can lead to quicker treatment and implementation of effective coping strategies.

EPILEPSY

As a long-term condition affecting both children and adults, epilepsy is a serious neurological disease that affects the brain, leading to recurrent sensory disturbances resulting in seizures that may include loss of consciousness (Smith et al., 2015a). These symptoms occur as a result of bursts of abnormal electrical activity within the brain, which are unpredictable, transient and affect physiological motor function. Whilst the clinical manifestation of seizure represents the immediate outcome, patients with epilepsy are subject to a raft of related side effects, including cognitive impairment, neuropsychiatric problems, stigma and factors often correlating with greater risk of lower socioeconomic status (Smith et al., 2015a).

Epilepsy is the third most common neurological disease in older adults (Smith & Tiwari, 2015), with 500,000 people in the UK receiving this diagnosis. A third of patients with a learning disability also have epilepsy, and individuals with epilepsy are also 20 times more likely to have a shorter life expectancy (Smith et al., 2015a). Seizure activity for patients with epilepsy is both unpredictable and frightening; therefore the GPN's knowledge of this complex disease is vital in supporting patients to manage and cope with this disease.

Diagnosis

An epilepsy specialist should make the diagnosis, and this will be primarily based on a detailed patient history and eyewitness accounts by observers of the seizure occurrence/manifestation (NICE, 2020). The use of neuroimaging and electroencephalogram (EEG) is only undertaken to support the diagnosis or establish the differential diagnosis in respect of epilepsy type, for example, if photosensitive epilepsy is suspected (NICE, 2020; SIGN, 2018). The use of neuroimaging may identify any structural abnormalities that cause certain epilepsies, with magnetic resonance imaging (MRI) being specifically indicated in the following patients:

- Patients who develop epilepsy before the age of 2 years or into adulthood
- Patients with an indication of a 'focal onset' based on history, examination or EEG
- Patients in whom seizures continue despite treatment with first-line medication

A computed tomography (CT) scan is useful in identifying underlying gross pathology if MRI is not available or contraindicated or in an acute situation. Other serological tests may be indicated in some instances, namely, plasma electrolytes, glucose and calcium levels. However, serological blood testing on a regular basis is not indicated as part of routine management. Adults with suspected epilepsy should have a 12-lead ECG, which may be requested in primary care to rule out cardiomyopathies (NICE, 2020).

Seizure Classification

Seizure classification is a critical part of diagnosing and managing epilepsy because an accurate classification will direct evidence-based care in relation to pharmacological treatment, investigations, prognosis and the appropriate provision of important information for patients and their families, including first aid management (SIGN, 2018).

Both NICE (2020) and SIGN (2018) provide guidance on seizure classification, drawing on the widely used and internationally accepted system provided by the International League Against Epilepsy (ILAE) (Fisher et al., 2017). Whilst the NICE (2020) and SIGN (2018) guidelines refer to the ILAE classification, the ILAE in 2017 amended its classification, terminology and definitions to provide transparent clinical language to support the accurate diagnosis of seizures and epilepsy syndromes (Fisher et al., 2017). The new ILAE 2017 classification (Fig. 11.1) involves determining 'seizure type' based on where the onset of the abnormal electrical discharge occurs within the brain:

- **Focal onset** – originates within one hemisphere, with abnormal activity limited to networks within this area
- **Generalised onset** – originates in some area of the brain and affects the bilaterally distributed networks
- **Unknown onset** – where the onset is missed or unclear

The ILEA's 2017 classification includes determining the 'epilepsy type', classified as focal, generalised, combined generalised and focal and unknown. Focal seizures are classified in relation to the patient's level of awareness, the most obvious motor or nonmotor feature and if this progresses to include a bilateral tonic-clonic seizure. Generalised seizures are classified according to motor or nonmotor presentations. This classification seeks to support decision-making and management by specialists in that patients may potentially present with

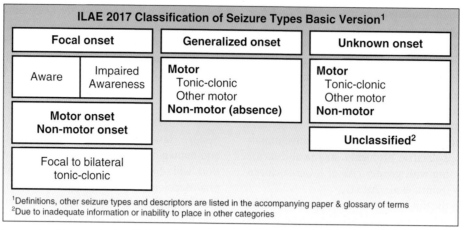

Fig. 11.1 ■ International League Against Epilepsy (ILAE) 2017 classification of seizure types, basic version. (From Fisher, R. S., Cross, J. H., French, J. A., Higurashi, N., Hirsch, E., Jansen, F. E.,...Scheffer, I. E. (2017). Operational classification of seizure types by the International League Against Epilepsy: Position paper of the ILAE Commission for Classification and Terminology. *Epilepsia, 58*(4), 522–530.)

multiple epilepsy types and may require further investigative tests (Fisher et al., 2017).

The following comprises a brief outline of the main categories within the ILEA 2017 classification (Fisher et al., 2017).

Focal-Onset Seizures (Formerly Classified as Simple Partial)

Focal Aware Seizures

Also known as 'auras', these types of seizures occur in one part of the brain and can cause abnormal sensations or a general feeling of strangeness that patients find difficult to describe in simple terms (National Health Service (NHS), 2017). Patients can therefore experience a range of sensory and physical symptoms, which may include unusual smells or tastes, tingling in their limbs, an intense feeling of fear or joy and stiffness or twitching in part of the body, and the patient is usually conscious during the episode. These symptoms can also be a warning sign that another type of seizure is about to happen.

Focal Impaired-Awareness Seizures (Formerly Classified as Complex Partial)

During this type of seizure, a more extensive part of the one side of the brain is affected, and the patient can lose their sense of awareness of what they are doing, and this can result in abnormal body movements such as smacking the lips, rubbing the hands, fiddling with objects or chewing or swallowing. Individuals will have no memory of the event.

Generalised Seizures (Formerly Tonic–Clonic Seizures)

Involving both parts of the brains simultaneously, a generalised seizure involves an initial tonic stage where the patient will be conscious and their muscles will become stiff, and at this point, the patient may collapse. This is rapidly followed by the clonic stage, where the person becomes unconscious, their limbs jerk, they may lose control of their bladder or bowel and they may bite their tongue or the inside of their cheek and might even have difficulty breathing, hence the need for first-aid interventions.

Epilepsy Emergency – Status Epilepticus

Status epilepticus is considered as a medical emergency that can develop when a patient has established epilepsy or during the initial presentation of the disease. A person can have a prolonged generalised tonic–clonic seizure or at least two back-to-back seizures without returning to consciousness. Rapid medical intervention is required to prevent neuronal damage, morbidity or death (Leitinger et al., 2015).

MANAGEMENT

Awaiting diagnostic confirmation from a specialist neurologist can be a difficult time for patients and families, and it is important they receive information to recognise a seizure, undertake first aid and the importance of reporting further episodes. The GPN can assist with this education because they may be the first point of contact and act as a conduit in referring patients to specialist epilepsy nurse-led intervention programs. They can also support patients in coping with the negative labelling epilepsy appears to invoke within society, which, because of a lack of understanding, results in stigmatisation and therein notably higher levels of psychosocial problems compared with the general population. Patients across the age span may need time and space to discuss how their epilepsy affects them and their families on a psychosocial level. Allowing them that space or referring them to specialist services that promote empowerment has been noted as beneficial (Aliasgharpour et al., 2013).

The GPN plays a crucial role in caring for patients with epilepsy and their families in promoting the best health outcomes via education, empowerment and self-management (Smith et al., 2015b); this is not without its challenges, and this may include discussion regarding sudden unexpected death in epilepsy (SUDEP). Whilst it is anticipated that this topic will have been discussed by a specialist neurologist/nurse within the acute setting at the point of diagnosis, ongoing discussion may occur, necessitating the provision of tailored information regarding SUDEP, support for optimising seizure control and awareness of nocturnal seizures (NICE, 2018a).

PHARMACOLOGICAL TREATMENT OF TONIC OR ATONIC SEIZURES

The cornerstone of treatment of generalised seizures is pharmacological (Nugent, 2020), and the following are common types of antiepileptic drugs (AEDs):

- Sodium valproate
- Carbamazepine
- Lamotrigine
- Levetiracetam
- Oxcarbazepine
- Ethosuximide
- Topiramate

The pharmacological treatment of epilepsy using AEDs is highly complex and determined following the classification of seizure and epilepsy typology. NICE provides detailed and regularly updated evidence-based guidance (https://www.nice.org.uk/guidance/cg137/chapter/Appendix-E-Pharmacological-treatment) on prescribing first-line treatment and, where required, adjunctive treatment, where monotherapy has proved unsuccessful in achieving seizure control (NICE, 2018a; SIGN, 2018). These evidence-based guidelines also detail prescribing contraindications, such as sodium valproate (Epilim) during pregnancy because there is a significant risk of fetal abnormality or developmental disorders (Gov.UK, 2019; Medicines and Healthcare Products Regulatory Agency, 2018). The GPN may be able to discuss this with women during pre-conceptual care and recommend referral to their neurology consultant or community midwife before conception. Women of childbearing age are only prescribed this medication if there is a pregnancy prevention programme in place (Gov.UK, 2019). Other types of epilepsy medication may also affect the efficacy of the oral contraceptive pill, so a higher dose of the pill will need to be prescribed. The GPN has an important role in ensuring that women with epilepsy, in their reproductive years, are fully aware of the wide-ranging implications and interventions necessary in attempting to become pregnant or in avoiding pregnancy.

Whilst medication is the cornerstone of management, this is a complex field requiring specialist input because nearly 40% of patients with epilepsy need to take more than one prescribed medication to control the disease (Smith et al., 2015b). Those with refractory epilepsy, that is, seizures that continue despite the use of a single or combination of antiepileptic medication, may need to take three or more drugs; consequently, polypharmacy is a common management feature.

Surgical Management

Surgery to remove the part of the brain that is triggering seizure activity is only considered if AEDs are ineffective in controlling seizures and if bespoke tests confirm that the seizures are caused by a problem in a small part of the brain that can be removed without causing serious effects (SIGN, 2018). There are several types of surgical interventions, which include the following:

- Resective surgery – removal of epileptogenic brain tissue
- Ablative surgery – minimally invasive, image-guided laser ablation of the epileptogenic brain tissue
- Disconnection surgery – involves severing of specific nerve pathways along which seizures spread

Despite the specific and individualised treatment options required in the management of epilepsy, caring for patients with a long-term condition involves structured patient-centred care, advice on lifestyle, involvement of specialist input and engagement with the wider multidisciplinary team (NICE, 2020).

MULTIPLE SCLEROSIS

MS is a chronic progressive neurological disease of the central nervous system in which inflammatory and neurodegenerative processes result in disability and a reduction in mortality of 7 to 10 years (Sawcer et al., 2011). The cause of the disease is not clearly understood, but researchers believe MS to be an autoimmune disorder that affects the central nervous system (Lassman, 2019). The immune system is thought to attack the myelin sheath that surrounds and protects the nerve fibres. There is an overproduction of the immunoglobulin (Ig) with oligoclonal bands, an environment of immune cell persistence and a disruption of the blood–brain barrier outside of the active lesions. This leads to inflammation and the presence of distributed glial scars (or sclerosis), which can be seen in pathology investigations. The damage is triggered by an unknown soluble factor in the cerebrospinal fluid (CSF), produced by the immune

system's CD8+ T cells or CD20+ B cells, which creates a toxic environment that activates microglia or macrophages (Lassman, 2019). These activated macrophages are thought to damage the myelin needed to support the nerves as they conduct electric signals efficiently, either directly or indirectly through microglia activation. Kremer et al. (2019) have suggested that the human endogenous W retroviruses (pHEV-W), particularly one of the proteins of the viral capsid that has been found to activate microglia in vitro, lead to MS. The enzyme GDP-L-fucose synthase has been found in pathology reports of patients with MS, leading researchers to consider it as a viable causative factor, particularly as patients on a strict diet have better control of their MS (Planas et al., 2018). As already mentioned, there are several possible causative factors, just as there are several risk factors for developing the disease.

Current thinking about the disease suggests that MS is not a single disease but, rather, a spectrum of disease courses, which worsen over time (Lassman, 2019). According to Thompson et al. (2018), there are four types of MS, which are accepted on a global scale, although there are also phenotypes in some of these groups:

- **Clinically isolated syndrome (CIS):** This type of MS is a single episode, where patients have symptoms for at least 24 hours. If the patient has another episode, the diagnosis is changed to relapse-remitting MS.
- **Relapse-remitting MS (RRMS):** This is the most common form of MS, affecting 85% of people with MS, and involves episodes of new or increasing symptoms, followed by periods of remission when symptoms partially or totally disappear.
- **Primary progressive MS (PPMS):** With this course of the disease, the symptoms worsen progressively with no remission, just periods of stability.
- **Secondary progressive MS (SPMS):** Patients will experience episodes of relapse and remission, but in the final stages, there is only a decline.

Signs and Symptoms

MS can affect nearly any part of the central nervous system, so the clinical presentation can vary (NICE,

2019). The four most common initial signs and symptoms are as follows:

- Optic neuritis
- Transverse myelitis, where there is focal inflammation within the spinal cord. This presents as sensory symptoms such as paraesthesia; urinary symptoms such as frequency, urgency or retention; and motor weakness below the level of the inflammation. Patients may present with Lhermitte's phenomena, which is a sensation of a tight band around the trunk at the level of the inflammation, or a shock-like sensation radiating down the spine, which is caused by neck flexion. These symptoms can develop over hours or days.
- Cerebellar-related symptoms, such as ataxia, vertigo, clumsiness, and dysmetria
- Brainstem syndromes, which can result in ataxia, eye movement problems or bulbar muscle problems, which can cause dysarthria or dysphagia

Diagnosis

If a patient has an undeferential diagnosis of MS, then within the primary care setting, serological tests can be obtained whilst referral to a consultant neurologist is being progressed and may include the following:

- Full blood count
- Erythrocyte sedimentation rate or C-reactive protein
- Liver function tests
- Renal function tests
- Calcium
- Glucose/HbA1c
- Thyroid function tests
- Vitamin B_1
- HIV serology

The process of diagnosis for MS should include clinical assessment and laboratory tests (NICE, 2018b). Stone (2016) stresses the importance of a full and appropriate history for any neurological disorder because it may lead to treatment during the process of assessment or lead to the appropriate treatment. The diagnosis for MS can be made on clinical grounds alone in secondary care, and MRI of the central nervous system can support and replace the clinical criteria in the McDonald Criteria of the International Panel on Diagnosis of MS (Polman et al., 2011). Studies have shown that MRI testing can help identify inflammation, demyelination, and neuro-axonal loss in MS (Filippi et al., 2019).

RISK FACTORS

There are a variety of risk factors for developing MS. Generally, people will be diagnosed between the ages of 20 and 40 years, and the disease is more common in countries with temperate climates, such as the UK, Scandinavia and Iceland. Women are also twice as likely to develop MS as men. There are also genetic factors because MS has been found to be a disease with a mutation inside the gene *NR1H3* (Wang et al., 2016). Smoking is also a risk factor for MS because smokers have been found to have more lesions and brain shrinkage than nonsmokers (Arneth, 2020). Exposure to viruses, such as Epstein-Barr virus (EBV), mononucleosis or human endogenous W retroviruses, may increase a person's risk of developing MS (Kremer et al., 2019).

Vitamin deficiencies are also risk factors; notably, a deficiency of vitamin D may make the immune system less effective, thereby increasing the risk of MS (Ascherio et al., 2014). Vitamin B_{12} is required for myelin synthesis, so a deficiency may increase the risk of neurological diseases, such as MS and epilepsy (Footitt et al., 2013).

ONGOING MANAGEMENT AND HEALTH PROMOTION

Patients with a diagnosis of MS should be under the care of a local MS team, and in keeping with managing neurological diseases, this should include the support of MS specialist nurses (Galea et al., 2015). Nonetheless, given the trajectory and age span of individuals affected by this disease, patients with MS may consult with the GPN, providing the opportunity for GPNs to support care delivery. Furthermore, GPNs may represent the link between acute and primary care, and care may involve MS teams liaising with the GPN and may extend to working alongside the MS team in supporting and empowering the person with MS to maintain overall good health in relation to exercise, healthful diet and smoking cessation (NICE, 2019). These issues are important because lifestyle choices can have detrimental effects on the progression of MS, as is the case with smoking. The recommendation regarding smoking cessation is in keeping with evidence-based studies that have shown that smoking roughly doubles the risk of developing MS and may adversely affect the course of the disease. Encouraging activity in the form of low-impact aerobic exercises and gradually increasing the intensity, duration and frequency have been shown to be an effective strategy in reducing fatigue in some adults with chronic autoimmune conditions such as MS.

Pharmacological Management

There is no known cure for MS, but there are treatments available that can modify the course of the disease and manage symptoms, ultimately improving the patient's quality of life. The aim of treatment is therefore to reduce the frequency and length of episodes of relapse, therefore slowing disability (NICE BNF, 2019a). There are several disease-modifying treatments used to treat MS. These include interferons such as beta-1a and beta-1b; the monoclonal antibodies natalizumab, alemtuzumab, ocrelizumab; and immunomodulators such as glatiramer acetate, mitoxantrone, fingolimod, teriflunomide, dimethyl fumarate and siponimod (NICE BNF, 2019b).

Management of a Relapse

If a patient suspects a relapse, then they may contact the surgery as their first point of call. Initial clinical assessment is required to exclude other possible causes, such as infection, particularly urinary tract and respiratory infections (NICE, 2019). The patient may need hospital admission if the relapse is severe or they become so incapacitated they cannot manage at home.

PARKINSON'S DISEASE

PD is the second most common neurodegenerative disorder, after Alzheimer's disease, in the UK (Worth, 2013). It is caused by a loss of nerve cells, particularly

the dopaminergic neurons in the pars compacta (SNpc) of the substantia nigra, part of the basal ganglia. Dopamine plays a vital role in regulating the movement of the body (NHS, 2019). The reasons for the damage to the dopaminergic neurons in the SNpc are unknown, but some theories suggest oxidative stress, inflammatory assault and mitochondrial inhibition (Breuer et al., 2013). There have also been several recent studies that have suggested a possible link between the human gastric pathogen *Helicobacter pylori* and PD (McGee et al., 2018).

Irrespective of causation, PD is an incurable and progressive disease, although the rate of progression can vary from patient to patient (Worth, 2013). Although the assessment and ongoing management of patients with PD will be overseen by acute specialist services, the GPN may encounter patients with PD and so needs to be aware of the trajectory of the disease, the signs and symptoms and the transitioning between these stages to ensure any unmet healthcare needs are addressed. There are four overlapping stages in establishing a diagnosis and ongoing management: diagnosis, maintenance, complex and palliative disease.

Signs and Symptoms

People with PD have increased muscle weakness because there is less activation of motor neurons and have the typical symptoms of tremor, stiffness, slowness, balance problems and/or gait disorders (NICE, 2017). Initially, they may present with nonmotor symptoms such as sleep disturbances, anosmia, anxiety and depression (Worth, 2013). Other symptoms may include an overactive bladder, urgency and nocturia as a result of the role of dopaminergic mechanism and its function in maintaining normal bladder control (Sakakibara et al., 2012). Hobson et al. (2010) indicate that 80% of patients with PD can develop psychiatric problems such as hallucinations and dementia, with a reduction in life expectancy.

Diagnosis

If PD is suspected, patients should be referred to a clinical specialist for assessment based on the Parkinson's Disease Society Brain Bank Clinical

Diagnostic Criteria (NICE, 2017). The diagnosis of PD should be reviewed regularly, every 6 to 12 months, and reconsidered if atypical clinical features develop because high rates of misdiagnosis of PD have been recorded (NICE, 2017).

Management of the Condition

The mainstay of treatment of PD is the pharmacological management of motor symptoms using dopamine agonists, levodopa and monoamine oxidase B (MAO-B) inhibitors (NICE, 2017). Patients can be prescribed a dopamine agonist, levodopa or MAO-B inhibitors if they are in the early stages of the disease and their motor symptoms are not affecting their quality of life. However, levodopa is recommended for people in the early stages of PD whose motor symptoms are affecting their quality of life (NICE, 2017; Worth, 2013). Levodopa is a naturally occurring amino acid that is used for PD symptoms and is metabolised to dopamine in the brain and is considered an effective drug for PD; however, prolonged use may result in side effects, including changes in motor function and dyskinesias (Worth, 2013). A working knowledge of medicine management within this field is important because patients may ask about treatment approaches and their potential side effects.

Some patients with PD may also be candidates for deep-brain stimulation and levodopa or levodopa–carbidopa intestinal gel if they have advanced PD and their symptoms are not adequately controlled by oral therapy (Chang et al., 2016; NICE, 2017). This is an emerging area of research looking at the long-term prognosis of these patients (Chang et al., 2016).

Alongside the patient's general practitioner and specialist Parkinson's nurse, the GPN is ideally placed to support the delivery of tailored care for individuals and their families (Hellqvist & Berterö, 2015). Most patients with PD will face increasing problems with their mobility, which often include difficulties with posture, balance, and walking, and as a result, patients can develop loss of independence and fear of falls or injury. Exercise is important in prolonging muscle strength and movement. Physiotherapy has been found to improve gait, transfers, balance and functional ability. Education and appropriate referral to occupational therapy, speech and language therapy and physiotherapy are therefore key in the management of these problems (NICE, 2017). The GPN can therefore support patients in accessing the appropriate multidisciplinary services to remain as active as possible. NICE (2017) recommends that patients with PD should have the following care:

- Clinical monitoring and medicine adjustment
- A continuing point of contact for support, which may include home monitoring and information about clinical and social matters of concern to people with PD and their family members and carers

SUMMARY

Although the vast majority of patients with neurological conditions will be continually or intermittently cared for by specialist services within the acute sector, the general practice setting remains the first point of contact for these patients. Consequently, the GPN represents a vital resource in caring and supporting people living with serious and complex neurological conditions.

REFERENCES

Aliasgharpour, M., Nayeri, N. D., Yadegary, M. A., & Haghani, H. (2013). Effects of an educational program on self-management in patients with epilepsy. *Seizure, 22*(1), 48–52.

Arneth, B. (2020). Multiple sclerosis and smoking. *The American Journal of Medicine, 133*(7), 783–788.

Ascherio, A., Munger, K. L., White, R., Köchert, K., Simon, K. C., Polman, C. H., & Edan, G. (2014). Vitamin D as an early predictor of multiple sclerosis activity and progression. *JAMA Neurology, 71*(3), 306–314.

Breuer, M. E., Koopman, W. J., Koene, S., Nooteboom, M., Rodenburg, R. J., Willems, P. H., & Smeitink, J. A. M. (2013). The role of mitochondrial OXPHOS dysfunction in the development of neurologic diseases. *Neurobiology of Disease, 51*, 27–34.

Camfield, P., & Camfield, C. (2011). Transition to adult care for children with chronic neurological disorders. *Annals of Neurology, 69*(3), 437–444.

Carrier, J. (2015). *Managing long-term conditions and chronic illness in primary care: A guide to good practice.* Routledge.

Chang, F. C., Kwan, V., van der Poorten, D., Mahant, N., Wolfe, N., Ha, A. D., ... Fung, V. S. (2016). Intraduodenal levodopa-carbidopa intestinal gel infusion improves both motor performance and quality of life in advanced Parkinson's disease. *Journal of Clinical Neuroscience, 25,* 41–45.

Fernie, B. A., Kollmann, J., & Brown, R. G. (2015). Cognitive behavioural interventions for depression in chronic neurological conditions: A systematic review. *Journal of Psychosomatic Research, 78*(5), 411–419.

Filippi, M., Brück, W., Chard, D., Fazekas, F., Geurts, J. J., Enzinger, C., ... & Schmierer, K. (2019). Association between pathological and MRI findings in multiple sclerosis. *The Lancet Neurology, 18*(2), 198–210.

Fisher, R. S., Cross, J. H., French, J. A., Higurashi, N., Hirsch, E., Jansen, F. E., ... Scheffer, I. E. (2017). Operational classification of seizure types by the International League Against Epilepsy: Position paper of the ILAE Commission for Classification and Terminology. *Epilepsia, 58*(4), 522–530.

Footitt, E. J., Clayton, P. T., Mills, K., Heales, S. J., Neergheen, V., Oppenheim, M., & Mills, P. B. (2013). Measurement of plasma B6 vitamer profiles in children with inborn errors of vitamin B6 metabolism using an LCMS/MS method. *Journal of Inherited Metabolic Disease: Official Journal of the Society for the Study of Inborn Errors of Metabolism, 36*(1), 139–145.

Galea, I., Ward-Abel, N., & Heesen, C. (2015). Relapse in multiple sclerosis. *British Medical Journal, 350,* Article h1765.

Hamiwka, L. D., & Wirrell, E. C. (2009). Comorbidities in pediatric epilepsy: Beyond 'just' treating the seizures. *Journal of Child Neurology, 24*(6), 734–742.

Hellqvist, C., & Berterö, C. (2015). Support supplied by Parkinson's disease specialist nurses to Parkinson's disease patients and their spouses. *Applied Nursing Research, 28*(2), 86–91.

Hickey, J. (2013). *Clinical practice of neurological & neurosurgical nursing.* Lippincott Williams & Wilkins.

Hobson, P., Meara, J., & Ishihara-Paul, L. (2010). The estimated life expectancy in a community cohort of Parkinson's disease patients with and without dementia, compared with the UK population. *Journal of Neurology, Neurosurgery, and Psychiatry, 81,* 1093–108.

Kremer, D., Gruchot, J., Weyers, V., Oldemeier, L., Göttle, P., Healy, L., Ho Jang, J., Xu, Y., Volsko, C., Dutta Trapp, B., Perron, H., Hartung, H., & Küry, P. (2019). pHERV-W envelope protein fuels microglial cell-dependent damage of myelinated axons in multiple sclerosis. *Proceedings of the National Academy of Sciences, 116*(30), 15216–15225. https://doi.org/10.1073/pnas.1901283116

Lassmann, H. (2019). The changing concepts in the neuropathology of acquired demyelinating central nervous system disorders. *Current Opinion in Neurology, 32*(3), 313–319.

Leitinger, M., Höller, Y., Kalss, G., Rohracher, A., Novak, H. F., Höfler, J., ... Trinka, E. (2015). Epidemiology-based mortality score in status epilepticus (EMSE). *Neurocritical Care, 22*(2), 273–282.

McGee, D. J., Lu, X. H., & Disbrow, E. A. (2018). Stomaching the possibility for a pathogenic role for *Helicobacter pylori* in Parkinson's disease. *Journal of Parkinson's Disease, 8*(3), 367–374.

Medicines and Healthcare Products Regulatory Agency. (2018). *Valproate medicines (Epilimɷ, Depakoteɷ): Contraindicated in women and girls of childbearing potential unless conditions of Pregnancy Prevention Programme are met.* https://www.gov.uk/drug-safety-update/valproate-medicines-epilim-depakote-contraindicated-in-women-and-girls-of-childbearing-potential-unless-conditions-of-pregnancy-prevention-programme-are-met

National Health Service. (2017). *Symptoms – Epilepsy.* https://www.nhs.uk/conditions/epilepsy/symptoms/

National Health Service. (2019). *Overview – Parkinson's disease.* https://www.nhs.uk/conditions/Parkinsons-disease/

National Institute for Health and Care Excellence. (2017). *Parkinson's disease in adults.* https://www.nice.org.uk/guidance/NG71

National Institute for Health and Care Excellence. (2019). *Multiple sclerosis.* https://cks.nice.org.uk/multiple-sclerosis

National Institute for Health and Care Excellence. (2020). *Epilepsies: Diagnosis and management.* https://www.nice.org.uk/Guidance/cg137

National Institute for Health and Care Excellence. (2021). *Quality Standard 198. Suspected neurological conditions: Recognition and referral.* https://www.nice.org.uk/guidance/qs198/resources/suspected-neurological-conditions-recognition-and-referral-pdf-75545788558021

NHS Digital (2019). *Indicators no longer in QOF (INLIQ).* https://digital.nhs.uk/services/general-practice-gp-collections/service-information/indicators-no-longer-in-qof-inliq

NICE BNF. (2019a). *Azithromycin.* https://bnf.nice.org.uk/drug/azithromycin.html#sideEffects

NICE BNF. (2019b). *Multiple sclerosis.* https://bnf.nice.org.uk/treatment-summary/multiple-sclerosis.html

Nugent, D. (2020). Neurological problems. In A. Staten & P. Staten (Eds.), *Practical general practice guidelines for effective clinical management* (7th ed., pp. 170–190). Elsevier.

Polman, C. H., Reingold, S. C., Banwell, B., Clanet, M., Cohen, J. A., Filippi, M., ... Lublin, F. D. (2011). Diagnostic criteria for multiple sclerosis: 2010 revisions to the McDonald criteria. *Annals of Neurology, 69*(2), 292–302.

Sakakibara, R., Tateno, F., Kishi, M., Tsuyuzaki, Y., Uchiyama, T., & Yamamoto, T. (2012). Pathophysiology of bladder dysfunction in Parkinson's disease. *Neurobiology of Disease, 46*(3), 565–571.

Sawcer, S., Hellenthal, G., Pirinen, M., Spencer, C. C., Patsopoulos, N. A., Moutsianas, L., ... Edkins, S. (2011). Genetic risk and a primary role for cell-mediated immune mechanisms in multiple sclerosis. *Nature, 476*(7359), 214.

Scottish Government. (2019). *Neurological care and support in Scotland: A framework for action 2020-2025.* https://www.gov.scot/publications/neurological-care-support-scotland-framework-action-2020-2025/

Scottish Intercollegiate Guidelines Network. (2018). *SIGN 143. Diagnosis and management of epilepsy in adults.* https://www.sign.ac.uk/media/1079/sign143_2018.pdf

Smith, G., Wagner, J. L., & Edwards, J. C. (2015a). CE: Epilepsy update. Part 1: Refining our understanding of a complex disease. *American Journal of Nursing, 115*(5), 40–47.

Smith, G., Wagner, J. L., & Edwards, J. C. (2015b). CE: Epilepsy update. Part 2: Nursing care and evidence-based treatment. *American Journal of Nursing, 115*(6), 34–44.

Smith, N., & Tiwari, D. (2015). Epilepsy in older people. *Reviews in Clinical Gerontology, 25*(1), 53–59.

Stone, J. (2016). Functional neurological disorders: The neurological assessment as treatment. *Practical Neurology, 16*(1), 7–17.

Thompson, A. J., Banwell, B. L., Barkhof, F., Carroll, W. M., Coetzee, T., Comi, G., ... Fujihara, K. (2018). Diagnosis of multiple sclerosis: 2017 revisions of the McDonald criteria. *The Lancet Neurology, 17*(2), 162–173.

Wang, Z., Sadovnick, A. D., Traboulsee, A. L., Ross, J. P., Bernales, C. Q., Encarnacion, M., ... Wright, G. (2016). Nuclear receptor NR1H3 in familial multiple sclerosis. *Neuron, 90*(5), 948–954.

Welsh Government. (2017). Neurological Conditions Delivery Plan. https://gov.wales/topics/health/nhswales/plans/neurological/?lang=en

Worth, P. F. (2013). How to treat Parkinson's disease in 2013. *Clinical Medicine, 13*(1), 93–96.

12 MANAGING MENTAL HEALTH CONDITIONS IN PRIMARY CARE

IVANO MAZZONCINI ■ CAROL McALANEY

MENTAL HEALTH PROBLEMS IN PRIMARY CARE

The high prevalence of mental health problems within the population is well documented. A survey by the Mental Health Foundation found that approximately two-thirds of adults have experienced a mental health problem in the UK, with only 13% of participants reporting positive mental health (Mental Health Foundation, 2017). Primary care represents an essential access point for people seeking help with their mental health, with 90% of mental health conditions managed entirely within primary care (Royal College of General Practitioners Primary Care Mental Health Steering Group, 2017). Consequently, the general practice setting will assess, treat and manage various subsections of the practice population who may present with a range of minor to complex mental health needs. The therapeutic interventions required may be singular and prescriptive; however, whilst these may involve a series of complex procedures, critical inquiry at the point of consultation is crucial to assessing and managing patients' health and wellbeing.

As front-line healthcare providers, the general practice nurse (GPN) can expect to encounter a wide range of mental health conditions presenting routinely in daily practice. Common factors that affect patients' mental wellbeing, such as work-related stress, bereavement, undertaking caring roles, chronic physical conditions and adverse life events, can be easily understood in terms of the struggles involved in juggling these life challenges and responsibilities. However, other presentations may be more unusual or complex and therefore difficult to comprehend and ultimately manage, such as bizarre behaviours, psychotic symptoms and suicidal ideation. These clinical scenarios can be challenging and ultimately necessitate further sensitive inquiry as part of holistic assessment. Furthermore, it is recognised that people with serious mental illness suffer health inequalities (NHS England, 2020) and, as such, have lower life expectancy, in the region of 15 to 20 years, in comparison to their peers (Chesney et al., 2014). This may be associated with the higher prevalence of multimorbidity in relation to cardiovascular and respiratory illness, metabolic syndromes and cancer diagnosis in this group (Ilyas et al., 2017). Higher levels of substance and alcohol misuse and social drift and lower levels of employment may also compound the healthcare challenges.

Caring for others means adopting a person-centred, holistic, values-based approach to care delivery that will not only consider an individual's physical needs but also their mental, emotional and social needs. Consequently, professional bodies, strategic planners, healthcare and social care professionals and third-sector organisations have recognised the mandatory need to consider, plan for, and develop services that interconnect and address complex relationships between physical, social and emotional health (UCL Institute of Health Equity, 2017). The World Health Organisation (WHO, 2018) establishes necessity in such practice; consequently, all levels of social care and healthcare are attempting to develop services that are integrated, seamless and reflective of the whole system. In Scotland, this has been realised at a legislative level with the introduction of the Public Bodies (Joint Working) (Scotland) Act 2014.

The current impetus to recognise and improve mental health has resulted in concerted efforts across the UK to raise the profile of mental wellbeing and address deficiencies within service provision (Public Health England, 2019). For example, within a Scottish context, the 10-year mental health strategy (Scottish Government, 2019) advocates developing integrated models of care that allow action at the earliest point to prevent the onset of serious mental illness, with healthcare and social care providers working together to provide this.

Mental health problems are common presentations within the primary care setting (Thomson, 2020), and GPNs thus play a vital role in supporting and empowering people. However, the practice nurse may feel apprehensive about navigating the consultation with patients presenting with apparent, or indicative, mental health problems and therein uncertainty around how best to manage them. This chapter aims to offer pragmatic guidance on a range of mental health issues and thus build confidence in asking what may be perceived to be difficult consultation questions to assess and manage mental health problems presenting in primary care.

ASSESSING AND SCREENING MENTAL HEALTH STATUS

It is important to acknowledge the symbiotic impact that mental health and emotional distress have on physical health (Mental Health Foundation, 2019). A clear example of this may be the patient who, during a consultation, complains of disturbed sleep, a common feature occurring across a range of mental health difficulties. Disturbances in hours slept or quality of sleep may subsequently affect concentration, interpersonal skills, energy and mood. Another factor to consider is that every individual's mental health will manifest in a unique way. Engle's (1977) classical biopsychosocial model (Fig. 12.1) continues to provide a contemporary understanding of how mental health affects individuals, based on the interplay of factors affecting a person's health. This model allows for a deeper understanding of a patient's presentation and usefully directs compassionate inquiry to better understand the patient experience by exploring the biological, psychological and social factors influencing health outcomes. The use of this model to structure the consultation may also support the GPN in care planning when helping to construct change strategies that may positively affect the patient's physical health.

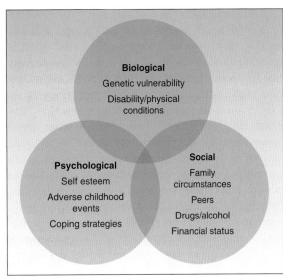

Fig. 12.1 ▪ Biopsychosocial model. (From Engel, G. (1977). *The need for a new medical model: A challenge for biomedicine* (1st ed.). American Association for the Advancement of Science.)

The use of the biopsychosocial model also reinforces the importance of the development of informal and formal links between primary and secondary care mental health services. For example, within one large Scottish Health Board, mental health annual review, summary and staying well plans are routinely shared with primary care. Furthermore, these information-exchange strategies have provided the opportunity to go beyond this perfunctory level of communication and spawned the development of links between nursing groups. The sharing of information may therefore act as a catalyst to help develop informal and formal links between general practice and mental health services, resulting in the forging of professional relationships to improve seamless partnership work (Mental Health Taskforce, 2016).

Assessment Tools

Standardised evidence-based screening tools and questionnaires also contribute to the assessment and identification of various mental health conditions (Peterson, 2015), such as the Core Net, PHQ-9 (Patient Health Questionnaire-9 item questionnaire) HADS (Hospital Anxiety and Depression Scale) and BDI (Beck Depression Inventory) GAD-7 (General Anxiety Disorder-7 item questionnaire). The application of these indicators of mental health wellbeing is used to aid decision-making, and usage will vary locally based on local guidelines and protocols. However, the National Institute for Health and Care Excellence (NICE) offers specific cautions regarding such tools, for example, the PHQ-9 provides straightforward questions that allow insight into the patient's mental health status and is commonly used in primary care in the UK as a validated tool to screen for depression; however, in the context of promoting evidence-based practice, the use of such tools should never replace clinical judgement. Nonetheless, such tools do inform and contribute to the assessment, identification and treatment of mental health conditions (Thomson, 2020). Using assessment tools/scales such as these will often require appropriate training to enable their application in practice.

COMMON MENTAL HEALTH PRESENTATIONS

NICE lists common mental health problems, including depression, generalised anxiety disorder (GAD), social anxiety disorder, panic disorder, obsessive-compulsive disorder (OCD), body dysmorphic disorder and posttraumatic stress disorder (PTSD). Serious mental illness includes psychosis, bipolar disorder and eating disorders. There are, however, common clinical indicators pertinent to these aforementioned mental health issues that may signal clinical cues within the consultation, which necessitate further inquiry as part of early intervention in assessing a patient's mental health status. For example, practitioners will routinely see patients whose appetite, diet and personal tastes can change as a result of the impact of physical illness or treatment. Whilst the discussion points that follow can and do apply, reflecting on the biopsychosocial model (see Fig 12.1) indicates that someone experiencing reduced appetite, for example, whilst receiving chemotherapy, may also be experiencing reduced appetite in the context of lowered mood.

Structuring the Consultation

The basis of nursing assessment for any condition utilises a range of communication and observation skills to collect, synthesise and interpret data. These processes can be aided by the use of Roper et al.'s (1996)

model for nursing, well known for its capacity to provide a framework for holistic care delivery (Holland & Jenkins, 2019). Despite the inherent challenges in fusing integrated mental health and physical health services, this nursing model's simple yet comprehensive structure allows the practitioner to focus and investigate, in a professional and curious way, how an individual manages, for example, sleeping, eating, walking and communicating with others. The Mental State Examination (Rocho Neto, 2019) is also routinely used in psychiatry and, additionally, is also likely to form the basis of every nursing interaction. It can be used to structure the consultation for mental health assessment within the primary care setting, in addition to the Roper et al. nursing model. This approach would enable a compressive and detailed assessment of an individual's appearance and behaviour, speech, mood, affect, thoughts, perceptions, cognitions, risks and judgements.

The Roper et al. model can enable the practice nurse's inquiry to move seamlessly between the physical, psychological and social domains and can also aid recognition of the patient's strengths and resilience skills on which health and wellbeing can be built (Holland & Jenkins, 2019). A nursing assessment, entailing a conversation with a focus on mental health, may nevertheless be difficult for a patient because of a fear of stigma or discrimination; consequently, diligence is necessary in providing patient-centred communication; using clear, nonclinical, normalising language; and being culturally sensitive. The following sections of this chapter focus on clinical presentations the GPN may routinely encounter.

Low Mood

Emotion, as a mental state affected by thoughts and feelings that affect behaviours, may be identified as fluctuating and subject to rapid changeable patterns throughout an individual's day/hour. However, low mood, as a discernible symptom, may be more consistent, and when persistent for over 2 weeks, it could be indicative of depression (American Psychiatric Association, 2017).

The biological effect of low mood on a patient's appetite commonly results in a reduced appetite, with less enjoyment from favourite foods or, conversely, overeating, particularly a high intake of sugar-rich, caffeinated foodstuffs. Box 12.1 details appropriate consultation

---

BOX 12.1

ASSESSING CHANGES IN APPETITE

- Have you noticed your appetite changing? Do you feel like eating more or less than usual?
- Are you enjoying your food?
- Have you noticed any changes in your weight? Are your clothes feeling loose?
- Do you find yourself eating more convenience foods and junk foods?

BOX 12.2

ASSESSING CHANGES IN SLEEP PATTERN

- How many hours do you think you sleep?
- Has anything changed in your sleep pattern over the past 2 weeks?
- Are you finding you want to sleep more?
- Are you finding it difficult to get to sleep?
- Do you feel you toss and turn throughout the night?
- Can you think about what may be stopping you from sleeping?
- Do you find your mind busy at night when you go to bed?
- People often find that when they lie down to go to sleep, their minds become active and worry about things; is this something you've noticed?
- Some people may experience unpleasant dreams or feel frightened during the night; do you experience this?
- Are you staying in bed longer or napping during the day? If so, how does this affect getting to sleep at night?
- Are you feeling rested?
- What do you do before bed?
- How do you prepare for sleep?
- Enquire about substance use, including frequency and amount.
- What medication do you use, and when do you take this?

---

questions to undertake inquiry concerning changes in appetite that may be a result of low mood.

Sleep disturbance is also common in depressed mood and all mental health conditions (Krystal, 2012). Sleep quantity and quality will be affected, and patients may report sleeping too much but 'never feeling rested', difficulty getting to sleep or staying asleep and waking frequently throughout the night. Initially, the consultation inquiry needs to eliminate the possibility of detrimental environmental and lifestyle factors, such as room temperature and diet, which includes asking about high sugar, caffeine and alcohol intake, which may affect sleep quality. There may also be physical reasons for disturbance, such as bladder control, and general inquiry will eliminate these variables. Some individuals may sleep longer than usual and not arise at their usual time. Prolonged use of illicit substances or misuse of prescribed substances may have a longer-lasting impact on sleep even when the substance was not recently used. For example, some of the paradoxical effects of medications may affect sleep; antidepressants may negatively affect sleep if taken at the wrong time of day. Box 12.2 indicates consultation questions to assess a patient's sleep pattern.

Low mood may also be accompanied by lowered energy levels. Although a physiological symptom, the impact may affect social roles and functioning, including intimacy, with reduced libido and interpersonal interactions, which adversely affect relationships. This symptom may also be related to disturbed sleep and appetite changes; however, it may also be related to loss of feelings of enjoyment, loss of volition or perhaps social withdrawal and reduced self-esteem. Box 12.3 indicates typical inquiry-based consultation questions to assess energy levels.

Feelings of hopelessness, worthlessness and lowering of self-esteem are key features of depressed mood

---

BOX 12.3

ASSESSMENT OF ENERGY LEVEL

- Do you have less energy than you used to?
- Are you feeling tired and that things require more of an effort?
- Have you stopped doing the things that you usually enjoy, like hobbies and seeing friends?
- Is there anything else stopping you from doing the things you usually would?

---

whereby patients may question and underestimate their ability to cope with things that they previously would have been able to positively address. There may be a sense of feeling overwhelmed in making simple decisions, performing actions or responding to others. There may be irritability and associated behaviour change, further lowering self-esteem with feelings of guilt and embarrassment. Box 12.4 indicates typical inquiry-based consultation questions to explore self-esteem in the context of low mood.

BOX 12.4
ASSESSING LEVELS OF ESTEEM

- Are you finding it difficult to make decisions that you usually would?
- Are you finding it difficult to maintain your day-to-day roles regarding work, family and social life?
- Can you tell me your key strengths and personal goals?
- What would you say were your strengths and goals 3 to 6 months ago or when you felt happier?
- What would a close friend or family member say about your strengths?

Anxiety

Anxiety is a healthy emotion in the short term that allows us to assess and manage our awareness of personal risk (Healthline, 2019). However, it can become a more frequent and prolonged experience with no obvious stimulus, with patients often describing their anxiety as 'coming from nowhere'. Anxiety may also become increasingly pronounced and affect all areas of daily living. Patients may find the emergence of idiopathic anxiety difficult and confusing to understand, and this will often be a prelude to the development of other mood-related issues, such as low mood and suicidality.

Some patients with anxiety-related difficulties may present to primary care with a range of biological complaints, including gastrointestinal disturbances, numbness or tingling or other unusual sensations in the body. They may describe dizziness, light-headedness or unusual feelings, such as the world or their presence in a situation seeming unreal, reflecting derealisation and depersonalisation (WHO, 2004). Individuals can appear physically restless and distracted, and these feelings may lead to a wide range of symptoms, which may include hyperventilation and tachycardia and may result in panic attacks, which are fearful and distressing. There will likely be complaints of disturbed sleep and appetite, gastrointestinal difficulties and perhaps a change in bladder/bowel habits. Consultation questions that permit exploration of biological changes are outlined in Box 12.5.

For some people, they may find it difficult to identify psychosocial factors that trigger their anxiety and instead will focus on the previously mentioned biological responses that they have no control over.

BOX 12.5
ASSESSING PHYSICAL SYMPTOMS

- When do these feelings/sensations happen, and how long do they last?
- Is there anything that makes it worse/better?
- How do you manage this when it happens?
- Do you remember when you first noticed this? What happened?

BOX 12.6
ASSESSING PSYCHOLOGICAL SYMPTOMS

- Do you find it difficult to switch off?
- Does this affect your concentration?
- Have you found yourself avoiding anything because of these feelings or thoughts?
- Do you find it difficult to come to appointments?
- Is there anything I can do to help you?

However, there will commonly be thoughts around the perception of danger, dread, overestimating risk, thinking the worst and underestimating their ability to cope with this. This may result in avoidance of perceived trigger situations, which, in turn, can have an isolating effect and significant impact on social roles.

Other anxiety disorders include PTSD and/or phobia (Anxiety UK, 2019). This may be challenging to assess in a care setting where clinical procedures and practices may cause significant distress and anxiety to a patient; for example, routine venepuncture may be a common cause of anxiety. It is important to approach this with compassion, particularly if information is available in the form of prior history, to be mindful of this type of interaction. Consultation questions that permit exploration of psychosocial issues are outlined in Box 12.6.

TREATMENT STRATEGIES FOR COMMON MENTAL HEALTH ISSUES

Treatment of common mental health conditions may include the use of pharmacological and/or nonpharmacological treatments. The former may include antidepressants or anxiolytics to treat anxiety. Medical treatments may offer significant relief in treating symptoms; however, they may also result in notable side effects, such as nausea, weight gain, and headaches. There can also be challenges where some antidepressants, for example, may trigger discontinuation or withdrawal syndrome (Davies & Read, 2019). This may result in increased agitation, restlessness and disturbed sleep and may be mistaken for a re-emergence of the mental health condition originally being treated. Being aware of this and the impact it may cause can help individuals to understand and make informed decisions about medical treatment.

Talking therapies is a broad term to describe a range of psychological evidence-based nonpharmacological treatments (Rethink Mental Illness, 2019). This type of therapy may be delivered on a one-to-one or group basis. The UK governments have committed to improving access to psychological therapies; however, the delivery of this type of intervention still varies greatly across localities. These therapies may be delivered by specific specialist service models, such as trauma or sexual assault, or be delivered by third-sector agencies. There are services available to support a wide range of difficulties associated with asylum, sexual assault, bereavement, stillbirth, postnatal mental health and carers' needs. A simple web search can provide a range of local services and organisations available. Within a mental health service, it would be common to have a local resource folder/repository where all available resources for patients can be added and updated to be used as required and shared with other professionals. It may be that in your local area, this may help support signposting in day-to-day practice.

The evidence-based treatment for common mental health problems is well established. NICE guidelines (2019) list steps for evidence-based intervention using a stepped-care model. Patients in contact with a GPN who potentially have a mental health issue should be assessed promptly to identify the problem, providing the earliest intervention. It may be that the patient only requires information and education regarding their symptoms, for example, sleep hygiene information, or relaxation techniques; however, they may require onward referral in lieu of medication and/or talking therapies or social prescribing. All primary care practitioners will have local guidelines for referring to mental health services. Voluntary organisations and social groups vary across the UK, and an awareness of local voluntary organisations and resources may support the GPN in directing patients towards helpful supports. Access to self-help websites is widely available throughout the UK, and well-known sites include Beating the Blues, Mood Gym and Living Life to the Full. These low-level self-directed cognitive–behavioural therapy (CBT) approaches allow for immediate access to low-level psychological therapies. For example, NICE guidelines (2019) identify CBT as useful in treating mild depression that is unlikely to respond to antidepressants; furthermore, exercise and CBT approaches are recommended to be most useful in treating mild to moderate depression. Awareness of local resources and directing towards evidence-based strategies by the GPN can ensure the earliest intervention with people at risk of developing mental health conditions.

EATING DISORDERS

Eating disorders constitute a wide and complex topic area, where patients may present a range of symptoms, from disturbed eating habits and preoccupation with food to extreme, life-threatening illness. The biological inferences suggest that people with disordered eating patterns are not likely to present with complaints of suffering from an eating disorder but instead present with biological features previously described in the context of low mood and anxiety. Consequently, patients may describe, in response to the questions noted in Box 12.7, reduced energy, reduced enjoyment and unpleasant physical sensations such as dizziness and palpitations.

The psychosocial impact of intentionally restricting food intake may have significantly changed a person's lifestyle, for example, becoming vegetarian or vegan with no prior interest or inclination to do so. Conversely, individuals may overeat with episodes of binging and then engage in reversing behaviours, such as purging by self-induced vomiting, use of laxatives,

---

BOX 12.7
ASSESSING EATING DISORDERS

- When, where and how often do you experience these symptoms?
- How much water do you drink per day?
- Have you noticed any change in your sleep, appetite or energy levels?

BOX 12.8
EATING DISORDER SYMPTOMS AND BEHAVIOURS

- Do you feel that your eating habits have changed recently?
- Do you feel you have lost/gained weight?
- What would be your ideal weight/size?
- How do you plan to reach this goal?
- Do you ever feel you have eaten too much/feel uncomfortably full?
- Is there anything you do to reduce this feeling?
- Have you ever taken laxatives, self-induced vomiting or skipped meals?

---

restriction and excessive exercise. Individuals may be overtly preoccupied with food and calorific values. Self-esteem is likely to be significantly reduced, and comorbid anxiety and depression are common (Eating Disorder Hope, 2019). Box 12.8 outlines typical questions to pursue inquiry.

As obesity becomes a global epidemic (WHO, 2019), the concepts surrounding eating disorders are changing, and primary care consultations focusing on nutrition may be increasing. Although medication is not usually indicated in treating eating disorders, a high level of comorbid mood disorder is likely, and therefore medication may well be prescribed. In terms of nonpharmacological strategies, NICE guidelines (2019) indicate a range of psychological treatments, including individual and family therapies. These would usually be delivered by specialist teams; however, at an early-intervention level, there may be consideration of involving the primary care mental health team (PCMHT) and self-help guides, such as Living Life to the Full: Overcoming Bulimia and the Beat Eating Disorder charity.

SERIOUS MENTAL ILLNESS

It is well recognised that people with serious mental illness are more likely to suffer from health inequalities and subsequent poor physical health and social outcomes (Mental Health Foundation, 2019). With increasing awareness of the importance of healthcare professionals addressing the physical health needs of those with serious mental illness (Nazarko, 2019), it is like that primary care practitioners will become more

involved in the monitoring and support of this population's health and wellbeing.

The GPN may encounter patients with a previous clinical diagnosis of bipolar disorder or psychotic illness who may present without any active symptoms; however, some may be experiencing a wide range of symptoms, including those described previously. Patients may experience a range of perceptual difficulties in all senses: sight, sound, taste and touch. Visual, auditory, olfactory, gustatory and tactile hallucinations may be linked to organic pathology or serious mental health problems and should be referred immediately to the general practitioner (GP) for further investigation. There may also be challenges in interacting with individuals experiencing active perceptual disturbances because concentration will likely be disturbed, and the ability to converse and interact will be affected. It may be difficult to follow the thought processes or more subtle in that only after initial contact do thought processes and experiences become more unusual. GPNs should thus be mindful that during a consultation, it may take time for a person to respond to questions, or they may have difficulty answering at all.

OCD may cause significant challenges for individuals seeking treatment. A patient may appear obsessive regarding cleanliness and have a range of rituals that are engaged in to reduce the stress caused by obsessional thought processes. Patients with personality disorder may present with a range of the features already described, such as depression or anxiety, and may also display perceptual disturbances. Box 12.9 details inquiry-based consultation questions that may elicit investigation.

BOX 12.9
ASSESSING SERIOUS MENTAL ILLNESS

- Have you ever had these experiences before today? How long has this been happening?
- Is there any other possible explanation for what you are thinking/feeling/seeing/tasting?
- Is there anyone you go to see because of these experiences? What do they say?
- Is there anything that has helped before?
- You appear to be taking some time to answer; is anything or anyone stopping you from answering?
- Do you believe anyone wants to hurt you?
- What can I do to help?

Treatment for Serious Mental Illness

A patient experiencing symptoms of a serious mental health condition should be assessed and referred immediately to the GP. If the patient is already engaged with mental health services, then making links with the care team can support the GPN in their interactions. In reciprocating, the GPN may note deterioration and alert the mental healthcare team to prevent a worsening mental state, allowing for early intervention and management. There is likely to be a local protocol in place for such interactions between teams.

NICE treatment pathways identify medications, such as antidepressants, mood stabilisers or antipsychotics, and as an adjunct to pharmacological interventions, there will also be psychological treatments, including family therapies. Social interventions may be available within the community treatment team or third-sector organisations. These may include group activities with the aim of increasing activity and improving quality of life.

Many community mental health teams will make a commitment to assessing and monitoring the physical health of this patient group. However, because there are higher rates of cardiovascular disease and diabetes in this patient group, it is likely that interaction will happen in general practice related to these conditions. It is therefore important to be mindful of the patient's mental health condition with sensitive inquiry.

SELF-HARM AND SUICIDE

Low mood, poor self-esteem and emotional distress are often accompanied by feelings of hopelessness and worthlessness, and the patient may feel they have limited or no control over events in their life. A patient may feel sufficiently desperate and feel the need to absent themselves from their current environment via a holiday or break. However, they may think about more insidious ways to feel better or reduce or control the feelings of distress, and this may lead to self-harming behaviours. Self-harm may present as a way of coping with these sensations, for example, harming as a strategy to ground the self in reality and refocus thoughts and feelings as a type of distraction from the ongoing emotional distress that may be present (Masuku, 2019). It may be related to low self-esteem as

a process of expressing hatred towards one's self. This scenario may also lead to thoughts of suicide.

Suicide is currently the most common reason for death in men under 35 in the UK (Atter, 2018), and 90% of suicides occur in people with pre-existing mental health conditions, including previous self-harm. Other factors that increase the risk of suicide and self-harm include unemployment, alcohol/drug dependency, physical illness and/or chronic pain, isolation and previous work within organisations/institutions such as care, prison and armed forces.

Bullying is a significant risk factor for poor mental health among children and teenagers, and of particular concern in this context is the use of technology, a common platform on which bullying occurs. Consultation questions, as indicated in Box 12.10, are representative of leading sensitive inquiry regarding self-harm and suicide.

ADVERSE LIFE EVENTS

Adverse life events may affect an individual's physical, emotional and mental wellbeing, the outcome of which may be associated with low mood and anxiety, and therein substance misuse may also be present. There may already be awareness by the GPN of a patient's adverse

---

BOX 12.10
ASSESSING SELF-HARM AND SUICIDE

- Do you ever feel overwhelmed by life?
- Have you thought about what might help you feel better?
- Have you found it hard to tell others how you are feeling?
- Sometimes when people feel this way, they might experience thoughts of self-harm or suicide; do you ever have thoughts like this?
- Is there anything that would make it more likely to act on these thoughts?
- What would stop you from acting on these thoughts?
- Do you have any plans to harm yourself?
- Whom would you tell if you find it difficult to manage these thoughts?
- Do you have any contact numbers that are useful, for example, mental health team or Samaritans?
- Do you ever feel frightened of anyone?
- Do you ever feel trapped or that there is no way out?

BOX 12.11
ASSESSING THE IMPACT OF
ADVERSE LIFE EVENTS

- Is there anything I could do to make this less distressing for you today?
- Can I explain why I need to do this in a particular way?
- Is there any reason why this might be difficult for you?

life events; however, the interaction via a values-based consultation may lead to this disclosure. It could simply be a patient feeling safe and secure enough to disclose such difficulties, or attending for a simple procedure or treatment, such as wound care, could result in a disclosure of domestic violence. A routine abdominal exam may trigger a reaction to touch or close proximity to another. These disclosures should be sensitively managed, and it is important to remain calm and enable a therapeutic environment of safety and concern to assess risks and make a plan for what will happen next. This may be encouraging the patient to contact the mental health service already involved or simply asking what they would like to happen next. It is also for consideration that some patients who have experienced trauma and/or interpersonal difficulties may feel confused and perhaps even irritable by someone showing them care and compassion. Being aware of potential responses allows the clinician, as indicated in Box 12.11, to navigate such professional interactions in a sensitive way.

RISK MANAGEMENT AND SAFETY NETTING

It can be difficult to navigate the nuances of mental health services because local provision varies throughout the UK. Similarly, the differing legal frameworks (Mental Health Acts) that the UK's constituent governments have in place to secure the compulsory admission of an individual to the hospital setting to safeguard them and protect others (Thomson, 2020). Common mental health problems are most likely to be treated within primary care, and although serious mental illness may be treated in secondary care, primary care has an essential role in early identification and intervention. It is of paramount importance to undertake assessment of risk by asking direct questions about thoughts and behaviours around

harming self or others. Questions should not be avoided but should be asked with the understanding that a plan must then be formulated. Where there is an immediate risk of harm, this will require referral for urgent or emergency assessment. Expression of suicidal thoughts may not necessarily indicate an immediate, same-day response; however, if there is the feeling that the patient cannot maintain their safety or the safety of others, accessing immediate intervention, usually via the GP, is paramount. Mental health teams will have associated out of hours/emergency care and crisis response team provision; however, service availability varies greatly across the UK, and it is therefore helpful to be aware of local policies and provisions for the presentation of crisis mental health issues. If a patient is already engaged with a mental health team, there may be a crisis plan already in place. A robust crisis plan will provide a sense of how the patient presents and what to do, including helpful resources and phone numbers.

Confidentiality in dealing with patient data is paramount; however, critical situations occur where patient information must be shared between healthcare practitioners to provide safe, effective holistic care. Reviewing local confidentiality guidelines offers reassurance and guidance in situations where a data breach may be necessary. Other services that may be useful for patients in this context include Samaritans and Breathing Space.

PROFESSIONAL ISSUES

GPNs engaging with and caring for patients with mental health difficulties in primary care settings may often feel challenged in terms of their professional competency and/or providing care within their individual comfort zone. However, being mindful of the need for early intervention is key in treating common mental health problems and intervening early in those patients demonstrating serious mental illness.

Professionally, clinical supervision will allow for space to discuss any professional/practice issues and should offer a safe, nurturing space that encourages personal and professional curiosity that allows for continuous development within the professional standards, as directed in the Nursing and Midwifery Council (NMC, 2018) Code. Similarly, shared education forums, complex case discussions and the support of a clinical supervision framework will also be useful. Not only will this enhance care delivery, but it will also support the re-validation process and professional development.

GPNs, with their sustained contact with a local population, are in a privileged position to help individuals suffering mental health issues and support them through very difficult periods in their lives. This, however, can place the nurse in situations that may challenge their own sense of safety, values and views. The inherent value of education, training and awareness sessions on mental health cannot be underestimated, and the advent of online learning can maximise the GPN's awareness and learning. As previously stated, having knowledge of local mental health teams and fostering links will not only optimise care planning but will also provide the necessary level of professional support for the GPN in dealing with patients presenting with mental health conditions and help to alleviate work-related stress.

SUMMARY

This chapter has provided insight into caring for people with or at risk of mental health issues and offered pragmatic guidance for GPNs seeking to build confidence in asking what may be perceived as difficult consultation questions to support nursing assessment and management. However, even at times where practitioners feel clinically unsure of patient presentations, maintaining a compassionate curiosity will enable the exploration of unmet health needs. Be curious and seek understanding, and this will be helpful in developing a plan; professional curiosity allows a level of clarity and understanding that supports values-based care.

Nurses will offer evidence-based mental health advice every day; however, there is also a need to be mindful of the professional's mental wellbeing. Being cognisant of maintaining healthy lifestyles and utilising support systems are important factors in managing the stress and demands of what can be an emotionally and physically challenging job on the front line of primary care.

REFERENCES

American Psychiatric Association. (2017). *Diagnostic and statistical manual of mental disorders* (5th ed.).

Anxiety UK. (2019). *Quick guide.* https://www.anxietyuk.org.uk/our-services/help-for-the-asian-community/quick-guide/

Atter, N. (2018). *Mental health awareness week – Suicide Prevention* [Blog]. British Psychological Society. https://www.bps.org.uk/blogs/bps-policy-unit/mental-health-awareness-week-suicideprevention

Chesney, E., Goodwin, G., & Fazel, S. (2014). Risks of all-cause and suicide mortality in mental disorders: A meta-review. *World Psychiatry, 13*(2), 153–160.

Davies, J., & Read, J. (2019). A systematic review into the incidence, severity and duration of antidepressant withdrawal effects: Are guidelines evidence-based? *Addictive Behaviours, 97*, 111–121.

Eating Disorder Hope. (2019). *Addressing underlying anxiety and depression in eating disorders.* https://www.eatingdisorderhope.com/blog/anxiety-depression-eating-disorders

Engel, G. (1977). *The need for a new medical model: A challenge for biomedicine* (1st ed.). American Association for the Advancement of Science.

Healthline. (2019). *Stress and anxiety: Causes and management.* https://www.healthline.com/health/stress-and-anxiety

Holland, K., & Jenkins, J. (2019). *Applying the Roper, Logan and Tierney model in practice* (3rd ed). Elsevier.

Ilyas, A., Chesney, E., & Patel, R. (2017). Improving life expectancy in people with serious mental illness: Should we place more emphasis on primary prevention? *British Journal of Psychiatry, 211*(4), 194–197.

Krystal, A. (2012). Psychiatric disorders and sleep. *Neurologic Clinics, 30*(4), 1389–1413.

Masuku, S. (2019). Self-harm presentations in emergency departments: Staff attitudes and triage. *British Journal of Nursing, 28*(22), 1468–1476.

Mental Health Foundation. (2017). *Surviving or thriving? The state of the UK's mental health.*

Mental Health Foundation. (2019). *Physical health and mental health.* https://www.mentalhealth.org.uk/a-to-z/p/physical-health-and-mental-health

Mental Health Taskforce. (2016). *The five year forward for mental health.* https://www.england.nhs.uk/wp-content/uploads/2016/02/Mental-Health-Taskforce-FYFVfinal.pdf

National Institute of Clinical Effectiveness. (2019). *Depression in adults: Recognition and management.* https://www.nice.org.uk/guidance/cg90/resources/depression-in-adults-recognition-and-management-pdf-975742638037

Nazarko, L. (2019). Improving the physical health of people with severe mental illness. *Nursing Times, 113*(8), 42–45. https://www.nursingtimes.net/roles/mental-health-nurses/improving-the-physical-health-of-people-with-severe-mental-illness-24-07-2017/

NHS England. (2020). *Advancing mental health equalities strategy.* https://www.england.nhs.uk/wp-content/uploads/2020/10/00159-advancing-mental-health-equalities-strategy.pdf

Nursing and Midwifery Council. (2018). *The code: Professional standards of practice and behaviour for nurses, midwives and nursing associates.*

Peterson, T. (2015). *Mental health assessment and screening tools.* Healthy Place. https://www.healthyplace.com/other-info/mental-illness-overview/mental-health-assessment-and-screening-tools

Public Bodies (Joint Working) (Scotland) Act 2014. http://www.legislation.gov.uk/asp/2014/9/pdfs/asp_20140009_en.pdf

Public Health England. (2019). *Wellbeing and mental health: Applying All Our Health*. https://www.gov.uk/government/publications/wellbeing-in-mental-health-applying-all-our-health/wellbeing-in-mental-health-applying-all-our-health

Rethink Mental Illness. (2019). *Mental illness and talking therapies*. https://www.rethink.org/advice-and-information/living-with-mental-illness/treatment-and-support/talking-therapies/

Rocha Neto, H., Estellita-Lins, C., Lessa, J., & Cavalcanti, M. (2019). Mental State Examination and its procedures – Narrative review of Brazilian descriptive psychopathology. *Frontiers in Psychiatry*, 10.

Roper, N., Logan, W. W., & Tierney, A. J. (1996). *The elements of nursing: A model for nursing based on a model for living*. Churchill Livingston.

Royal College of General Practitioners Primary Care Mental Health Steering Group. (2017). *RCGP position statement on mental health in primary care*. http://www.infocoponline.es/pdf/RCGP-PS-mental-health.pdf

Scottish Government. (2019). Mental health strategy 2017–2027. https://www.gov.scot/publications/mental-health-strategy-2017-2027/

Thomson, D. (2020). Psychiatric problems. In A. Staten & P. Staten (Eds.), *Practical general practice guidelines for effective clinical management* (7th ed., pp. 313–339). Elsevier.

UCL Institute of Health Equity. (2017). *Psychosocial pathways and health outcomes: Informing action on health inequalities*. Public Health England.

World Health Organisation. (2004). *ICD-10: International statistical classification of diseases and related health problems: Tenth revision, 2nd ed.*

World Health Organisation. (2018). *Integrating health services: Brief*. https://apps.who.int/iris/handle/10665/326459

World Health Organisation. (2019). *Controlling the global obesity epidemic*. https://www.who.int/nutrition/topics/obesity/en/

13

MANAGING MINOR ILLNESS IN PRIMARY CARE

EILEEN P. MUNSON ■ SUSAN F. BROOKS

INTRODUCTION

The demands and challenges of contemporary healthcare practice evidence that more than ever, the National Health Service (NHS) and general practice services are working at full capacity. It is therefore vital for general practice nurses (GPNs) to possess the core skills of how to assess, diagnose and manage commonly presenting minor illness. The GPN needs to have the knowledge base and be competent to advise regarding over-the-counter (OTC) products and (if a nonmedical prescriber to prescribe) pharmacological treatments. For those unable to prescribe, the practice may work from patient-specific directive protocols, or it may require that the patient call back for the prescription once signed by a general practitioner (GP). Each general practice will be individual in the way it manages and coordinates its services to ensure that patients are seen or advised regarding minor illness. The key competency in the management of minor illness is using evidence-based decision-making to identify any 'red flags' among the various clinical presentations.

This chapter will focus on common minor illnesses that present in general practice, where minor illnesses are essentially nonurgent conditions, often self-limiting, but commonly presenting. This contrasts with other chapters, which have addressed presentations such as exacerbation of asthma (Chapter 8) and sexual and reproductive health (Chapter 15). In addition, Chapter 6 addresses the nuances of consultation, which should be applied when seeing patients who present with minor illness that may be self-limiting but may require intervention and/or referral. This

chapter details the practical management of common minor illness presentations that the GPN may encounter and offers some bespoke guidance on aspects of history taking (complementary to that already offered in Chapter 6), differential diagnosis and evidence-based models to support and develop practice in managing minor conditions.

The process of assessing a patient who presents with undifferentiated symptoms requires skilled history taking with exploration of the person's ideas, concerns and expectations about their condition. Many GPNs develop these skills through attending accredited programmes of study as well as observation of skilled and experienced colleagues. Safety is always the most important aspect of any consultation, acting in the patient's best interest and using up-to-date evidence to practise effectively (Nursing and Midwifery Council (NMC), 2018). Sometimes a GPN will not be able to ascertain a differential diagnosis, and referral to a senior colleague or specialist is essential for the preservation of safety. Regardless of experience and competency, the practice of 'safety netting' is key to consulting with people who are experiencing symptoms that may worsen and require urgent medical attention.

The following sections will utilise structure to assist in the recognition of minor illness conditions and consider key points for history taking (using a suggested framework to guide the process; see Chapter 6), possible differentials and management advice. Details of how to conduct physical examinations are not within the scope of this text, and the reader is encouraged to refer to recommended resources, such as *Macleod's Clinical Examination* (Innes et al., 2018), and to consider enrolling for academic development of the necessary skills through an accredited and assessed module of study at a higher education institution.

RESPIRATORY CONDITIONS

Upper Respiratory Tract Infection

Upper respiratory tract infection (URTI) is an umbrella term for illnesses that are generally minor and consist of coryza (acute inflammation of the respiratory mucosa) often aligned with the common cold, sore throats and coughs, which are common presentations within primary care (Arroll, 2011).

Aetiology

Coryza is commonly attributed to rhinovirus (30%–50%), with coronavirus, adenovirus and influenza virus attributed to most other causes. The National Institute for Health and Care Excellence (NICE, 2016a) purports that no pathogens are isolated in 20% to 30% of colds because of multiple viruses. URTI is viral in aetiology and affects the upper airways. The upper respiratory tract extends from the tympanic membranes to the tracheal carina; the upper bronchi are often infected by the same viruses.

Signs and Symptoms

The symptomology of coryza is usually short-lived, lasting an average of 7 to 10 days, with a sore throat, coughing, rhinorrhoea and nasal congestion and low-grade fever less than 38°C. Individuals may present

---

BOX 13.1
UPPER RESPIRATORY TRACT INFECTION SYMPTOMS

- Sore throat
- Cough
- Shortness of breath
- Nasal congestion
- Rhinorrhoea
- Sneezing
- Facial pain
- Fever
- Fatigue
- Myalgia
- Headache
- Malaise
- Irritability
- Otalgia
- Hearing loss
- Anosmia

---

with various symptoms, which can contribute to several differential diagnoses (see Box 13.1).

History Taking

See Box 13.2 for a suggested framework for taking a history of URTI.

Examination

It is advisable to include a set of physical observations with a minimum of temperature, respiratory rate, blood pressure and radial pulse.

The relevant structures should be examined – nose, throat, ears, cervical lymph nodes (see standard text for physical examination, such as Innes et al. (2018)). Auscultation of the anterior and posterior chest wall would be clinically indicated if coughing is the main symptom, but this requires competence in physical assessment, as discussed previously.

BOX 13.2
SUGGESTED FRAMEWORK FOR TAKING A HISTORY OF UPPER RESPIRATORY TRACT INFECTION (URTI)

Initial approach to the patient: introduction, identification, explanation of role, consent to proceed

Exploration of clinical features: the onset and duration of symptoms, their character and timing, along with any precipitating and relieving factors

Associated features to exclude 'red flags': sputum consistency and colour, haemoptysis, weight loss, chest pain, pyrexia (systemic upset), wheeze (allergy, asthma), ankle oedema (possible cardiac condition), calf tenderness (deep vein thrombosis (DVT)), cough for

>3 weeks, contact with COVID-19 or other respiratory viruses

Past medical history: which is usually available in general practice

Drug history: to include immunosuppressants, combined oral contraceptive pill, OTC and recreational

Allergies: drugs and sensitivities

Social: who is at home, occupation, alcohol, smoking

Investigations: not usually required for URTI unless symptoms worsen or fail to resolve

Management

It is important to explain the likely diagnosis of a URTI and provide reassurance that it has an expected duration of 7 to 10 days.

Explain the rationale for treatment, which is supportive, as antibiotics are not prescribed for viral infections because they do not treat or reduce the duration of symptoms (Kenealy & Arroll, 2013; NICE, 2016a). Self-management advice includes OTC paracetamol and ibuprofen at recommended doses and frequency to alleviate myalgia and fever. The evidence base for the use of antihistamines is limited, as is the use of anecdotal remedies such as steam inhalation, throat lozenges, vapour rubs or gargling with saltwater or nasal saline drops (NICE, 2016a). Wiest's (2011) research demonstrated that vitamin supplements and antihistamines have no proven benefit for shortening the duration of cold symptoms. The GPN should warn the patient that OTC decongestants can result in an unwanted sympathomimetic effect of rebound congestion and insomnia. These drugs should be particularly avoided in patients with diabetes, hypertension, hyperthyroidism, glaucoma, prostatic hypertrophy and ischaemic heart disease and in those taking antihypertensives and antidepressants (British National Formulary (BNF), 2020).

Time should be taken to include health-promotion measures that will relieve the symptoms (such as rest and increasing fluid intake), prevent recurrence and spread (such as frequent hand washing and isolating at home) and behaviour changes such stopping smoking if appropriate. The need for a seasonal influenza vaccination may be indicated once the patient is well (Public Health England (PHE), 2020).

Take-home advice should reiterate the self-care measures previously described and also include clear instructions to return or seek alternative medical support if the symptoms do not resolve or worsen.

Acute Pharyngitis

Acute pharyngitis is characterised by the rapid onset of sore throat and pharyngeal inflammation (with or without exudate). There is usually an absence of cough but often nasal congestion and discharge. It can be caused by a variety of viral and bacterial pathogens, including group A *Streptococcus* (GAS), as well as fungal pathogens (*Candida*). Bacterial pharyngitis is more

TABLE 13.1	
Viral Pharyngitis – Typical Symptomology	
Virus	**Symptom**
Rhinovirus	Coryza
Adenovirus	Pharyngoconjunctival fever
Parainfluenza	Hoarseness, croup
Herpes simplex type 1 and 2	Gingivitis and stomatitis
Respiratory syncytial virus	Hoarseness, wheezing
Epstein-Barr virus (infectious mononucleosis)	Fatigue, cervical lymphadenopathy, fever
Coronavirus	Viral upper respiratory infection symptoms
Cytomegalovirus	Fatigue, cervical lymphadenopathy, fever
Influenza	Flu-like symptoms

common in winter (or early spring), whereas enterovirus infection is more common in the summer and autumn. Generally, this is a self-limiting condition with resolution within 2 weeks.

Aetiology

The viral aetiology includes several pathogens that make pharyngitis clinically indistinguishable from those caused by group A beta streptococcal pharyngitis (Table 13.1). Bacterial causes of acute pharyngitis include GAS, which accounts for approximately 5% to 15% of adults presenting with pharyngitis and up to 30% in children (Van Brusselen et al., 2014).

Signs and Symptoms

Signs and symptoms include fever, lack of cough, tonsillar exudate (unilateral or bilateral), fatigue, tender cervical adenopathy and headache.

History Taking

See Box 13.3 for a suggested framework for taking a history of acute pharyngitis.

Examination

Nose, throat – grading the tonsils and looking for exudate in crevices of tonsil beds (Fig. 13.1)
Ears – for any associated signs of infection
Cervical lymph nodes (Fig. 13.2)

BOX 13.3

**SUGGESTED FRAMEWORK FOR
TAKING A HISTORY OF ACUTE
PHARYNGITIS**

Initial approach to the patient: introduction, identification, explanation of role, consent to proceed

Exploration of clinical features: the onset and duration of symptoms, their character and timing, along with any precipitating and relieving factors. Incubation period can be as short as 24 hours, peaking in 5 days, with coryza symptoms that can last up to 2 weeks.

Associated features to exclude 'red flags': malaise, chills, fever, cough, dyspnoea, neck stiffness, photophobia, headache, dysphagia or dyspepsia

Past medical history: recurrence of the same problem, asthma requiring steroid inhalers – consider oral *Candida* infection

Drug history: to include immunosuppressants, combined oral contraceptive pill, over-the-counter (OTC) and recreational drugs

Allergies: drugs and sensitivities

Social: who is at home if care is required, occupation in relation to Fit to Work note, alcohol, smoking advice if relevant

Investigations: not usually required for pharyngitis unless symptoms worsen or fail to resolve

Management

Some medical centres now offer a rapid antigen test (RAT) for the detection of GAS, which gives the advantage of immediate point-of-care testing. Testing should be used only when the clinical symptoms are consistent with GAS disease because it can give false-positive results, potentially leading to inappropriate prescribing of antibiotics. Cohen et al.'s (2016) Cochrane review established that RAT is 70% to 90% sensitive and 95% specific compared with throat culture. However, Barakat et al. (2019) identified that the rapid antigen detection tests have a lower specificity in children recently treated for GAS. He also suggests that children should have a throat swab culture where the test result is negative to exclude any potential risk of rheumatic fever after GAS.

'Red flags' such as drooling and/or dysphonia (muffled or 'hot potato' voice), especially with dysphagia, warrant immediate attention to exclude the following:

■ Epiglottitis
■ Trismus (spasm of jaw muscles indicative of tetanus)
■ Peritonsillar abscess (quinsy)
■ Unilateral neck swelling indicative of various underlying pathologies
■ Retropharyngeal infections
■ Submandibular infections (possible acute cellulitis, mumps)
■ Diphtheria

In addition, neutropenic and immunocompromised patients (including those taking prescribed carbimazole; see BNF (2020) regarding bone marrow suppression) with a persistent sore throat may need hospital admission for treatment of the infection.

Viral pharyngitis can usually be managed with supportive measures, such as increasing fluids, small nutritious meals and rest. Analgesia, such as ibuprofen or paracetamol, is the main option for pain relief. OTC throat sprays or gargles can be effective in soothing throat pain. Reinforce that the normal duration is 7 to 10 days and that antibiotics are not prescribed for viral infections because they do not treat or shorten the length of time of experiencing symptoms.

Take-home advice should reiterate the self-care measures described previously and also include clear instructions to return or seek alternative medical support if the symptoms do not resolve or worsen, especially if the patient is exhibiting any of the 'red flags' listed earlier.

Tonsillitis

Tonsils are glands that are oval-shaped lymphatic tissue. Their primary role is to act as a filter to trap bacteria and viruses entering the body via the mouth and sinuses. A secondary role for the tonsil is to stimulate the immune system to produce antibodies to fight off infection. When infection occurs, they swell and become enlarged as a result of inflammation. The enlarged tonsils are graded on a scale of 1 to 4 or A to E, depending (see Fig. 13.1) on where they are situated in relation to the uvulae.

Aetiology

Viral pathogens include rhinovirus, coronavirus, parainfluenza, herpes simplex I and Epstein-Barr virus, which causes infectious mononucleosis, commonly known as *glandular fever*. These viral infections can be clinically indistinguishable from group A beta

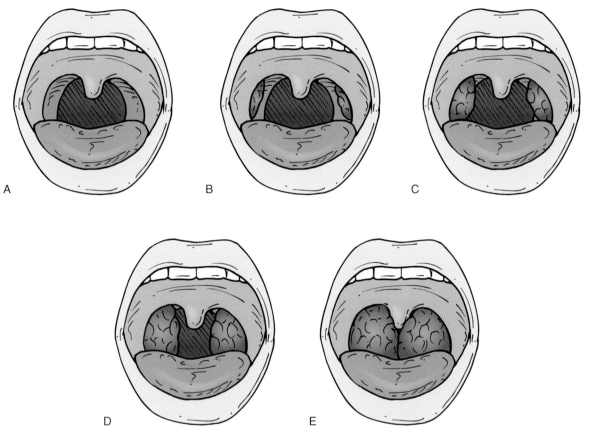

Fig. 13.1 ■ Tonsil grading. (A) Surgically removed tonsils. (B) Tonsils hidden within tonsil pillars. (C) Tonsils extending to the pillars. (D) Tonsils are beyond the pillars. (E) Tonsils extend to midline. (From Friedman M, Tanyeri H, et al. Clinical predictors of obstructive sleep apnea. Laryngoscope. 1999;109[12]:1901-1907.)

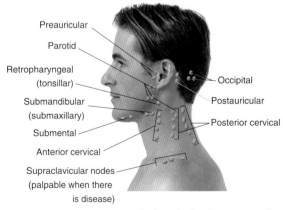

Fig. 13.2 ■ Examination of the lymph glands. (From Ball, J. W., Dains, J. E., Flynn, J. A., et al. [2019]. Seidel's guide to physical examination [9th ed.]. St. Louis: Elsevier.)

streptococcal infections, the typical bacterial cause of tonsillitis. A systematic review by Spinks et al. (2013) purported that group A beta-haemolytic streptococci (GABHS) infection accounts for approximately 20% of adults presenting with tonsillitis, but the incidence is age dependent. Spinks et al.'s evidence has established that GABHS is responsible for 15% of cases in children younger than age 3, 50% of cases between ages 4 and 13, and 10% of cases in adults.

Signs and Symptoms

Signs and symptoms include a burning/scratching sensation at the back of the throat, dysphagia, neck pain and other symptoms that may accompany sore throat, such as coughing, sneezing, laryngitis halitosis, fever, fatigue and lymphadenopathy.

History Taking

See Box 13.4 for a suggested framework for taking a history of tonsillitis.

Examination

Lymph Nodes. The initial examination starts with palpation of the lymph nodes of the face and neck. Standing behind the patient, the practitioner commences the examination with the postauricular glands and concludes with the cervical chain with the supraclavicular node (see Fig. 13.2). When palpating, the practitioner should use the tips of the fingers in a circular motion, paying attention for evidence of raised nodes that feel like small peas; note should be made of any tenderness of the specific node area on palpation, including estimated size, consistency and whether the margins of the node are smooth or irregular.

Tonsils. To gain a clear visualisation of the back and roof of the mouth, it is important to get the individual to relax and hyperextend their head back as far as possible with a wide-open mouth. Using a pen torch and a tongue depressor if required, the practitioner should be able to clearly view if the tonsils are enlarged and inflamed and grade them from grade 1 to 4, recording the findings in the notes (Fig. 13.3). The grading determines the severity of the tonsillitis and helps contribute to the overall assessment.

A record should be made if a petechial rash on the roof of the mouth is present, which can denote a streptococcal infection requiring a penicillin-based antibiotic (NICE, 2018f). The uvula should be central, not deviating to the right or left or touching the tonsillar beds. The tonsils should be examined for any exudate, which may be evident in the cervices of the tonsil beds. In addition, the following evidence-based assessment tools can assist the GPN in decision-making regarding the management of tonsillitis. The Centor assessment criteria (Centor et al., 1981) score the symptoms of tonsillar exudate, tender anterior cervical lymphadenopathy or lymphadenitis, history of fever (over 38°C) and the absence of cough with a maximum score of 4 but note only a 32% to 56% likelihood of isolating streptococcus with a score of 3 or 4. More recently, the FeverPAIN tool (NICE, 2018a) has become a useful decision-making aid requiring the practitioner to score symptoms in patients seeking advice for medical intervention within 3 days of the start of symptoms. The criteria include a fever (38.5°C) during the past 24 hours, exudate on the tonsil bed, severely inflamed tonsils and absence of a cough or symptoms of a cold.

Management

Because Spinks et al. (2013) found that only 20% of tonsillitis in adults was caused by GABHS requiring antibiotics (usually from the beta-lactamase group, such as phenoxymethylpenicillin), education in self-care measures to relieve the symptoms of a sore throat and associated problems is vital. OTC local antiseptic gargles in the form of sprays or lozenges, such as benzydamine or benzocaine and lidocaine, can anecdotally help, but evidence for their use is limited (Farah & Visinitini, 2018). Throat lozenges containing local anaesthetics, such as benzalkonium chloride and hexylresorcinol, can help stimulate the salivary flow, which helps soothe the throat, with the caution to use the

---

BOX 13.4

SUGGESTED FRAMEWORK FOR TAKING A HISTORY OF TONSILLITIS

Initial approach to the patient: introduction, identification, explanation of role, consent to proceed

Exploration of clinical features: the onset and duration of symptoms, their character and timing, along with any precipitating and relieving factors. Onset can be within 24 hours. Presence of unilateral symptoms may indicate a quinsy or peritonsillar abscess, where a collection of pus develops between the back of a tonsil and the wall of the throat. If there is difficulty opening the mouth, *do not examine* but seek urgent medical assistance because a differential diagnosis could be epiglottitis or trismus.

Associated features to exclude 'red flags': drooling, dysphonia, dysphagia, extreme fatigue, stridor, dehydration

Past medical history: recurrence of the same problem, asthma requiring steroid inhalers –consider oral *Candida* infection

Drug history: to include immunosuppressants, combined oral contraceptive pill, over-the-counter (OTC) and recreational drugs

Allergies: drugs and sensitivities

Social: who is at home, occupation in relation to Fit to Work note; alcohol intake and smoking are risk factors for tonsil cancer (also human papilloma virus (HPV)).

Investigations: not usually required for tonsillitis unless symptoms worsen or fail to resolve

maximum dose for no longer than 3 days. Oral analgesia, such as paracetamol, is the first-line choice for pain relief. Self-care advice includes avoiding hot drinks to limit pain; however, this must be balanced with ensuring adequate hydration.

Advice to be given at the end of the consultation would include reassurance that a sore throat tends to be self-limiting, lasting around 7 days whether antibiotics are used or not. As always, the individual must be cautioned to seek urgent medical advice if they develop difficulty breathing, drooling, dysphagia or become systemically unwell. Urinary problems could indicate post-streptococcal glomerulonephritis and need urgent investigation.

For people with severe recurrent tonsillitis (a frequency of more than seven episodes per year for 1 year, five per year for 2 years, or three per year for 3 years, and for whom there is no other explanation for the recurrent symptoms), referral to an ear, nose and throat (ENT) specialist is advised because this cohort may benefit from tonsillectomy (NICE, 2018f).

OPHTHALMIC CONDITIONS

Conjunctivitis

Conjunctivitis is a common condition affecting the thin layer of tissue covering the eye; this thin layer is called the *conjunctiva,* and conjunctivitis is the inflammation and redness associated with this. There are three main types, and this section will address each individual condition.

Aetiology

Conjunctivitis can be allergic, viral or bacterial and does not always need treatment because it often resolves without intervention (NICE, 2018b). It is classically characterised by irritation, itching and a sensation of grittiness in the eye, often with watering or discharge. Allergic conjunctivitis is commonly seen seasonally in patients and is associated with immunoglobulin E (IgE) hypersensitivity resulting from hayfever allergens. Viral conjunctivitis is caused by adenovirus in 65% to 90% of cases, making it the most common type of conjunctivitis. Herpes simplex causes 1.3% to 4.8% of cases, with varicella zoster, molluscum contagiosum, Epstein-Barr, coxsackie and enteroviruses being other causes (NICE, 2018b).

Signs and Symptoms

Allergic and viral conjunctivitis symptoms include itchiness, redness of the conjunctiva and watery discharge and sometimes photophobia.

Bacterial conjunctivitis is the second most common cause of conjunctivitis, accounting for 50% to 75% cases (NICE, 2018b), with various sources, including *Haemophilus influenzae, Streptococcus pneumoniae* and *Moraxella catarrhalis* (main causes in children), as well as *Staphylococcus aureus, Chlamydia trachomatis* and *Neisseria gonorrhoea.* Bacterial conjunctivitis symptoms can persist for up to 4 weeks. Symptoms are usually unilateral, with one eye having a red conjunctiva, with watery discharge in the early stages, leading to a mucopurulent discharge and sticky eyelashes, which tend to be worse in the morning (see Fig 13.3).

Ophthalmia neonatorum presents in newborns within the first 30 days of life. The causes of infection may be bacterial, chlamydial or viral. Organisms responsible may include adenoviruses, *Escherichia coli, C. trachomatis, N. gonorrhoea,* herpes simplex and *Pseudomonas* (Alfonse et al., 2015). *N. gonorrhoea* can present at any time from delivery through the first 7 days, whilst *C. trachomatis* usually presents within the first 14 days. Since 2010, ophthalmia neonatorum is no longer a notifiable disease (College of Optometrists, 2020b).

Ophthalmia neonatorum symptoms include sticky eyes with mucopurulent discharge, which can present at any time in the first 4 weeks of life. Profuse discharge and/or swollen eyelids with surrounding cellulitis should be referred immediately for specialist assessment.

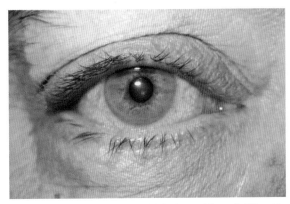

Fig. 13.3 ■ Infective conjunctivitis. (From Bonewit-West, K., & Hunt, S. (2021). *Today's medical assistant: Clinical and administrative procedures* (4th ed.). Elsevier.)

History Taking

See Box 13.5 for a suggested framework for taking a history of conjunctivitis.

Examination

Examination (of both eyes even if only one is affected) may be conducted as follows (NICE, 2018b):

Conjunctiva – look for injection, chemosis (swelling), follicles, papillae and membranes. Pull on lower eyelid and evert upper lid using a cotton wool tip to examine the conjunctiva.

Follicles (small yellowish elevations of lymphocytes) can be viewed on the palpebral conjunctiva associated with adenovirus and chlamydia.

Papillae (small conjunctival elevations with central vessels) can be associated with allergic conjunctivitis and contact lens intolerance.

BOX 13.5
SUGGESTED FRAMEWORK FOR TAKING A HISTORY OF CONJUNCTIVITIS

Initial approach to the patient: introduction, identification, explanation of role, consent to proceed (parental consent if appropriate)

Exploration of clinical features: the onset and duration of symptoms, their character and timing, along with any precipitating and relieving factors. Onset can be within 24 hours. Unilateral or bilateral. Discharge – watery or mucopurulent.

Associated features to exclude 'red flags': herpes simplex or zoster in or around the eye orbit (vesicles), systemic illness, changes to vision with reduced visual acuity, painful eye(s), neonates with a red sticky eye within first 30 days of birth, profuse mucopurulent discharge, history of trauma, headaches, photophobia

Past medical history: recurrence of the same problem, concomitant skin conditions such as eczema or psoriasis. Associated systemic conditions such as rheumatoid arthritis, HIV, systemic lupus erythematous and reactive arthritis.

Drug history: to include immunosuppressants, chemotherapy, combined oral contraceptive pill, over-the-counter (OTC) and recreational drugs

Allergies: drugs and sensitivities, especially to pollen

Social: occupational risk factors, contact lens wearer, contact with others who have eye infections

Investigations: not usually required for conjunctivitis unless symptoms worsen or fail to resolve

---

Conjunctival membranes (yellow/white layer of fibrin to underlying conjunctival tissue) can form in severe viral or bacterial infections and cause complications such as conjunctival scarring and severe dry eye.

Cornea – look for ulceration and opacities.

If available (and following specific training), consider evaluation of the cornea with a Wood's lamp and fluorescein staining to identify pathology such as corneal dendrites in herpes simplex virus corneal ulcers.

Sclera – look for localised or widespread oedema and erythema, which indicate a serious cause, such as scleritis.

Pupil – assess shape, size and pupillary reaction (with a pen torch) and look for asymmetrical or unreactive pupils.

Visual acuity (using a Snellen chart) and visual fields – compare with previous measurements of visual acuity, if possible.

Eyelids – look for discharge, swelling, inflammation, malposition, nodules, loss of lashes (may indicate sebaceous gland carcinoma), vesicles (herpes) or blepharitis.

Herpes simplex (HSV) – may present as unilateral red eye with vesicular lesions on the eyelid.

Herpes zoster – assume ocular involvement if lesions are present on the tip of the nose (Hutchinson's sign).

Periorbital area – look for swelling and erythema, which may indicate orbital or periorbital cellulitis. Periorbital cellulitis can develop from conjunctivitis in young children.

Lymph nodes – look for regional lymphadenopathy.

Investigations

Swabs are not routinely taken but may be appropriate if the patient needs to be referred after failing to respond to initial treatment. Severe purulent discharge (which may indicate gonococcal infection) or conjunctivitis in neonates warrants urgent referral, where swabs will be taken in secondary care. In summary, if seeing a baby under the age of 1 month with sticky eyes, referral to a specialist must be made if the eyes are red as well as sticky or if any of the other concerning features are present. If there are no concerning features, then swabs can be taken for bacterial culture, gonorrhoea and chlamydia.

Management

- Viral and allergic conjunctivitis treatment includes mast cell stabiliser eye drops, such as sodium cromoglycate, and antihistamine eye drops, such as antazoline sulphate (or oral antihistamines), sometimes combined with sympathomimetics.
- Noninfectious/Nonallergic conjunctivitis treatment is mainly eye lubricants/artificial tears.
- Bacterial conjunctivitis treatment includes chloramphenicol and fusidic acid.
- Ophthalmia neonatorum treatment includes topical and oral antibiotics under specialist care.

Individuals can be advised regarding bathing eyes that have discharge or crusting of the eyelashes to use water that has been boiled and cooled to gently clean away debris with lint-free cotton. The eyes should be wiped from the inside of the eye outwards in one clear movement and the piece of cotton disposed of immediately, always treating each eye separately. Contact lenses should not be worn until any infection has cleared.

With regards to work or school attendance, PHE (2017) and Public Health Wales (PHW, 2020) state that there is no requirement to avoid these unless the individual is feeling particularly unwell. Individuals should be advised to exercise caution, which may include remaining at home if working in an environment near others and sharing computers or other equipment such as telephones until the eye infection has cleared.

Corneal Abrasions/Foreign Body in the Eye

Corneal abrasions are defined as an abrasion in the cornea resulting from a foreign body (object or substance) in the eye.

Aetiology

Corneal abrasions usually occur from occupational or leisure pursuits. Occupational pursuits include construction work where drilling, hammering and metal from steel splinters or iron filings to splinters and sawdust from carpentry can damage the eye. Leisure and sport activities include those where dust, dirt or even grass when mowing the lawn can end up in the eyes because of windy weather (Drummond, 2020). Any high-velocity injuries should be referred immediately to an emergency eye service and should be treated as a penetrating injury until proven otherwise.

Signs and Symptoms

Trauma, with the size of the abrasion varying according to the severity of trauma

Lid oedema and erythema

Conjunctival hyperaemia

Corneal epithelial defect (visual when stained with fluorescein)

Corneal oedema beneath defect

Visual loss (as a result of epithelial disruption and stromal oedema)

History Taking

See Box 13.6 for a suggested framework for taking a history of corneal abrasions/foreign body in the eye.

BOX 13.6

SUGGESTED FRAMEWORK FOR TAKING A HISTORY OF CORNEAL ABRASIONS/FOREIGN BODY IN THE EYE

Initial approach to the patient: introduction, identification, explanation of role, consent to proceed (parental consent if appropriate)

Exploration of clinical features: the onset and duration of symptoms, including eye pain, which may range from mild irritation resulting from an eyelash in the eye to severe pain from a chemical splash. Other causes of pain may include lacrimation/blepharospasm. Note any precipitating and relieving factors. Onset may be reported after a specific eye trauma. Unilateral or bilateral symptoms.

Associated features to exclude 'red flags': visual acuity reduction or loss; discharge – watery, bloody or mucopurulent; red eye; swelling of the eyelid or vesicles around the eye; photophobia; corneal opacity. Irregular, dilated or nonreactive pupils; hypopyon (pus within in the anterior chamber) or hyphema (blood within the anterior chamber).

Past medical history: recurrence of the same problem, any concurrent ocular conditions

Drug history: to include immunosuppressants, chemotherapy, combined oral contraceptive pill, over-the-counter (OTC) and recreational drugs

Allergies: drugs and sensitivities

Social: occupational/leisure risk factors, contact lens wearer

Investigations: may be required for corneal abrasion, so referral for specialist care is highly likely.

Examination

If the eye trauma is a result of a chemical injuries, then immediately irrigate the eye using copious amounts of water (or normal saline if available) to neutralise the ocular surface, which can be a vital procedure to prevent permanent visual loss.

Having determined how the injury was caused, ruling out chemical injury and penetrating trauma, the initial examination should include an assessment of the eye guided by the history. This needs to be focused, and the following list acts as a guide (adapted from the College of Optometrists (2020a)):

- Inspection of the entire eye orbit for swelling or redness. Check the pupil for regularity and the sclera for injection. Check for any obvious external abnormalities such as cystic lesions. Eversion of the eyelid (tarsal plate) may be carried out to examine the underside of the lid(s) and to check the eyelashes, which may be the cause of the foreign body in the eye.
- Palpation of the adjacent sinuses for any tenderness. Palpation of the temporal artery, looking for tenderness with or without loss of pulsation.
- Check eye movements by asking the patient to follow a finger movement writing the letter *H* and check if there is any pain associated with the movements as well as observing for diplopia. Check the pupils for equal reaction to light and accommodation.
- Check visual acuity using a Snellen chart if there is any alteration of vision.
- Exclusion of corneal foreign body. Do not touch foreign bodies that are in or near the cornea because there is an increased risk of permanent loss of vision; refer to a specialist immediately (NICE, 2017a). If a foreign body is present, its size and location should be established and recorded.
- If a foreign body has been removed by the patient, there is no need to use fluorescein drops because an abrasion may have been caused during removal.

Management

Urgent same-day referral to an ophthalmological specialist will be dependent on history and examination findings.

- If temporal arteritis is suspected, then urgent discussion with vascular surgeons is necessary.
- In the case of a suspected penetrating foreign body in the eye, protruding from the eye globe, urgent referral is needed.
- In all chemical injuries, immediate referral is needed (after irrigation of the eye using copious amounts of water or normal saline if available, to neutralise the ocular surface).
- If periorbital cellulitis is suspected, an urgent maxillo-facial review is needed.
- If an intracranial bleed or other pathology is suspected, urgent admission for computed tomography (CT)/magnetic resonance imaging (MRI) and neurological assessment is required.

Abrasions of the cornea are common, usually being caused by a minor accidental injury, for example, by a finger, mascara brush or contact lens, or by a speck of foreign matter under the upper eyelid. There are also medical conditions that make abrasions more likely, for example, dystrophy, in which the surface tissue of the cornea (the epithelium) is more delicate than usual, or when the cornea is exposed by failure of the normal blink reflex or when its sensitivity to touch is reduced by damage to its nerves (sometimes associated with diabetes or following ocular shingles).

Superficial corneal abrasions usually heal quickly and completely, but if the injury is deeper or contaminated by foreign material and possibly infected, referral to an ophthalmologist is recommended.

EAR CONDITIONS

Earwax

Cerumen is a naturally occurring substance consisting of slough and epithelial cells. Cerumen acts as a protective agent that cleans and lubricates the external auditory canal. As ageing occurs, it gets drier, and hence the potential increases for impaction, which can lead to impaired hearing and discomfort. Impacted cerumen is evidently not an illness but is included in this chapter as a commonly presenting issue in general practice.

Aetiology

The amount of cerumen produced is thought to be genetically determined. The incidence of impaction in children is around 10%, attributed to children having smaller ear canals, and 3% to 6% in adults. This rises to 35% in those over 65 years old and is associated with the increased hair in the ear canals (BMJ, 2019).

Signs and Symptoms

Signs and symptoms include itching and a sensation of fullness in the ear, difficulty hearing, otalgia and occasionally high-pitched tones causing tinnitus or hearing-aid feedback.

History Taking

See Box 13.7 for a suggested framework for taking a history of impacted cerumen.

Examination

Inspect the external auditory meatus, noting redness, swelling or discharge.

BOX 13.7

SUGGESTED FRAMEWORK FOR TAKING A HISTORY OF IMPACTED CERUMEN

Initial approach to the patient: introduction, identification, explanation of role, consent to proceed (parental consent if appropriate)

Exploration of clinical features: the onset and duration of symptoms, including reduced hearing with unilateral or bilateral effect, sudden or gradual onset, otalgia, any attempts to remove cerumen, otorrhoea

Associated features to exclude 'red flags': associated symptoms of tinnitus, dizziness and vertigo could indicate inner ear problems/other pathology. Recent irrigation causing pain or discharge (possible otitis externa, otitis media or internal infection after irrigation or perforation of the ear canal or tympanic membrane)

Past medical history: recurrence of the same problem, any concurrent aural conditions, including use of hearing aids

Drug history: to include immunosuppressants, chemotherapy, combined oral contraceptive pill, over-the-counter (OTC) and recreational drugs

Allergies: drugs and sensitivities, especially to any OTC wax-removal products

Social: occupational/leisure risk factors affecting ears, such as ear defenders/headset use

Investigations: unlikely for impacted cerumen

Inspect the ear canal for inflammation and possible foreign bodies.

Palpate the pinna and tragus of the ear up and down – if pain is present, this suggests external otitis media.

Palpate the mastoid area posterior to the pinna. If this area is painful, it is suggestive of mastoiditis.

In adults, gently but firmly hold the helix and pull it up and back; this straightens the external auditory canal.

In children, gently and firmly hold the earlobe and pull it down and back to straighten the external ear canal.

Commence the otoscopic examination:

- Inspect ear each individually, commencing with the less symptomatic ear, starting externally and proceeding internally, taking notes of findings regarding any redness, swelling or discharge, including its colour and consistency.
- Note the tympanic membrane colour; a clear light-white colour with a light reflection on the attic membrane is a normal sign. The handle of the lateral part of the malleus may also be seen. A red, yellow or cloudy appearance can be a sign of infection. Record if the tympanic membrane is bulging, and observe if there is any evidence of a perforation. This must be done before and after ear irrigation because it is a common cause of litigation.

Management

Cerumenolytic agents can be used to break down the cerumen to clear the ear canals. There is insufficient evidence to demonstrate that one agent is superior than the other (Aaron et al., 2018; BMJ, 2019) but the two main types available are as follows:

Water-based agents – including acetic acid, docusate sodium, saline solutions and hydrogen peroxide, which work by hydration and fragmentation of the corneocytes in the cerumen.

Oil-based agents – cerumenolytic ear drops such as oil (olive, mineral, almond, sunflower) are recommended as a first-line treatment to either soften cerumen, before irrigation, or to facilitate the natural removal of the wax from the ear (NICE, 2016b).

Millward (2017) purposed that whilst there are numerous preparations available, some can increase the risk of dermatological reactions, and the use of normal saline or water may cause swelling of keratin or organic foreign bodies in the external auditory meatus, which could render the patient more deaf. In addition, the patient should be encouraged to discuss the selection of OTC preparation(s) with the pharmacist and with attention to any known sensitivities or allergies (e.g., to nuts, should almond oil be considered).

It is therefore vital that the GPN examines and fully visualises the tympanic membrane and/or contents of the ear canal, assesses the findings and documents these, along with any advice given for referral or treatment.

Take-home advice includes discouraging the use of cotton buds and reminders that the ear is a self-cleaning system. OTC preparations will often successfully soften cerumen sufficiently for it to exit the ear canal, but medical advice can be sought if problems persist. Ear irrigation or micro-suction procedures are rarely carried out in general practice now, but local referral to a specialist service can be made.

Otitis Externa

Acute otitis externa (AOE) is defined as inflammation of the external ear canal involving the pinna and/or the skin within the ear canal (meatus). It affects people of all age groups but peaks in the 7- to 12-year-old age group and declines in incidence among people over 50 years of age (Staten, 2020).

Aetiology

It is commonly caused by bacterial infections, which may be localised or diffuse in the form of a furuncle or boil. Otitis externa can be precipitated by ear trauma (from scratching, use of cotton buds, foreign body), swimming (especially in polluted or chemical-contaminated water) or pre-existing skin conditions such as eczema or psoriasis.

Signs and Symptoms

Rapid onset within 48 hours is possible, with a combination of the following: pain (otalgia), itching, discharge (otorrhoea), furunculosis (localised cartilaginous infected hair follicle) and hearing reduction or loss

History Taking

See Box 13.8 for a suggested framework for taking a history of otitis externa.

Examination

See the earlier examination section under 'Earwax'.

Management

OTC analgesia, such as ibuprofen or paracetamol, can be prescribed/advised according to age. For infections of the pinna, which is commonly affected by eczema, topical corticosteroid creams or antibiotic creams such as fusidic acid may be prescribed, but prolonged use should be avoided. For superficial cases of otitis externa, the first-line treatment of acetic acid 2% spray or cream can be prescribed, which acts as antifungal and antibacterial treatment and can be used for a maximum of 2 weeks, in adults and children aged over 12 (BNF, 2020).

BOX 13.8
SUGGESTED FRAMEWORK FOR TAKING A HISTORY OF OTITIS EXTERNA

Initial approach to the patient: introduction, identification, explanation of role, consent to proceed (parental consent if appropriate)

Exploration of clinical features: the onset and duration of symptoms, including reduced hearing with unilateral or bilateral effect, sudden or gradual onset, otalgia, otorrhoea, itching, any recent piercings of the external auditory meatus, recent ear irrigation or injury

Associated features to exclude 'red flags': associated symptoms of tinnitus, dizziness and vertigo. Recent irrigation causing pain or discharge – colour and consistency (possible otitis externa, otitis media or internal infection after irrigation or perforation of the ear canal or tympanic membrane). Perichondritis, mastoiditis, hearing loss.

Past medical history: recurrence of the same problem; any concurrent aural conditions; any concurrent skin conditions, such as eczema, psoriasis or seborrheic dermatitis; long-term conditions such as diabetes or HIV

Drug history: to include immunosuppressants, chemotherapy, over-the-counter (OTC) and recreational drugs

Allergies: drugs and sensitivities, metals

Social: occupational/leisure risk factors affecting ears, such as ear defenders/headset use/swimming.

Investigations: possible swab for microscopy, culture and sensitivity

Those with signs of cellulitis, otorrhoea or deafness resulting from occlusion may require systemic antibiotic therapy. For staphylococcal infections, a penicillin such as flucloxacillin should be prescribed, or alternatively, ciprofloxacin should be prescribed if pseudomonal infection is present, especially in immunocompromised patients or those with diabetes (BNF, 2020).

Several topical ear drops are available for the treatment of otitis externa, but they should be discontinued after a maximum of 7 days, and medical reassessment is required if there is no improvement. To enhance the effectiveness of ear drops, the tragus can be manipulated to aid them to reach deeper within the ear canal.

Antibiotics should be avoided unless there is systemic illness or persistent symptoms for 4 or more days. For those requiring oral antibiotics, the NICE (2018e) prescribing pathway should be followed.

Advise to avoid getting soap or shampoo into the ear canal when bathing and to avoid scratching or cleaning the ears using cotton buds. When drying the external meatus, individuals should avoid using cotton buds or the corner of towels because these can push any infection deeper into the canal. Swimming should be avoided until the otitis externa has healed completely.

Chronic or repeated otitis externa would warrant referral to a specialist ENT consultant.

Acute Otitis Media

Acute otitis media (AOM) is described as inflammation of the middle ear that can be caused by viral or bacterial infections. Common causative pathogens include *Streptococcus pneumoniae*, respiratory syncytial virus (RSV) and rhinovirus. Symptoms can develop over a short period of time, especially in children, who may present with effusion, a collection of fluid in the middle ear cavity that does not always indicate infection but can cause considerable pain and reduction in hearing (NICE, 2018d).

Signs and Symptoms

Signs and symptoms include itching, otalgia, otorrhoea and deafness, and associated symptoms seen in infants are sleeplessness, tugging at ear, cough, poor feeding, irritability and fever.

History Taking

See Box 13.9 for a suggested framework for taking a history of otitis media.

BOX 13.9

SUGGESTED FRAMEWORK FOR TAKING A HISTORY OF OTITIS MEDIA

Initial approach to the patient: introduction, identification, explanation of role, consent to proceed (parental consent if appropriate)

Exploration of clinical features: the onset and duration of symptoms, including reduced hearing with unilateral or bilateral effect, sudden or gradual onset, otalgia, otorrhoea, itching, recent ear irrigation, ear injury

Associated features to exclude 'red flags': associated symptoms of tinnitus, dizziness and vertigo. Recent irrigation causing pain or discharge – colour and consistency (possible otitis externa, otitis media or internal infection after irrigation or perforation of the ear canal or tympanic membrane). Perichondritis, mastoiditis, hearing loss, fever with systemic illness, anorexia. Severely unwell patients need assessment for meningitis, intracranial abscess, sinus thrombosis and facial nerve paralysis.

Past medical history: recurrence of the same problem, any concurrent aural conditions, any aural surgery such as grommet insertion

Drug history: to include immunosuppressants, chemotherapy, over-the-counter (OTC) and recreational drugs

Allergies: drugs and sensitivities

Social: occupational/leisure risk factors affecting ears, such as ear defenders/headset use/swimming.

Investigations: possible swab for microscopy, culture and sensitivity

---

Examination

See the examination section under 'Earwax' earlier in the chapter. Include a full set of observations, and use the National Early Warning Score (NEWS2; Royal College of Physicians, 2017) if the patient is severely unwell before immediate referral.

Management

Patients may require regular analgesia, such as paracetamol or ibuprofen, at the correct maximum dosage for age.

Otitis media usually resolves in 60% of patients in 24 hours, and most patients will not require antibiotics, which only reduce pain at day 2 and do not prevent deafness (NICE, 2018e). Antibiotics should be avoided unless the patient is systemically unwell and has had symptoms for 4 or more days or in children with bilateral infection and aged under 2 years old or a child with perforation and/or discharge in the ear canal (NICE, 2016b).

If the individual requires antibiotics, the first-line drug of choice is a penicillin (amoxicillin). For those individuals who are allergic to penicillin, clarithromycin can be prescribed (NICE, 2018e). Advice should be given to take the full course of treatment prescribed and to dispose of any ear drops left over after the completion of treatment. Topical antibacterial drops or spray may be given to children over age 12 and to adults but should be discontinued after a maximum of 7 days.

Safety netting is key to review patients whose symptoms may not resolve, and clear instructions must be given regarding follow-up should any of the following occur:

- An increased smelly discharge from the ear
- Excessive pain/tenderness of the ear not resolved by OTC analgesia
- Developing a high temperature and feeling unwell

URINARY CONDITIONS

Lower Urinary Tract Infections

Urinary tract infections (UTIs) are caused by bacteria and rarely by fungi or viruses that involve the kidneys, bladder (cystitis), or urethra. If a UTI is not diagnosed early enough or treated, it can lead to inflammation of the urethra or even pyelonephritis and sepsis (Pope, 2020). Complicated UTIs are those seen in patients with higher risk of complications because of recurrent infections, structural abnormalities, catheterisation, diabetes or immunosuppression (NICE, 2018c).

Aetiology

In 70% to 90% of uncomplicated lower UTI cases, *Escherichia coli* is the causative pathogen, but other organisms, such as *Staphylococcus saprophyticus*, *Proteus mirabilis* and *Klebsiella* species, can be identified less frequently (NICE, 2018c).

Signs and Symptoms

In adults, signs and symptoms include dysuria; urinary urgency, nocturia and urinary frequency; vaginal/

penile discharge; loin, suprapubic and/ or back pain; and haematuria (check if not menstruating; check last menstrual period (LMP) to exclude pregnancy).

Children younger than 3 months (NICE, 2017c) commonly present with fever, vomiting, lethargy, irritability, poor feeding and failure to thrive. Less common signs and symptoms include abdominal pain, jaundice, haematuria and offensive urine. If UTI is suspected, refer urgently to paediatric specialist care and send a clean-catch urine sample for urgent microscopy and culture.

History Taking

See Box 13.10 for a suggested framework for taking a history of lower UTI.

Examination

A full set of observations should be taken, including temperature, pulse, respiratory rate and blood pressure (in adults).

Abdominal examination is required to establish if there is suprapubic tenderness and to exclude abdominal masses (if the GPN has competency in abdominal examination, for referral to GP if not). Appendicitis may also present as dysuria, so it is important to assess all clinical findings and refer as appropriate.

A urine sample should be inspected for cloudiness, offensive smell and visible haematuria.

Dipstick urinalysis is considered as the first diagnostic test to observe for haematuria, nitrites and leucocytes on the test strip (All Wales Medicines Strategy Group (AWMSG), 2018; PHE, 2019).

AWMSG (2018) purports that noncloudy urine is thought to have 97% negative predictive value and thus does not warrant antibiotics unless the patient is particularly unwell or displays risk factors for resistance.

- If nitrite plus blood or leucocytes are present, AWMSG (2018) states this indicates a 92% chance of infection, and absence of all three indicates a 72% chance of no infection.
- If both leukocyte esterase and nitrite are positive, treat as a UTI and start antibiotic as per the national guidelines (NICE, 2018g).
- If both leukocyte esterase and nitrite are negative, UTI is unlikely. But if symptoms persist, re-take a sample.

BOX 13.10

SUGGESTED FRAMEWORK FOR TAKING A HISTORY OF LOWER URINARY TRACT INFECTION

Initial approach to the patient: introduction, identification, explanation of role, consent to proceed (parental consent if appropriate)

Exploration of clinical features: the onset and duration of symptoms, including dysuria, frequency/urgency of micturition, offensive odour to urine, haematuria, pyuria, fever, low abdominal/suprapubic pain, nausea/vomiting, balanitis and vulvitis/vulvovaginitis

In children, symptoms may include fever, vomiting, lethargy, irritability, poor feeding and failure to thrive and, less commonly, abdominal pain, jaundice, haematuria, nappy rash, dermatitis and offensive urine. Check frequency of wet nappies/pants/accidental incontinence.

Associated features to exclude 'red flags': associated symptoms of systemic illness, including high temperature, tachycardia, increased respiratory rate, confusion or other signs of sepsis. Poor stream/retention, especially in older men when prostatic enlargement should be considered. Pyelonephritis (fever and loin pain).

In men: epididymitis (scrotal pain, oedematous and tender epididymis), urethritis (urethral discharge, frequency and dysuria); consider a sexually transmitted infection (STI) in sexually active men. Referral for genitourinary assessment where symptoms persist despite treatment for urinary tract infection (UTI). Meatal stenosis (congenital or acquired post-circumcision). Acute prostatitis (acute-onset fever, frequency, urgency and dysuria). Urological cancer (unexplained persistent haematuria in men over 45 after treatment

should be referred using a cancer referral pathway for an appointment within 2 weeks or nonurgent referral for those aged over 60 (NICE 2017b)).

In children: referral to secondary care if temperature of 38°C or higher in an infant younger than 3 months of age; rigors; tachycardia; pale/mottled/ashen/blue skin, lips, or tongue. Unresponsive social cues, not smiling, decreased activity. Not waking, or if roused, not staying awake. Weak, high-pitched or continuous cry and/or grunting. Nasal flaring, respiratory rate >60 breaths/minute. Moderate or severe chest indrawing. Reduced skin turgor, bulging fontanelle.

Past medical history: recurrence of symptoms; any concurrent urological problems, such as renal colic, calculi or pyelonephritis; past surgical intervention; urinary catheter in situ; diabetes. Pelvic inflammatory disease in women.

In children, previous suspected or confirmed UTI, vesico-ureteric reflux, poor growth, constipation

Drug history: to include immunosuppressants, chemotherapy, over-the-counter (OTC) and recreational drugs

Allergies: drugs and sensitivities

Social: occupational/leisure risk factors – prolonged travel/unusual destinations, poor fluid intake.

Investigations: mid-stream clean-catch urine sample for microscopy, culture and sensitivity in atypical presentations, all men, children/young people under 16 years and pregnant women (NICE, 2018c)

- If leukocyte esterase is positive and nitrite is negative, send a urine sample for microscopy and culture.
- If leukocyte esterase is negative and nitrite is positive, treat as a UTI, as per guidelines for age-appropriate antibiotic.
- If the dipstick result is negative but the symptoms suggest a UTI, the probability of disease is still relatively high.
- Microhaematuria in the absence of UTI requires further evaluation to determine the aetiology

Management

Paracetamol or ibuprofen can be recommended to treat any fever and as an analgesic for pain. Antibiotics may be required for all men, pregnant women and

children initially empirically as per NICE (2018c) guidelines and then as guided by results of microscopy, culture and sensitivity from the midstream specimen of urine (MSU) sample. Resistance to many agents is increasing, particularly in the elderly (>65 years). A higher risk of resistance is associated with those who are care home residents, have had recurrent/resistant UTIs, have been hospitalised for >7 days in the last 6 months, or have experienced recent travel to areas of high antimicrobial resistance (outside northern Europe and Australasia).

Encourage increased intake of oral fluids (approximately 2 L per day in adults) to avoid feeling thirsty and to keep urine pale, encourage regular voiding and educate on wiping from front to back with good hygiene. Treat any constipation if present, and encourage a daily shower rather than a bath. Children in nappies should be changed regularly. Evidence from systematic reviews has indicated that cranberry juice is ineffective in the treatment of an acute attack of cystitis and should not be used by patients taking anticoagulants (NICE, 2018g).

Treatment (Adapted From NICE 2018c)

It is recommended that practitioners consult the full guidelines for antibiotic prescribing as recommended in the current BNF and BNF for Children.

Alkalising agents such as potassium citrate can be useful in burning dysuria to give relief of discomfort in mild UTIs. However, evidence for the effectiveness is weak because no systematic reviews or randomised controlled trials (RCTs) have provided data on cranberry products for UTI in men, nonpregnant women and children (NICE, 2018g).

In nonpregnant women, consider a backup/delayed antibiotic prescription if presenting with mild symptoms of short duration because treatment ideally should be based on an MSU result. With a backup antibiotic prescription, advise why an antibiotic is not needed immediately and to use the prescription if there is no improvement in 48 hours or symptoms worsen at any time.

With all antibiotic prescriptions, advise regarding possible adverse effects of antibiotics, which can include diarrhoea and nausea, and make sure the patient knows how to seek medical help if symptoms worsen at any time, do not improve within 48 hours of taking the antibiotic or if the patient becomes very unwell.

Offer men an immediate prescription and consider a differential diagnosis if symptoms are not resolving in the first 24 to 48 hours after having been treated with a first-line antibiotic.

Assess the need for referral in the case of men for urological assessment for those having frequent re-occurrence.

Antibiotics should be changed if the microorganism is resistant to the prescribed antibiotic on urine culture result, and safety netting is of paramount importance, alongside antimicrobial stewardship in prescribing and carefully communicated advice for self-care.

SUMMARY

The management of minor illness in general practice continues to be an important and developing role for GPNs. People can present on a daily basis with a wide breadth of conditions, some of which can be self-limiting without any intervention and some of which may indicate illness and pathology that is far from minor. The reference to reliable sources of evidence, such as the BNF and NICE guidelines, will always be necessary, as well as liaison within the primary care team and senior colleagues for the most important feature of patient safety and practising within levels of competency. The GPN's role in developing skills of history taking and physical assessment cannot be underestimated as a vital part of the primary care team and service delivery. This can be through opportunistic consultations in the treatment room but increasingly through services designed to meet the needs for urgent or same-day care. However, the impact of managing care in the context of the current COVID-19 pandemic has resulted in considerable change away from face-to-face consultations and towards assessment of patients now being conducted using online methods, all of which adds considerable challenge to the safe and effective process of managing minor illness.

This chapter has explored a range of common minor illnesses that often present within general practice settings and endeavoured to indicate a systematic and evidence-based approach to managing these for early-career GPNs and those developing into these roles in primary care settings.

REFERENCES

Aaron, K., Cooper, T. E., Warner, L., et al. (2018). Ear drops for removal of ear wax. *Cochrane Database of Systematic Reviews, 2018*(7), Article CD012171.

Alfonse, S. A., Fawley, J. D., & Alexa Lu, X. (2015). Conjunctivitis. *Primary Care, 42*(3), 325–345. https://doi.org/10.1016/j.pop.2015.05.001

All Wales Medicines Strategy Group. (2018). *All Wales Antimicrobial Guidance Group. Primary care empirical urinary tract infection treatment guidelines.*

Arroll, B. (2011). Common cold. *Clinical Evidence (BMJ), 3*(1510), 1–27.

Barakat, A. J., Evans, C., Gill, M., et al. (2019). Rapid strep testing in children with recently treated streptococcal pharyngitis. *Pediatric Investigation, 3*(1), 27–30.

British National Formulary. (2020). *Treatment summary.* https://bnf.nice.org.uk/treatment-summary/ear.html

British Medical Journal. (2019). *Cerumen impaction.* https://bestpractice.bmj.com/topics/en-us/1032

Centor, R. M., Witherspoon, J. M., Dalton, H. P., et al. (1981). The diagnosis of strep throat in adults in the emergency room. *Medical Decision Making, 1*(3), 239–246.

Cohen, J. F., Bertille, N., Cohen, R., et al. (2016). Rapid antigen detection test for group A streptococcus in children with pharyngitis. *Cochrane Database of Systematic Reviews, 2016*(7), Article CD010502. http://onlinelibrary.wiley.com/doi/10.1002/14651858.CD010502.pub2/full

College of Optometrists. (2020a). *Corneal abrasions.* https://www.college-optometrists.org/guidance/clinical-management-guidelines/corneal-abrasion.html

College of Optometrists. (2020b). *Ophthalmia neonatorum.* https://www.college-optometrists.org/guidance/clinical-management-guidelines/ophthalmia-neonatorum.html

Drummond, A. (2020). Eye problems. In A. Staten & P. Staten (Eds.), *Practical general practice guidelines for effective clinical management* (7th ed., pp. 371–381). Elsevier.

Farah, B., & Visintini, S. (2018). *Benzydamine for acute sore throat: A review of clinical effectiveness and guidelines. CADTH rapid response report: Summary with critical appraisal.* https://www.ncbi.nlm.nih.gov/books/NBK537954/

Innes, J. A., Dover, A. R., & Fairhurst, K. (Eds.). (2018). *Macleod's clinical examination* (14th ed.). Elsevier.

Kenealy, T., & Arroll, B. (2013). Antibiotics for the common cold and acute purulent rhinitis. *Cochrane Database of Systematic Reviews, 2013*(6), Article CD000247.

Millward, K. (2017). Ear care – An update for nurses (part 2). *Practice Nursing, 28*(8), 332–337.

National Institute for Health and Care Excellence. (2016a). *Common cold. NICE clinical knowledge summaries.*

National Institute for Health and Care Excellence. (2016b). *Earwax.* https://cks.nice.org.uk/earwax.

National Institute for Health and Care Excellence. (2017a). *Corneal abrasion.* https://cks.nice.org.uk/corneal-superficial-injury

National Institute for Health and Care Excellence. (2017b). *Suspected cancer: Recognition and referral* (NICE Guideline NG12). https://www.nice.org.uk/guidance/ng12

National Institute for Health and Care Excellence. (2017c). *UTI in children and young people* (National Institute for Health and Care Excellence Guidance CG054). https://guidance.niceorg.uk/CG054

National Institute for Health and Care Excellence. (2018a). *Centor and FeverPain score. NICE clinical knowledge summaries.*

National Institute for Health and Care Excellence. (2018b). *Conjunctivitis-infective.* https://cks.nice.org.uk/conjunctivitis-infective

National Institute for Health and Care Excellence. (2018c). *Lower urinary tract infection.* https://www.nice.org.uk/guidance/ng109/resources/visual-summary-pdf-6544021069

National Institute for Health and Care Excellence. (2018d). *Otitis media.* https://cks.nice.org.uk/otitis-media-acute

National Institute for Health and Care Excellence. (2018e). *Otitis media prescribing pathway* (NG91). https://www.nice.org.uk/guidance/ng91/resources/visual-summary-pdf-4787282702

National Institute for Health and Care Excellence. (2018f). *Sore throat-acute.* https://cks.nice.org.uk/sore-throat-acute

National Institute for Health and Care Excellence. (2018g). *Urinary tract infection (lower): Antimicrobial prescribing guideline. Evidence review.* https://www.nice.org.uk/guidance/ng109/documents/evidence-review

Nursing and Midwifery Council (NMC). (2018). *The code.* https://www.nmc.org.uk/globalassets/sitedocuments/nmc-publications/nmc-code.pdf

Pope, L. (2020). Urinary and renal problems. In A. Staten & P. Staten (Eds.), *Practical general practice guidelines for effective clinical management* (7th ed., pp. 340–353). Elsevier.

Public Health England. (2017). *The Spotty Book Notes on infectious diseases in schools and nurseries.* South West Health Protection Team.

Public Health England. (2019). *Diagnosis of urinary tract infections. Quick reference tool for primary care for consultation and local adaptation.* https://assets.publishing.service.gov.uk/government/uploads/system/uploads/attachment_data/file/829721/Diagnosis_of_urinary_tract_infections_UTI_diagnostic_flowchart.pdf

Public Health England. (2020). *Annual flu programme.* https://www.gov.uk/government/collections/annual-flu-programme

Public Health Wales. (2020). *About the notification of infectious disease in Wales.*

Royal College of Physicians. (2017). *National Early Warning Score (NEWS2).* https://www.rcplondon.ac.uk/projects/outputs/national-early-warning-score-news-2

Spinks, A., Glasziou, P. P., & Del Mar, C. B. (2013). Antibiotics for sore throats. *Cochrane Database of Systematic Reviews, 2013*(11), Article CD000023.

Staten, A. (2020). Ear, nose and throat problems. In A. Staten & P. Staten (Eds.), *Practical general practice guidelines for effective clinical management* (7th ed., pp. 354–370). Elsevier.

Van Brusselen, D., Vlieghe, E., Schelstraete, P., De Meulder, F., Vandeputte, C., Garmyn, K., Laffut, W., & Van de Voorde, P. (2014). Streptococcal pharyngitis in children: To treat or not to treat? *European Journal of Paediatrics, 173*(10), 1275–1283.

Wiest, E., & Jones, J. S. (2011). Towards evidence-based emergency medicine: Best BETs from the Manchester Royal Infirmary. BET 1: Use of non-sedating antihistamines in the common cold. *Emergency Medicine Journal, 28*(7), 632–633.

14

THE PRACTICE NURSE'S ROLE IN OPTIMISING CHILD HEALTH

PAT COLLIETY

INTRODUCTION

This chapter examines key concepts supporting working with children and young people (CYP). Definitions of childhood and CYP's legal rights are explored, and the issue of consent to treatment is discussed. There is an overview of children's psychological development and how this influences communication with CYP.

Safeguarding and child protection are defined and discussed in the context of the role of the general practice nurse (GPN) and the wider multidisciplinary team.

CYP's physiological norms are outlined, and common reasons for consulting a GPN, such as skin complaints, nutrition and immunisation, are discussed. The role of the GPN as a practitioner and as a member of the multidisciplinary team is explored.

Finally, the need for a child-friendly environment to ensure high-quality care for CYP and their families is discussed.

CARING FOR CHILDREN

What Is a Child?

In Scotland, once a child turns 18, they are legally an adult, although in some contexts, such as child protection orders and children's hearings, a child is defined as someone who is under the age of 16 years. In England, Northern Ireland and Wales, a child is a person who has not yet had their 18th birthday (National Society for the Prevention of Cruelty to Children (NSPCC), 2019a). However, this is not as simple as it sounds because children mature emotionally and cognitively at different rates, and the age of consent for different aspects of life varies within and between the

four countries of the UK. A reflection of this is that it is more usual to refer to 'children and young people' (CYP) than 'children' because this encompasses the wide range of differences between them.

In recent years there has been a massive increase in our understanding of the neuro-development of CYP. When this is combined with knowledge of children's cognitive development, particularly the seminal work of Jean Piaget (Piaget & Inhelder, 1972), it can be seen that CYP vary enormously in their level of physical, intellectual and emotional maturity, and this needs to be taken into account when working with them.

Brain development begins in utero and continues into adulthood, with the simpler neural connections and skills being developed first, then the more complex. By the time the child is 6 years old, 95% of brain development is complete. There is a second spurt in brain growth at about age 10 to 12, and in adolescence, there is pruning of some synapses and strengthening of others. New connections can be made throughout life, and unused connections are pruned from the brain (Harvard Centre on the Developing Child, 2019).

This process begins at the back of the brain, the occipital region, and the prefrontal cortex, at the front of the brain, is the last part to be remodelled, and this process can continue into early adulthood. The prefrontal cortex is responsible for decision-making, problem solving and impulse control. While it is being developed, adolescents may rely on the amygdala, which is associated with impulses, emotions, aggression and instinctive behaviour, to make decisions (Blakemore, 2018).

CHILDREN AND YOUNG PEOPLE'S PHYSIOLOGICAL DEVELOPMENT

The physiology of CYP is different from adults, and the range of normal for blood pressure, heart rate and respiratory rate will vary with their age. Table 14.1 gives an overview of the range of readings for CYP at different ages.

CHILDREN'S PSYCHOLOGICAL DEVELOPMENT/WAYS OF THINKING

Cognitive development is rapid during childhood and adolescence, and there is a range of theories of CYP's cognitive development, as shown in Table 14.2.

When communicating with CYP, it is useful to consider Piaget's theory of cognitive development because he argues that children think in very different ways from adults. For the first 2 years of life, all learning is based on experience; what the child experiences, the child learns. From 7 to 11, they can problem solve but cannot hypothesise and so would find it difficult to answer a 'what if' question. From 11 onward, children can think in abstract terms and hypothesise. They are also able to think about multiple variables and consider multiple outcomes (Cowie, 2019).

It can be seen how Piaget's theory can be used to guide communication with young children. For example, it would be difficult to ask a child of 3 years how they think their actions may affect another person because they cannot conceptualise in this way. Equally, asking a child who has not reached the formal operations stage to consider a hypothetical scenario would be difficult for the child. It is much better to give concrete examples that they can relate to.

CONSENT

The previously described concepts are important when considering the concept of consent. Decisions have to be made by healthcare professionals (HCPs) about CYP's capacity to consent, so an understanding of the way children think helps in this process.

Across the UK, it is generally accepted that a child becomes an adult on their 18th birthday (Children Act 1989), and they have autonomy over their healthcare decisions. Additionally, young people aged 16 and 17 years can, to a more limited extent, make decisions about medical issues independently from their parents. Although rare, their decisions may be overruled by a person with parental authority if it is deemed that it is in the young person's best interests to do, for

TABLE 14.1			
Range of Physiological Readings for Children and Young People			
Age	Respirations	Heart rate	Blood Pressure
Neonate (under 28 days)		100–205	Diastolic 35–53 Systolic 67–84
Infant (1 month to 1 year)	30–53	100–190	Diastolic 37–56 Systolic 72–104
Toddler (1–2 years)	22–37	98–140	Diastolic 42–63 Systolic 86–106
Pre-school (3–5 years)	20–28	80–120	Diastolic 46–72 Systolic 89–112
School age (6–11 years)	18–25	75–118	Diastolic 57–76 Systolic 97–115
Adolescence	12–20	60–100	Diastolic 61–80 Systolic 102–120

Adapted from Novak, C., & Gill, P. (2018). Pediatric vital signs reference chart. *Peds Cases.* https://www.pedscases.com/pediatric-vital-signs-reference-chart)

TABLE 14.2
Cognitive Development Theories

Developmental Theory	Key Concepts	Associated Concepts
Psychosexual Freud	Child progresses through stages of psychosexual development to reach maturity Oral (0–1 years) Anal (1–3 years) Phallic (3–5 years) Latent (5 years–puberty) Genital (adolescence)	Fixation Libido Ego Superego Id Oedipus and Electra complexes Penis envy
Cognitive Piaget	Child progresses through stages of cognitive development Sensorimotor (0–2 years) Pre-operational (2–7 years) Concrete operational (7 years–adolescence) Formal operations (adolescence onward)	Object permanence Symbolic thought Operational thought Abstract thought
Social learning Bandura	People learn from each other	Observation Imitation Modelling Scaffolding
Behaviourism Skinner Pavlov	Behaviour is learned through interaction with the environment	Stimulus–response

example, if refusing treatment would lead to mental or physical harm (Care Quality Commission (CQC), 2018).

A landmark ruling was made in *Gillick v. West Norfolk & Wisbech Area Health Authority and Department of Health and Social Security* (1985). The judgement from the case set out criteria to determine if a child has the capacity to consent to treatment, and this is known as the 'Gillick test' to determine if the child is 'Gillick competent'. A child under the age of 16 can consent to treatment if they demonstrate sufficient intelligence and understanding to fully understand the proposed treatment. This includes understanding why the treatment is needed, what effects and risks it may have, what the success rate is and if there are any alternatives to the treatment. The child needs to be deemed Gillick competent for each treatment decision. If the child is not deemed to be Gillick competent, then consent is sought from the person who has parental responsibility for the child. If an HCP

accepts that a child is Gillick competent and the child consents, a person with parental responsibility cannot overrule that consent. However, if a child with Gillick competence refuses treatment, then consent may be obtained from a person with parental responsibility. This raises important ethical issues; for example, if a child of 15 refuses consent for travel vaccines and a parent insists that the vaccine is given, legally this is correct, although not ethically. The GPN should try to find out why the child is refusing – it could be a needle phobia – and try to reach a solution other than forcibly injecting the child.

The term *Fraser guidelines* is often used interchangeably with *Gillick competence* despite Fraser guidelines being used specifically to determine if a child can consent to sexual health or contraceptive advice and treatment. The guidelines are clear that the HCP should encourage the young person to talk to their parents about their sexual health or allow the HCP to do so on their behalf. However, if the young person refuses to do so, then advice and treatment can be given if the young person is very likely to either begin to or continue to have sexual intercourse without contraceptive treatment. Also, if the treatment is in the young person's best interest, their mental or physical health is likely to suffer unless they receive the advice or treatment and they have sufficient intelligence and maturity to understand the treatment and any implications of it.

With regard to Scots law, and in relation to healthcare decisions, the Age of Legal Capacity (Scotland) Act 1991 details that individuals over the age of 16 years have the presumptive capabilities of adults, and those under 16 years require evidential testing. Consequently, practitioners must establish that an individual capably understands the nature and possible consequences of procedural treatment. This demonstrates similarities with Gillick competence in establishing CYP's capability to provide valid consent.

If the previously outlined criteria are not met, then the HCP has grounds to break confidentiality. There are also grounds if there is any suspicion that the child is being pressurised to seek advice and treatment or they are being sexually exploited.

Although there is not a specific lower age for either Fraser guidelines or Gillick competence to be used, it is not seen as safe or appropriate for a child younger than 13 years to consent to treatment without involving someone with parental responsibility (CQC, 2018). This should be borne in mind when working with young people in settings such as general practice surgeries and walk-in centres because the young person may be attending by themselves, without a responsible adult, and the GPN will have to make a decision about whether or not they are competent to give consent.

CHILD PROTECTION AND SAFEGUARDING

Safeguarding is protecting children from harm and promoting their welfare, and child protection is part of this and focuses on protecting CYP who either are suffering or are at risk of suffering significant harm (NSPCC, 2019b). Child abuse or neglect is where a child or young person's welfare has not been protected, and so they are not safeguarded and are in need of child protection. All CYP need safeguarding; individual children and young people may require child protection.

Safeguarding is defined as follows in *Working Together to Safeguard Children* (Department for Education (DfE), 2018):

- Protecting children from maltreatment
- Preventing impairment of children's health or development
- Ensuring that children are growing up in circumstances consistent with the provision of safe and effective care
- Taking action to enable all children to have the best outcomes

This document outlines practitioners' responsibilities in relation to safeguarding and states that a child-centred approach is crucial and that the child must remain the focus when decisions are being made about them and that practitioners need to work in partnership with them and their families. It notes that the risk to the child may come from within their family and that the needs of the child must come first.

It also notes that no single practitioner has a full view of a child and their life. A recurrent theme in child death reviews has been poor communication between practitioners and agencies. It is important that practitioners understand that 'safeguarding is everyone's responsibility' (DfE, 2018, p. 10). This means that practitioners have to understand each other's roles, and they are clear about their role in safeguarding. As well as reading the statutory guidance in *Working Together* (DfE, 2018), GPNs need to make themselves aware of their local guidance and safeguarding procedures. Within each practice, there should be a safeguarding lead. If a GPN has any safeguarding concerns, these should be discussed with the safeguarding lead and fully documented in the records.

The NSPCC (2019c) identified categories of abuse: physical, psychological/emotional, neglect, child sexual exploitation, domestic abuse, bullying and cyberbullying, female genital mutilation and sexual abuse. Sometimes there are obvious physical signs that suggest that there is a safeguarding issue, such as bruising in a pre-mobile child or an injury that is inconsistent with the caregiver's explanation of how the injury occurred. Often, however, it is much less obvious, and this is why it is vital to raise any concerns. The NSPCC has published a list of common signs, as shown in Box 14.1.

The signs themselves do not mean that there is a safeguarding issue, but they are signs that something is happening in that CYP's life that needs further investigation. It is also important to assess the behaviour of caregivers; if there is anything in their behaviour that raises concerns about their ability to care for children, this needs to be escalated.

The legal age of consent to have sex is 16 years old in the UK. GPNs, as a result of their role in contraception and sexual health and screening, will have contact with young people who are sexually active. The law aims to protect children from exploitation rather than penalise under-16s who are having mutually consensual sex. However, being underage should always be seen as a possible indicator of child sexual exploitation. The law clearly says that no one under the age of 13 years can legally consent to sexual activity, whether or not they are deemed to be Gillick competent, so anyone who engages in sexual activity with a child under the age of 13 is breaking the law and should always be referred to child protection services (CQC, 2018).

It is also illegal to pay or arrange for the sexual services of a child, or to take, show or distribute indecent images of a child. It is also illegal for someone in a position of trust to engage in sexual activity with a child or young person under the age of 18 years who is in the care of that organisation (Sexual Offences Act 2003).

BOX 14.1
COMMON SIGNS INDICATING SAFEGUARDING CONCERNS

- Unexplained changes in behaviour or personality
- Always choosing to wear clothes that cover their body
- Becoming withdrawn
- Becoming uncharacteristically aggressive
- Poor bond or relationship with a parent
- Running away or going missing
- Knowledge of adult issues inappropriate for their age
- Seeming anxious
- Lacks social skills and has few friends, if any

From National Society for the Prevention of Cruelty to Children. (2019c). *Spotting the signs of child abuse.* https://www.nspcc.org.uk/what-is-child-abuse/spotting-signs-child-abuse/

If a young person under the age of 16 discloses something that raises safeguarding concerns, if they are not Gillick competent, the GPN must raise what the young person has disclosed as a safeguarding concern using the safeguarding process. If the young person is Gillick competent but their disclosure requires further action, either to protect them or if it is in the public interest, the GPN must still escalate the issue to the safeguarding lead within the general practice or, if they are not available, the multiagency safeguarding hub (MASH), which will offer advice and guidance (CQC, 2018).

Practitioners should try to gain consent to share information with other practitioners and/ or organisations where there is a safeguarding concern. It is deemed good practice to be open and transparent about concerns with those involved, unless doing so would endanger the child or young person. However, if consent is not given, either by the child or young person or their caregiver, then the practitioner can break confidentiality if it is in the best interest of the child (DfE, 2018). If a child or young person says that they want to disclose an issue, but it is confidential, caution is required in promising to keep this confidential because this may well be a promise that, as a registered practitioner, the GPN cannot keep.

Safeguarding is complex and can be distressing for the GPN. It is therefore important for GPNs to know who the safeguarding lead is and ensure familiarity with the local policies and procedures. If there are any concerns, GPNs should seek advice and keep meticulous records. GPNs should protect their own professional and personal wellbeing by attending/seeking clinical supervision. Safeguarding is everybody's business, which means that GPNs are part of a team, so support should be sought from that team.

VACCINATION AND IMMUNISATION

The UK has a well-developed and robust immunisation system. Immunisation is the process whereby a person becomes immune or resistant to an infectious disease by the administration of a vaccine, which stimulates the body's immune system to protect the recipient against the disease (World Health Organisation (WHO), 2019).

Public Health England (PHE) and National Health Service (NHS) Health Scotland publish a routine immunisation schedule every year (NHS Scotland, 2019; PHE, 2019a), which sets out at what age vaccines should be given. The schedule starts at 8 weeks of age, which is when passive immunity from the mother's antibodies starts to wane, and for children, goes up to 14 years of age or year 9.

NHS Digital publishes an annual report of vaccination coverage, and in the report covering 2019/20, their summary concluded that coverage for all routine vaccination in children aged 12-24 months and 5 years has decreased. In Scotland, although the immunisation uptake rates were slightly higher, there were still declines in the uptake rates for all the immunisations (Information Services Division, National Services Scotland, 2019).

In August 2019, PHE reported that although the WHO had declared in 2017 that the UK had eliminated measles (an absence of circulating measles, high coverage of vaccine and robust reporting systems) in 2019, that was no longer the case, and the transmission of measles had been re-established (PHE, 2019a). For the vaccine to be effective, two doses are required, and although take-up of the initial dose has met the WHO target of 95% at age 5 years, take-up of the second dose is only 87.4%. At a population level, this has had an impact on achieving herd immunity, which is where enough people in the community are immune to an infectious disease so that it cannot spread through the population. In the case of measles, 19 out of 20 people need to be immune.

The reasons for the variation in vaccination take-up rates are complex. Factors such as reporting of flawed studies and the influence of social media, where 'anti-vaxxers' circulate misinformation about vaccination, need to be considered. It is important, therefore, that when engaging with CYP and their families, HCPs can competently advise on vaccines and are able to provide evidence-based information.

Consent is needed for immunisations to be given. For infants and younger children, the parent or person with parental responsibility gives this. For older children, the issues discussed previously are relevant, in terms of both consent and psychological development. When seeking consent and explaining what will happen, it is important to be aware of how they understand the world. For example, a child who is in middle childhood is just beginning to hypothesise. They would find it very difficult to think about what might happen, rather than the more concrete what will happen (Cowie, 2019).

For all healthcare interactions, it is important that the HCP involves CYP in discussions about them and that those conversations are open and honest. CYP should be listened to and their views respected. They usually want to know about any interventions and illnesses, any risks, possible pain or discomfort and who will be involved in their care (General Medical Council (GMC), 2019). zIn fact, they need the same information that you would give an adult, but provided in an age-appropriate way.

When communicating with CYP, appropriate language needs to be used, as well as other forms of communication, for example, pictures, stories and using toys to explain what is happening or may happen to a child. The surroundings of a conversation are also important to a child; a stark clinical room may be intimidating, so having toys or books on hand for these consultations can be of great benefit in putting the child more at ease. For older CYP, think about whether it would be beneficial to see the child or young person without their parent. They may need advice or help that they do not feel that they could ask for if their parent was present (GMC, 2019).

ALLERGIES

It is estimated that 1 in 4 people in the UK are affected by an allergy at some time in their lives. Children are particularly prone to allergies, some of which disappear as the child develops; others are lifelong. An allergen is a substance, food or drink that stimulates the body to have a reaction to it. The most common allergens include pollen (hay fever), animal hair or flakes of skin, insect stings and bites, latex, some medicines, household chemicals and food (NHS, 2018).

There is a difference between food intolerance and food allergy. *Food intolerance* is a term that describes a range of adverse reactions to food, including allergic reactions, where the body's immune system reacts inappropriately to food. The severity of the reaction can range from mild to potentially fatal. It is important that people are properly tested for food allergies and intolerances before making dramatic dietary changes because they may affect their nutritional balance.

This is even more important for children, whose nutritional needs are different from those of adults, such as the need for vitamin supplements and either breast milk or formula milk only until the age of 6 months. After this, there is the gradual introduction of solid food and, from the age of a year, the introduction of whole cow's milk or alternative milk. If a parent believes that their child is allergic to a food, such as milk or eggs, it is important that this is investigated so that a nutritionally balanced diet can be planned, ensuring that the removal of a group of food types does not inadvertently mean that the child becomes nutritionally deficient. It is also possible that dietary change before investigation could make diagnosis more difficult, for example, with coeliac disease.

Although the majority of allergies are mild and can be self-managed, some are severe and even life threatening. In 2015 it was reported that 21 million adults, or between a quarter and a third of adults in the UK, have at least one allergy, and half of under 18s have one or more allergy. A total of 900 million pounds per year is spent on allergies in primary care (Pillai, 2015), which illustrates how important this issue is to GPNs. Adults can buy a range of over-the-counter (OTC) medicines, such as antihistamines or decongestants, to help them to manage their allergies. Although OTC remedies are available for children, it is important that parents know what it is that their child is either intolerant or allergic to, so it is more appropriate to refer a child to an HCP who is trained in dealing with childhood allergies rather than suggest OTC medications for a child.

The multidisciplinary team plays a critical role in dealing with potential and actual allergies. The general practitioner (GP) is key in diagnosing allergies and formulating a plan of care for the child with other members of the team. GPNs will see children on a regular basis during the first few months of life for immunisations, and this may be the point at which parents voice their concerns. Health visitors have in-depth knowledge of infant and child nutrition, and many are also prescribers. School nurses have high levels of knowledge and skills in relation to school-age children and dealing with health needs, such as allergies, in a school setting. Community children's nurses may also be involved if a child has a severe allergy and is at risk

of anaphylaxis, where training within a school in relation to the use of an epi-pen may be needed. EPIPEN AUTO-INJECTOR 0.3MG (Child (body weight 26 kg and above) or EPIPEN JR AUTO-INJECTOR 0.15MG (Child (body weight 15–25 kg) (Joint Formulary Committee, British National Formulary 2021).

OBESITY AND EATING DISORDERS

Obesity and eating disorders are becoming more prevalent amongst CYP in the UK. The National Child Measurement Programme (NCMP) measures the weight of children in reception and in year 6. The figures for 2017 to 2018 show that there is a significant downward trend in boys in reception compared with previous years but a significant upward trend for girls in reception and both girls and boys in year 6. The prevalence for underweight shows a downward trend for boys and girls in reception and girls in year 6. There are differences between areas of most and least deprivation, with a higher prevalence of obesity in the most deprived areas (PHE, 2019b).

It is not uncommon for older children and young people to be concerned about eating, their shape and their weight. When these concerns become obsessive, they may turn into an eating disorder, the two most common of which are anorexia nervosa and bulimia nervosa. Both of these disorders are more common in girls, but boys may also suffer from them. It may be difficult to spot these disorders, but signs such as weight loss or unusual weight change are clear indicators.

Obesity and eating disorders need to be managed by a multidisciplinary team. Health visitors work with parents of infants and children to the age of 5. They have expert knowledge of infant and child nutrition, including the establishment and maintenance of breastfeeding. School nurses have in-depth knowledge and skills in working with school-age children and can advise on healthy eating and mental health issues. The GP would be key in diagnosing and referring the child or young person where necessary, for example, to a dietician, who has a clear role with their expertise in nutrition and dietetics. Where necessary, the child or young person may be referred to a specialist service, such as child and adolescent mental health services or an eating disorder team.

SKIN

Parents often present to general practice with concerns about their child's skin, such as cradle cap, nappy rash or eczema. Cradle cap is a noninfectious and noncontagious skin condition that presents as patches of greasy and yellow crusts on the infant's head and less commonly on the eyebrows, the nappy area and the nose. When the crusts flake, the skin underneath may look red. The advice from NHS online is to use either baby oil or vegetable oil (not peanut oil because of the risk of allergy) to soften the crusts and to wash the baby's hair regularly using baby shampoo. In the vast majority of cases, it does not need medical attention. However, if it does not resolve after a few weeks, spreads all over the baby's body or shows signs of being infected, the parents should be advised to seek advice from their GP.

Another very common problem is nappy rash, where the skin around the nappy area is irritated by contact with urine and faeces. Keeping the area clean and dry is essential, and there is a range of barrier creams available to reduce contact between the baby's skin and the urine and faeces. In the vast majority of cases, it is a minor condition that can be managed by the parents. However, if the rash does not respond, the parents should consult an HCP, who may prescribe steroids to reduce the inflammation, antibiotics if the skin has become infected or an antifungal cream if the area is infected with *Candida* (thrush).

It is estimated that about 20% of children have some form of atopic eczema. In 80% of cases, this develops before the age of 5, but many develop it in the first year of life. It may resolve as the child gets older, with half of all cases showing improvement by the age of 11 and two-thirds by the age of 16 (NHS Inform, 2019). The severity of symptoms varies, but they are characterised by redness and itchy, dry and cracked skin. There may also be secondary infection where the skin has been damaged by the patient's scratching.

Eczema may be self-managed with the application of emollients and avoidance of triggers. However, many people seek advice and treatment from their GP or other HCPs, such as a GPN, nurse practitioner, health visitor or school nurse. An HCP with appropriate knowledge and skills would be able to diagnose it, and a prescriber would be able to prescribe emollients, steroids or antihistamines. They would also be able to help to identify triggers and refer to a specialist service if needed.

Parents may also consult an HCP about sunburn. If a baby or young child has sunburn, medical advice should be sought because their skin is more delicate than an adult's, and they could become dehydrated very quickly. Once the initial sunburn has been treated, the parents should be educated about sun safety for their child; for example, using a sunscreen with a high sun-protection factor (SPF), wearing a hat, covering up and staying in the shade.

Acne is a very common condition in adolescence and is caused by blocked sebaceous glands in the pores of the skin. Sometimes, the normal skin bacteria (*Propionibacterium acnes*) multiply in the oil buildup and cause inflammation and the formation of pus-filled spots. Treatment depends on the severity, and widely ranging products are available OTC. However, where the skin does not respond to self-treatment, an HCP should be consulted to diagnose the condition and prescribe appropriate treatment. This may consist of topical treatments such as benzoyl peroxide to cleanse the skin or topical antibiotics. Systemic antibiotics may also be prescribed. Most cases improve with treatment and also as the patient ages. Where there is no improvement, referral to a specialist service may be needed.

Acne can be very distressing, affecting body image and self-esteem. Patients may need referral to school nurses, who are skilled in supporting young people with mental health needs, or a specialist service, such as Children and Adolescent Mental Health Services (CAMHS).

WHAT IS A CHILD-FRIENDLY ENVIRONMENT?

For a range of reasons, GPNs are very likely to come into contact with infants and CYP. Understanding their physical and psychological development is key to effectively working with them, as is knowledge of the wider multidisciplinary team that supports patients and families. It is also important to understand the concept of family-centred care, where the HCP considers the child as both an individual and part of a family unit. Decisions need to be made in partnership, and the family is the unit of care.

One could argue that any healthcare environment needs to be child-friendly, that is, free of environmental hazards and having a range of appropriate stimuli and activities. Keeping objects out of the reach of infants and young children may seem obvious but is critical; young children explore their environments through touch, so it is vital to ensure that what they touch is safe to touch! It is also essential that information is available in a way that is appropriate for their stage of development; storybooks and pictures can be very helpful. Toys and pictures have the double use of being a stimulus to keep the child occupied and also a means of distraction. If a child becomes distressed, it may be possible to use distraction to help them through the situation, such as books, music, controlled breathing and games. Many of these techniques are simple and can be applied in any setting; if more complex and in-depth interventions are required, the family may need to be referred to a hospital play specialist or a play therapist.

A child-friendly environment needs an appreciation of CYP's needs and the resources to meet them, whether they are physical, intellectual or emotional. Key to this is an appreciation that CYP are not adults on a smaller scale; there are physical and psychological differences that make working with them both challenging and fascinating and highly rewarding.

SUMMARY

This chapter has explored the salient issues for GPNs in caring for CYP in general practice. Research regarding the physiological, developmental and psychological needs of CYP has provided the context for effective and compassionate care that is tailored to the individual and considers safeguarding as a priority for these vulnerable members of society. The GPN's role within the multidisciplinary team has been considered, acknowledging the opportunities for developing a welcoming and child-friendly environment, along with efficient, evidence-based care provision for whole families.

REFERENCES

Age of Legal Capacity (Scotland) Act 1991. https://www.legislation.gov.uk/ukpga/1991/50/contents

Blakemore, S. J. (2018). The neuroscience of the teenage brain [Video]. https://www.youtube.com/watch?v=yQXhFa8dRCI

Care Quality Commission. (2018). Nigel's surgery 8: Gillick competency and Fraser guidelines. https://www.cqc.org.uk/guidance-providers/gps/nigels-surgery-8-gillick-competency-fraser-guidelines

Children Act 1989. http://www.legislation.gov.uk/ukpga/1989/41/section/17

Cowie, H. (2019). From birth to sixteen (2nd ed.). Routledge.

Department for Education. (2018). Working together to safeguard children. https://assets.publishing.service.gov.uk/government/uploads/system/uploads/attachment_data/file/779401/Working_Together_to_Safeguard-Children.pdf

General Medical Council. (2019). Ethical guidance. 0–18 years: Guidance for all doctors. Communication. https://www.gmc-uk.org/ethical-guidance/ethical-guidance-for-doctors/0-18-years/communication

Gillick v West Norfolk & Wisbech Area Health Authority, UKHL 7 (17 October 1985). Available via (BAILII) in The Law Reports (Appeal Cases) [1986] AC 112. http://www.bailii.org/uk/cases/UKHL/1985/7.html

Harvard Centre on the Developing Child. (2019). Brain architecture. https://developingchild.harvard.edu/science/key-concepts/brain-architecture/

Information Services Division, National Services Scotland. (2019). Childhood immunisation statistics. https://www.isdscotland.org/Health-Topics/Child-Health/Publications/2019-03-26/2019-03-26-Childhood-Immunisation-Report.pdf

Joint Formulary Committee. (2021). British National Formulary. http://www.medicinescomplete.com

National Health Service. (2018). Allergies. https://www.nhs.uk/conditions/allergies/

National Society for the Prevention of Cruelty to Children. (2019a). A child's legal rights. Legal definitions. https://www.nspcc.org.uk/preventing-abuse/child-protection-system/legal-definition-child-rights-law/legal-definitions/

National Society for the Prevention of Cruelty to Children. (2019b). Safeguarding children and child protection. https://learning.nspcc.org.uk/safeguarding-child-protection/

National Society for the Prevention of Cruelty to Children. (2019c). Child abuse and neglect. https://learning.nspcc.org.uk/child-abuse-and-neglect/

NHS Digital. (2020). Childhood vaccination coverage statistics–England 2019-2020. https://digital.nhs.uk/data-and-information/publications/statistical/nhs-immunisation-statistics/england---2019-20

NHS Inform. (2019). Atopic eczema. https://www.nhsinform.scot/illnesses-and-conditions/skin-hair-and-nails/atopic-eczema

NHS Scotland. (2019). Immunisation. http://www.healthscotland.scot/health-topics/immunisation/pregnancy-and-baby-immunisations

Piaget, J., & Inhelder, B. (1972). *The psychology of the child*. Basic Books.

Pillai, P. (2015). *General overview of allergy in the UK*. Guy's and St. Thomas' NHS Foundation Trust. https://www.guysandstthomas. nhs.uk/resources/membership/health-seminars/2015/20150929-allergy-presentations.pdf

Public Health England. (2019a). *The routine immunisation schedule*. https://www.guidelines.co.uk/immunisation-and-vaccination/ phe-uk-immunisation-schedule-green-book-chapter-11/454744.article

Public Health England. (2019b). *Trends in children's body mass index between 2006 to 2007 and 2017 to 2018*. https://app.box. com/s/hbddn16digjdhs24ocha6u40x9j9xsqh

Public Health Scotland. (2020). *Childhood immunisation statistics Scotland*. https://beta.isdscotland.org/find-publications-and-data/population-health/child-health/childhood-immunisation-statistics-scotland/23-june-2020/

Sexual Offences Act 2003. https://www.legislation.gov.uk/ ukpga/2003/42/section/74

World Health Organisation. (2019). *Immunization*. https://www. who.int/topics/immunization/en/

15

THE PRACTICE NURSE'S ROLE IN PROMOTING SEXUAL AND REPRODUCTIVE HEALTH

ALISON MACLEOD CRAIG

INTRODUCTION

The reduction in transmission of sexually acquired infection and prevention of unplanned and unwanted pregnancy are public health priorities. Sexual and reproductive healthcare (SRH) is a firmly embedded aspect of the role of the general practice nurse (GPN) that is most commonly associated with the provision of contraceptive care, cervical screening and low-risk testing for sexually transmitted infections (STIs). Along with the general practice setting, SRH services manage more complex and higher-risk clinical presentations and in some instances also provide a range of highly specialist medical gynaecology, abortion, gender and HIV outpatient care. In the last two decades there have been significant technological advances, economic drivers and new evidence that have led to a reconfiguration of the way in which SRH services are delivered.

This chapter, in addressing the SRH of adults, provides information that will enable practice nurses to develop the confidence to assess risk for STI and, where appropriate, offer testing and manage common and significant presentations. It also provides information and links to the most up-to-date evidence-based guidance on contraception and touches on emerging fields of practice, such as the provision of pre-exposure prophylaxis for HIV (PrEP) and transgender healthcare.

CERVICAL SCREENING AND GENERAL PRACTICE NURSES

Essential skills for GPNs have included cervical screening (Health Education England, 2017), and the

training to acquire the necessary knowledge and skills for competence has often been part of their early development in the role. The National Health Service (NHS) Cervical Screening Programme Guidance for the training of cervical sample takers (Public Health Agency, 2016) outlines that training for sample takers should include a theoretical programme followed by a period of supervised practice and assessment of clinical competency. Across the UK, training for sample takers is similarly offered by the Northern Ireland Cervical Screening Programme (Public Health Agency, 2016; NHS Education for Scotland, 2012), NHS Education for Scotland and Cervical Screening Wales.

The aim of cervical screening programmes is to reduce the incidence of and morbidity and mortality from invasive cervical cancer. Whilst cervical screening saves lives, as an invasive procedure, it also has the potential to cause both physical and psychological harm to women invited. This reinforces the imperative for quality assurance of training, assessment of competency and regular updating through continued professional development (CPD).

Training standards for sample takers have been key to the success of cervical screening programmes, which have had a significant impact on cervical cancer mortality since commencement in 1988, saving an estimated 5000 lives a year (Public Health England (PHE), 2019), and the education pathway has been updated to reflect developments in liquid-based cytology and human papilloma virus (HPV) testing as the primary screen following the introduction of a vaccination programme for young adults (PHE, 2020). The Clinical Professional Group for

Cervical Screening Education and Training (CSET) emphasises the need for initial high-quality training, supervision and assessment of a required minimum standard, ensuring adherence to a common core of learning for all sample takers. Training providers require accreditation to validate the quality and rigour of their programmes. GPNs need to have protected time and funding to access their initial training for competency and then the requisite supervision and assessment in practice with an experienced cervical screening mentor and assessor. The attainment of a certificate of completed training and recommended record keeping are the starting point, with the requirement for sample takers to undertake a minimum of 3 hours of update training every 3 years thereafter.

The desired positive outcomes of the NHS Cervical Screening Programme can only be protected by consistent and ongoing investment in GPNs (and other practitioners). Their service provision for eligible women (and trans men with a cervix) who access general practice is key to cervical screening and also to sexual and reproductive health when the nature of such consultations may be an ideal opportunity for GPNs to assess risk for STI, contraception and, where appropriate, offer testing and manage common presentations.

SEXUALLY TRANSMITTED INFECTIONS

The World Health Organisation (WHO) website (WHO, 2019) provides a helpful summary of global trends in STI rates and evidence of change as programmes of vaccination begin to take effect. STIs are spread predominantly by sexual contact, including vaginal, anal and oral sex. Additionally, many STIs can also be transmitted from mother to child during pregnancy and childbirth. In women, repeated or untreated infection can lead to chronic pain and infertility and can cause serious obstetric and neonatal complications in pregnancy.

The principles of STI management include early diagnosis, testing, early initiation of treatment and partner notification to break the chain of infection. STI risk assessment should be included as part of routine clinical history taking in general practice, with a low threshold for initiating STI testing in primary care (Pope, 2020).

History Taking

After eliciting a comprehensive history (see Chapter 6) of presenting symptoms, including medication, obstetric and gynaecological history and contraceptive use, a detailed sexual history should be taken. An assessment of 'lifetime' risk will indicate whether testing for blood-borne viruses (BBVs) is indicated. Throughout this chapter, the word *women* is used specifically in relation to 'cis women' – a term used to denote women whose gender identity matches the sex they were assigned at birth.

For contact(s), current and within the last 3 months, important factors affecting risk include the relationship status, partner gender, the types of sex that took place, use of condoms, the partner's place of origin and consent to sex. Questioning should be private, sensitive, inclusive and direct, avoiding euphemisms. This can feel intrusive or awkward, particularly in a general practice setting where patients may not present with an open and specific concern about STI. Box 15.1 provides some helpful suggestions about how to approach this.

Examination

Examination should be performed in all patients with symptoms. Nurses can perform female genital examination where they have demonstrated the necessary competence (Royal College of Nursing (RCN), 2016) and, in accordance with the Code of the Nursing and Midwifery Council (NMC, 2018), secure and document consent to perform an intimate examination for the specific purpose of eliciting signs of infection. Patients should be advised that this examination is not for the purpose of gynaecological investigation. Box 15.2 outlines the components of examination.

In undertaking genital examination, the GPN should be aware of the possibility of some patients from certain ethnic groups (Africa, Asia and Middle East) presenting with female genital mutilation (FGM) or indicating risk of the same; this is discussed later in the chapter.

Testing for STI

Nucleic acid amplification testing (NAAT) is widely available for the diagnosis of *Chlamydia trachomatis*, *Gonorrhoea*, herpes simplex (HSV), and increasingly for *Trichomonas vaginitis* (TV) and for early syphilis (ulcers) (Pope, 2020). When culture or microscopy are required, the swabs required will depend on the

---

BOX 15.1
SEXUAL HISTORY TAKING

1. Start with open questions: 'Tell me...'; 'Tell me about that...'; 'So tell me the story...'
2. Use well-known anatomical terms (e.g., 'vagina' rather than 'vulva'): 'So you mean on the lips of your vagina?'
3. Personal values might affect questions; for example, the question 'When was your last previous partner?' assumes serial monogamy. Use inclusive words such as 'partner' rather than 'boyfriend'.
4. Consider more open questions to establish detail: 'Tell me more about how this pain developed...'; 'What is the discharge like?'
5. A simple framing statement before taking the history avoids a sense of apology or embarrassment: 'So, thinking about your sex life...'; 'Some questions about your sex life...'; 'Just so I know what tests to do, tell me...have you or your partners ever injected drugs?'
6. A focus on events helps avoid subliminal personal bias or heteronormative assumptions: 'When did you last have sex, any sort of sex?'
7. A range of possible answers allows the 'unacceptable' response to be given: 'Was that a one-off thing, with a regular partner, or something else?'; 'Have your partners been men, women or both?'; 'Was that oral sex, vaginal sex, anal sex...or all of them?'; 'So that was without a condom?'; 'Do you ever use condoms?'; 'When did you last have sober sex?'; 'When did you last have sex with anyone else/any other partner?'
8. The partners' place of origin is a major determinant of STI risk: 'So was he/she from [this town/city] or elsewhere?'; 'Any partners from outside the UK?'
9. Balance gentleness with directness: 'So did everything happen with your consent...or perhaps not?'
10. Innocent inquisitiveness can reveal social/cultural factors: 'I really don't know much about which dating apps people use to meet up; can you tell me more?'

BOX 15.2
GENITAL EXAMINATION

INSPECT:
Pubic hair and surrounding skin for pubic lice and skin rashes

MEN:
Scrotum, perianal area, shaft and glans penis with retraction of foreskin for warts, ulcers, erythema or excoriation. Urethral meatus for any discharge or swelling, and check the scrotum /testes for any tenderness or swelling.

WOMEN:
Labia, clitoris, introitus, perineum and perianal area for warts, ulcers, erythema or excoriation
Skene's and Bartholin's glands for any discharge or swelling, vaginal walls and cervix for erythema, discharge, warts, ulcers, contact bleeding or raised lesions. *Consider bimanual pelvic examination to assess cervical motion tenderness and adnexal tenderness or masses.*

- CT/GC NAAT from other sites of potential exposure (throat and/or rectum) in women or men who have sex with men (MSM)
- HSV and syphilis NAAT if ulcers or fissures are seen
- Blood sample for syphilis and HIV serology with hepatitis B testing if they or any of their sexual partners are from areas of high prevalence (e.g., sub-Saharan Africa or Asia). Hepatitis C testing should also be undertaken if there is any history of injecting drugs.

Management of STIs in General Practice

Some STIs lend themselves well to management in general practice, whereas others are better dealt with in specialist settings where on-site microscopy is available and where treatment options, antibiotic resistance, follow-up and more complex partner notification can all be addressed. Partner notification is important to break the chain of infection. There are three options: 'patient referral', in which the patient agrees that they will tell their recent partner(s) themselves; 'provider referral', in which recent partner(s) details are passed to health advisers working in sexual health centres so that they can establish contact; and

laboratory facilities available locally and the presenting symptoms. Tests consist of the following:

- CT/GC NAAT
  - Men – urine sample (first 20 ml voided)
  - Women – self-obtained lower vaginal swab

'conditional referral', where provider referral is initiated by health advisers if patient referral has not occurred after an agreed period has elapsed. Enhanced partner-notification strategies include providing patients with antibiotic treatment for partner(s) or with pharmacy vouchers for treatment and the use of innovative web or mobile apps to allow patients to inform partner(s) while preserving anonymity. Patients are advised to abstain from sex until they and their partner(s) have completed treatment.

STI Infections – Signs, Symptoms and Management

The following list provides brief information about the main STIs, causes, common signs and symptoms, management approaches and when to refer to sexual health services. For more extensive explanation on specific infections and treatment details, GPNs are advised to refer to evidence-based guidance found on the British Association for Sexual Health and HIV (BASHH) website. A link to this website is provided in Box 15.3.

Chlamydia

Chlamydia (CT) is caused by the bacterium *C. trachomatis* and is the most commonly reported curable bacterial STI in the UK, with the highest prevalence rates in 15- to 24-year-olds. If untreated, infection may resolve spontaneously, with up to 50% of infections resolving approximately 12 months from initial

---

BOX 15.3
SEXUAL AND REPRODUCTIVE HEALTHCARE (SRH) RESOURCES

British Association of Sexual Health and HIV (BASHH)	Guidance and patient information leaflets for sexually transmitted infection (STI) and bloodborne viruses. Tailored training courses in STI and HIV designed for both primary care and more specialist providers of sexual healthcare: https://www.bashh.org/events-education/training-courses-and-meetings/
Royal College of General Practitioners (RCGP)	Free access to short modular online learning with a primary care focus: https://elearning.rcgp.org.uk/
National HIV Nurses Association	Free access to nursing modules designed for those working in the field of HIV – the introductory module would be useful for practice nursing: https://www.nhivna.org/NHIVNA-HIV-nursing-modules
Faculty of Sexual and Reproductive Health	Training options include the Diploma in Sexual and Reproductive Healthcare and Letters of Competence in subdermal contraceptive device implant (SDI) and intrauterine contraception (IUC) – competency based, with practical components and assessed suitable for those who want to offer contraceptive care in general practice: https://www.fsrh.org/education-and-training/
Faculty of Sexual and Reproductive Health	Guidance, standards and resources for all methods of contraception, including the UK Medical Eligibility Criteria for Contraceptive Use (UKMEC): https://www.fsrh.org/standards-and-guidance/current-clinical-guidance/
Lothian Sexual and Reproductive Health Service	Informative short films on IUC and abortion and IUC patient checklist: https://www.lothiansexualhealth.scot/
E-Learning for Health (ELFH)	Offers a range of free online modular courses in SRH free of charge, some of which are essential prerequisites for competence-based FSRH training: https://portal.e-lfh.org.uk/ Register
Faculty of Sexual and Reproductive Health	Useful summary of drug interactions with hormonal contraception: https://www.fsrh.org/standards-and-guidance/documents/ceu-clinical-guidance-drug-interactions-with-hormonal/

diagnosis (BASHH, 2018). Infection is often asymptomatic in men and women, and although this is unlikely to signal significant risk to their own health, they can unwittingly transmit infection to sexual contacts. Alternatively, women may complain of vaginal discharge, postcoital or intermenstrual bleeding, dysuria, and pain. Examination might elicit cervicitis with contact bleeding and pelvic or cervical motion tenderness. Men may have urethral discharge or dysuria. Complications are rare but include pelvic inflammatory disease, infertility, ectopic pregnancy, reactive arthritis for both men and women and epididymo-orchitis or lymphogranuloma venereum (LGV) (a genotype of chlamydia) that causes severe ano-rectal symptoms in men. Rectal symptoms, conjunctivitis and (rarely) sore throat can denote infection in extra-genital sites.

Historically, a 1-g single dose of azithromycin (SDA) has been the standard treatment for uncomplicated CT; however, doxycycline 100 mg twice a day for 7 days is now recommended (in nonpregnant individuals) for uncomplicated urogenital, pharyngeal and rectal CT infections, with a test of cure (TOC) for diagnosed rectal infections. This is due to the emergence of Mycoplasma genitalium (MGen) as a significant coinfecting pathogen, which shows evidence of macrolide resistance. SDA has been shown to be less effective than doxycycline for rectal CT in women and MSM. Undertreated rectal *Chlamydia* infection can contribute to reinfection rates (BASHH, 2018).

Gonorrhoea

Gonorrhoea (GC) is caused by the Gram-negative bacterium *Neisseria gonorrhoeae*. Common sites of infection are the urethra, endocervix, rectum, pharynx and conjunctiva. Transmission is by direct inoculation of infected secretions from one mucous membrane to another. The majority of infection is uncomplicated, but very rarely, GC can cause pelvic inflammatory disease, prostatitis or epididymo-orchitis or become disseminated, affecting other organs. It is known to facilitate transmission and acquisition of HIV, and the emergence of antimicrobial resistance is a worldwide concern. Symptoms appear within 2 to 5 days of infection and include mucopurulent urethral or endocervical discharge, dysuria and tender, swollen testes. Rectal infection is usually asymptomatic but presents in men with perianal itch/discomfort and/or anal

discharge, and 30% of women have asymptomatic rectal infection irrespective of anal sex. Pharyngeal infection is usually symptomless.

Whilst the principal role of general practice is the detection of GC infection, treatment of index patients (i.e., first known case) and their contacts can be complex, and it is important to consider sites of infection for sampling, treatment regimen and TOC. Partner notification is crucial, and testing, treatment and follow-up of partners can be time consuming. It is recommended that the patient is referred for treatment to their nearest sexual health clinic (Pope, 2020). The prevalence of ciprofloxacin resistance in the UK is high, so currently, treatment is with ceftriaxone unless antimicrobial sensitivity to ciprofloxacin is already known. Due to the risk of antimicrobial resistance, sexual health centres continue to provide TOCs and monitor for treatment failure.

Herpes Simplex Virus

Herpes simplex virus 1 (HSV-1) is the usual cause of oral herpes, whereas herpes simplex virus 2 (HSV-2) is associated with ano-genital infection and is more likely to cause recurrent symptoms. The majority of individuals will not develop symptoms with HSV-2. Incubation ranges from 2 days to 2 weeks. Prior infection with HSV-1 tends to make the symptoms of the first infection with HSV-2 less severe. The recurrence rate of HSV-2 is four times that of HSV-1, with a median recurrence rate of four recurrences per annum, which decreases over time. The virus becomes latent in local sensory ganglia, periodically reactivating to cause symptomatic lesions or asymptomatic, but infectious, viral shedding. See Table 15.1 for signs and symptoms (Clutterbuck, 2018).

It is important to confirm infection and determine the type of infection. Swabs should be taken from the base of the anogenital lesion. All MSM presenting with proctitis should have a rectal swab taken for the detection of HSV. Serological testing for HSV type-specific antibodies can be used to diagnose HSV infection in the absence of symptoms; however, its value in screening is not established and not recommended. Serology may be helpful in particular situations, for example, recurrence of genital disease with unknown cause or advising asymptomatic partners of patients with genital herpes, such as women who are planning a pregnancy or are pregnant.

	TABLE 15.1	
	Herpes Simplex Virus (HSV) Signs and Symptoms	
Symptoms	**Signs**	**Complications**
Painful ulceration	Blistering and ulceration of the external genitalia or perianal region (cervix/rectum)	Super-infection of lesions with *Candida* and strepto-coccal species (typically occurs in the second week of lesion progression)
Dysuria		
Vaginal or penile discharge	Tender inguinal lymphadenitis, usually bilateral in first episode and then favouring one side or another in recurrence	Autonomic neuropathy, resulting in urinary retention
Systemic fever and myalgia, usually in primary infection	Lymphadenitis in around 30% of patients	Autoinoculation to fingers and adjacent skin (e.g., on thighs)
		Aseptic meningitis

Management

- Saline bathing and simple oral analgesia are often sufficient.
- The use of topical anaesthetic agents may be useful, especially before micturition. Oral antiviral drugs are indicated within 5 days of the start of the episode, while new lesions are still forming, or when systemic symptoms persist.
- Antiviral medication is used for 5 days, irrespective of product, reducing the severity and duration of episodes.

Recurrence. Recurrences are usually self-limiting and generally cause minor symptoms. Episodic or suppressive oral antiviral medication may be considered in an attempt to reduce the severity and duration of recurrent episodes. Topical agents are less effective, and using these in combination with oral agents is of no benefit. For patients with complications or those who cannot tolerate oral medication, intravenous therapy may be indicated.

Genital Human Papilloma Virus

Genital human papilloma virus (HPV; warts) infection is common and benign, with 90% caused by HPV types 6 or 11. Usually asymptomatic, infection resolves spontaneously within a year. A quadrivalent vaccine (HPV types 6/11/16/18) for boys and girls is delivered through the routine UK schools vaccination programmes, primarily aimed at preventing cervical cancer (British National Formulary (BNF), 2020). From April 2018, all MSM aged 45 years and under attending sexual health or HIV clinics became eligible for HPV vaccination; furthermore, clinicians can utilise clinical judgement in considering vaccination for individuals with a similar risk profile to this population, including MSM aged over 45 years, sex workers and HIV-positive men and women (PHE, 2018; Scottish Government, 2017). The incubation period for HPV is between 3 weeks and 8 months.

Transmission:

- Most often via sexual contact
- Perinatal transmission possible
- Transfer from hand to genitals possible in children
- No evidence of transmission from fomites (articles/objects)

Presentation:

- Single or multiple soft 'cauliflower-like' growths of varying size (broad based or pedunculated, flat or pigmented)
- Lesions soft and firm on moist, non–hair-bearing skin and keratinised on dry and hairy skin
- Can occur at any genital or perigenital site and are common at sites of trauma (e.g., shaving)
- Irritation or discomfort, bleeding
- May be seen incidentally at time of examination in the vagina, cervix, urethral meatus and anal canal

Usually, a clinical diagnosis is made from recognition of characteristic lesions. Rarely, biopsy may be required to confirm the diagnosis in atypical lesions or in cases that do not respond to treatment. The practice nurse should, however, be aware of the possibility of lesions being neoplastic, and in this instance, a biopsy is indicated where clinical features raise suspicion.

Management

- Condoms reduce the risk of acquisition and may reduce recurrence when both partners are infected.
- Condoms can be weakened by imiquimod (used in the treatment of genital warts).

- Smokers may respond less well to treatment than nonsmokers.
- Avoid shaving of pubic hair.
- Several treatment attempts are usually needed before warts subside.
- If psychological distress is apparent, referral for counselling may be appropriate.
- No changes to routine National Cervical Screening Programmes are recommended.

Treatment. All treatments have significant failure and relapse rates and can cause local skin reaction. People with low numbers of small warts, irrespective of type, should be advised to allow them to resolve spontaneously. Soft, nonkeratinised warts respond well to topical treatments, whereas keratinised lesions may be better treated with ablative methods such as cryotherapy, excision and electrocautery. Very large lesions should be considered for surgical treatment. Topical applications include podophyllotoxin, imiquimod and catephen. Review is recommended at the end of a treatment course.

Warts in the vagina, cervix, anal canal or urethral meatus will often not require treatment. Ablative or surgical treatment, where required, should be carried out in a specialist setting. Colposcopy is not routinely recommended unless the diagnosis is in doubt. In pregnancy, treatment is not required except to minimise the number of lesions present at delivery to reduce neonatal exposure. Caesarean section is not normally indicated. Cryotherapy, excision and ablative methods are the preferred options.

Trichomonas vaginalis

TV is a flagellated protozoon; in women, it is found in the vagina, urethra and paraurethral glands, and in men, infection is usually of the urethra. Symptoms will affect more than half of men and women.

Women

- Vaginal discharge – scant or profuse (yellow frothy in <30%)
- Vulvitis, vaginitis, itch, dysuria
- Rarely – lower abdominal discomfort, vulval ulceration, 'strawberry cervix'

Men

- Urethral discharge (rarely purulent)/irritation and/or dysuria and frequency
- Rarely – balanoposthitis or posthitis

Treatment is usually metronidazole, either a 2-g single dose or 400 to 500 mg twice daily for 5 to 7 days. It is best to refer men to a sexual health clinic for differential diagnosis and appropriate screening for other STIs as appropriate. Persistent/recurrent TV is due to inadequate therapy, reinfection, or resistance. TV is associated with preterm delivery and low birth weight, but asymptomatic screening in pregnancy is not recommended.

Syphilis

Syphilis is caused by the spirochete bacterium *Treponema pallidum*. Transmission is by direct contact with an infectious lesion or via vertical transmission in pregnancy. Approximately one-third of sexual contacts of infectious syphilis will develop the disease. Amongst MSM, transmission may occur at extragenital sites through oral-anal or genital-anal contact. Infection is commonest among young, white MSM and is often associated with HIV coinfection. The role of primary care is to identify risk and have a low threshold for initiating screening amongst heterosexual and MSM populations. Patients can often present with symptoms if they are subtle and fleeting. A comprehensive sexual history may reveal risk factors, and direct questioning about any previous history of testing, diagnosis or treatment of syphilis can be helpful. Table 15.2 outlines the stages of syphilis infection.

Interpretation of test results is difficult, and specialist expertise is needed to confirm the diagnosis, distinguish between current and past infection, determine the stage of disease and monitor treatment success. Penicillin treatment is undertaken in sexual health clinics by sexual health advisers who also pursue partner notification, risk reduction and behaviour change to minimise risks of reinfection. Patients are advised of the possibility of penicillin reaction, including anaphylaxis, and are advised to avoid all sexual contact and exposure of other people to active lesions until the diagnosis is excluded or they have confirmation of effective treatment. For patients who cannot or refuse to attend a sexual health service, advice should be sought as to testing and treatment and ongoing management within primary care. A local referral pathway for pregnant women with suspected syphilis is crucial.

Human Immunodeficiency Virus (HIV)

HIV in the UK is predominantly prevalent amongst MSM or related to migration from countries where

TABLE 15.2

Stages of Syphilis Infection

Stage	Primary	Secondary	Latent	Late (Tertiary)
Features	Incubation usually 21 days (range 9–90)	Untreated, 25% will develop secondary in syphilis 4–10 weeks after initial chancre Multisystem	Secondary syphilis resolves within 3 months and enters asymptomatic latent stage Approximately 25% develop recurrence of secondary disease during the early latent stage	Occurs in around one-third of untreated patients 20–40 years after initial infection
	Chancre (ulcer) Typically anogenital,* single, painless, indurated with clean base, nonpurulent Resolves over 3–8 weeks	Widespread rash may be itchy; can affect palms and soles Mucous patches (buccal, lingual and genital) Condylomata lata (highly infectious) Hepatitis Splenomegaly Glomerulonephritis Neurological complications		Benign growths (gummata) can affect organs Cardiovascular and neurological complications

*Extra-genital sites may have multiple painful lesions.

the infection is endemic. The bulk of HIV prescribing and monitoring is done in specialist sexual health or HIV centres. The role of GPNs in relation to HIV is primarily that of early detection, which depends on comprehensive sexual history and a low threshold for testing. Primary care providers are encouraged to publicise the 'U=U' (undetectable = untransmittable) campaign, aiming to raise awareness that effective treatment resulting in an undetectable viral load means HIV is no longer sexually transmittable, highlighting the benefits of early detection and antiretroviral therapy (Gupta et al., 2020).

■ Post-exposure prophylaxis for HIV following sexual exposure (PEPSE): GPNs should be aware of where patients can access PEPSE locally because this treatment is effective if started up to 72 hours after exposure. The probability of HIV transmission varies with the characteristics of the exposure, that is, how infective the source was, how susceptible the person exposed is, how frequent the exposure was and what type of sex took place. Clinical algorithms are used to calculate individual risk, and PEPSE is recommended if the risk of transmission is high (>1:1000). A sexual health specialist will discuss with individuals in detail what their risk is and whether PEPSE should be considered.

■ Pre-exposure prophylaxis for HIV (PrEP): Consideration should also be given to whether PrEP might be relevant to reduce the risk of acquisition of HIV amongst any HIV-negative MSM having regular condomless anal sex. PrEP can be accessed from the NHS in Scotland and Northern Ireland and via enrolment in studies in NHS Wales (PrEPared Project) and NHS England (PrEP Impact Trial). Patients can be advised to look at the 'I want PrEP now' website (https://www.iwantprepnow.co.uk/prep-on-the-nhs/) for detailed information about how to access this as it is rolled out across the UK-wide NHS.

Vaginal Discharge – Non-STI

Women frequently seek advice from GPNs about perceived abnormal vaginal discharge. Common causes include bacterial vaginosis (BV) and candidiasis, STIs and aerobic organisms such as *Escherichia coli* and group B *Streptococcus*. Very commonly what is perceived as an abnormal vaginal discharge is actually a variation in the pattern of normal physiology, which is, however, sometimes associated with psychosexual problems and depression. Rarely does it indicate carcinoma. The majority of women with vaginal discharge can be managed entirely within the general practice setting once an STI has been ruled out.

A comprehensive history is essential in the differential diagnosis of abnormal discharge, which will include ascertaining the following:

- Duration of and associated symptoms
- Colour, amount and odour of discharge
- Vulval pain and deep dyspareunia
- Menstrual cycle variation (copious, clear and stretchy discharge at ovulation)
- Recent sexual history
- History of tampon use

Additionally, conducting a speculum examination or digital vaginal examination to elicit the cause of vaginal discharge may identify the presence of a foreign body, which may be tucked into the posterior fornix. Careful examination should be undertaken, and this includes identifying any abnormal appearances suggesting malignancy. Table 15.3 summarises findings on clinical examination.

Bacterial Vaginosis

BV is caused by the overgrowth of anaerobic organisms within the vagina or when the pH is altered by over-washing or the use of perfumed products. Odour may be worse after sex (seminal fluid has a high pH). Syndromic management is appropriate in routine presentations of BV without the need for microscopy.

Management of BV involves the avoidance of soaps and perfumed products. Soap substitutes can be bought over the counter or prescribed. Probiotics, either oral or vaginal, and vaginal acetate gel can be useful. Antibiotic treatment in nonpregnant women is given only if they complain of symptoms. Typically this consists of oral metronidazole 400 mg twice daily for 7 days or local application of clindamycin cream (2%), one applicator full for 7 days.

In pregnancy, BV may increase the risk of midtrimester miscarriage; however, routine screening is not recommended. Treatment is recommended for asymptomatic pregnant women, especially if they are less than 20 weeks' gestation and have other risk factors for preterm delivery; avoid 2-g stat metronidazole and treat with 400 mg BD for 7 days or intravaginal therapies. Metronidazole does, however, enter breast milk, affecting the taste.

Vulvovaginal Candidiasis

Vulvovaginal candidiasis (VVC; thrush) is a fungal infection caused by yeasts from the genus *Candida* and is one of the most common presentations observed by the practice nurse when undertaking cervical screening. Yeasts are part of the normal flora of the respiratory, gastrointestinal and female genital tracts, with overgrowth leading to infection. There are over 20 *Candida* species causing infections in humans, of which *Candida albicans* is the most common (80%–89%). The definitive diagnosis of VVC is made by finding yeast hyphae/pseudohyphae or spores on microscopy; however, a presumptive diagnosis can be made if the history and examination suggest VVC.

Management involves the avoidance of soaps and perfumed products, use of soap substitutes and antifungal treatment. Fluconazole, given in a single oral dose of 150 mg, is as effective as clotrimazole pessaries in the treatment of candidiasis and is the treatment of choice (contraindicated in pregnancy).

TABLE 15.3		
Vaginal Discharge: Clinical Examination		
Condition	Discharge	Associated Signs +/−
BV	Homogenous white/milky coats walls of vagina or pooling at introitus Fish-like odour Litmus paper pH >4.5 – sample from the lateral vaginal walls to avoid the naturally alkali cervical secretions	Odour more noticeable after sex Vaginal mucosa possibly mildly oedematous
VVC	Thick/crumbly, 'cottage cheese–like' Adheres to vaginal wall	Itch Vulval erythema/fissuring discomfort

BV, Bacterial vaginosis; *VVC*, vulvovaginal candidiasis.

REPRODUCTIVE HEALTH – CONTRACEPTION

There is a range of contraceptive methods available to suit the diverse needs of women of childbearing age. Some are more effective than others and have different side-effect profiles and contraindications, so contraceptive risk assessment and contraceptive counselling are crucial to guide choice. It is essential that those GPNs who offer contraceptive advice and prescription/supply are appropriately trained and that they are familiar with the UK Medical Eligibility Criteria (UKMEC), which are produced and updated by the Faculty of Sexual and Reproductive Healthcare (FSRH, 2016). The UKMEC, as detailed in Table 15.4, have four categories for contraceptive use for each method, which are important when assessing the suitability and safety of a method for an individual.

Methods of Contraception

No method of contraception should be ruled out solely on the basis of age. There are, however, a multitude of risk factors to consider, but women should have the widest choice possible and should have access to the most effective methods. FSRH provides comprehensive, evidence-based guidance on each method, underpinning assessment, and advice for patients is available on its website. The FSRH also offers specific guidance on drug interactions and on starting and switching methods safely (see resources in Box 15.3).

Long-Acting Reversible Contraception

Long-acting reversible contraception (LARC) methods are highly effective compared with other methods and are reversible, unlike sterilisation. They should be widely promoted, and within Scotland, the rollout of postpartum LARC is under way after research demonstrated the feasibility and acceptability of midwives providing these methods in the first 10 days postpartum (Cameron et al., 2017; Cooper & Cameron, 2018). It is hoped this will significantly reduce the risk of unplanned pregnancy and reduce abortion rates in the long term.

Intrauterine Contraception

There are two types of intrauterine contraception (IUC): copper intrauterine devices (CU-IUD) and levonorgestrel intrauterine systems (LNG-IUS). CU-IUDs release copper ions that are toxic to sperm and ova and also cause an endometrial inflammatory response. The LNG-IUS thickens cervical mucus, inhibiting sperm transport, and thins the endometrial lining of the uterus. Both types of IUDs inhibit ovulation and reduce the likelihood of uterine implantation.

A comprehensive medical and sexual history should be carried out as part of the routine assessment to assess suitability for the use of IUC. Because a CU-IUD is effective immediately after insertion, it can be inserted at any time in the menstrual cycle, if it is reasonably certain the woman is not already pregnant. If a woman has had unprotected sexual intercourse (UPSI), a CU-IUD can be inserted as a means of emergency contraception (EC), providing it is inserted before implantation begins (see the later section on emergency contraception). The LNG-IUS can be inserted on days 1 to 7 of the menstrual cycle without the need for additional contraception, but if inserted later in the cycle, additional contraceptive precautions

TABLE 15.4
Definition of UK Medical Eligibility Criteria for Contraceptive Use (UKMEC) Categories

Category 1	A condition for which there is no restriction for the use of the method
Category 2	A condition where the advantages of using the method generally outweigh the theoretical or proven risks
Category 3	A condition where the theoretical or proven risks usually outweigh the advantages of using the method. The provision of a method requires expert clinical judgement and/or referral to a specialist contraceptive provider because use of the method is not usually recommended unless other more appropriate methods are not available or not acceptable
Category 4	A condition that represents an unacceptable health risk if the method is used

From Faculty of Sexual and Reproductive Health, 2016 UK Medical Eligibility Criteria for Contraceptive Use (UKMEC) (updated 2019) https://www.fsrh.org/ukmec/ Accessed (30.04.20). Reproduced under licence from FSRH. Copyright © Faculty of Sexual and Reproductive Healthcare.

are required for 7 days. The need for STI testing before insertion should be assessed within the context of obtaining the sexual history. Asymptomatic women who are at risk of pregnancy need not wait for STI test results or receive antibiotic prophylaxis as long as firm arrangements for prompt treatment of an STI are in place should tests prove positive (FSRH, Clinical Effectiveness Unit, 2019).

Counselling for IUC insertion should include the following:

- The CU-IUD lasts between 5 and 10 years, or until menopause if fitted at, or after, age 40 and can be used as EC. It is the only effective hormone-free method of contraception. It can cause heavier, longer and more painful periods, so it may not be suitable for women who have heavy menstrual bleeding.
- The LNG-IUS lasts for 5 years (7 years if fitted at or after age 45). Typically it causes erratic bleeding in the first 3 to 6 months but then induces amenorrhoea or scant infrequent bleeds and so is useful in the treatment of menstrual disorders. It can also be used as endometrial protection in hormone replacement therapy.
- Efficacy – pregnancy rate of 0.2% to 0.6%
- Expulsion 1 in 20 (most common in first year of use)
- Infection 1 in 200
- Perforation: up to 2 in 1000 (6-fold higher risk in breastfeeding women)
- Women should be offered instruction on how to check for the IUC and advised that if the threads cannot be felt, then additional contraception should be used until the IUC can be confirmed in situ. Women should be advised to seek medical assistance at any time if they develop symptoms of pelvic infection, pain, abnormal bleeding, late menstrual period (CU-IUD), and nonpalpable threads or can feel the stem of the IUC.
- The overall risk of ectopic pregnancy is reduced with the use of IUC when compared with using no contraception. If pregnancy occurs with an IUC in situ, the risk of an ectopic pregnancy is increased. Users should be informed about symptoms of ectopic pregnancy, and it should be considered in women who present with abdominal pain, especially in connection with a change in bleeding pattern.

The recognised UK training to fit IUCs is the Letter of Competence provided by the FSRH. Fitters should maintain competence and attend regular updates (see SRH resources outlined in Box 15.3).

Subdermal Contraceptive Device Implant

The subdermal contraceptive device implant (SDI) is the most effective method of contraception, comparable to vasectomy (pregnancy rate <0.01%). It is a progestogen-only method whereby etonogestrel acts to prevent ovulation. It also prevents sperm transport by altering the cervical mucus and possibly prevents implantation by thinning the endometrium. The SDI lasts for 3 years and has few contraindications or associated health risks. Local anaesthesia should be administered before insertion and removal. Health professionals who insert or remove SDIs should be appropriately trained, maintain competence and attend regular updates. The FSRH offers a training package with a Letter of Competence (see SRH resources in Box 15.3).

There is no need for routine follow-up after insertion, but women should be advised to seek advice if they cannot feel their implant or it appears to have changed shape, if they notice any skin changes or pain around the site of the implant or they become pregnant. Approximately 25% of women will have prolonged or frequent bleeding with the SDI, and those who are eligible may be offered combined oral contraception (COC) cyclically or continuously for 3 months (outside the product licence) for control. A reduction in the duration of contraceptive efficacy amongst women with a high body mass index (BMI) cannot be completely excluded. It is good practice to inform women, however, that although the manufacturer recommends consideration of earlier replacement in 'heavier' women, there is no direct evidence to suggest this is necessary, and it can be discussed on an individual basis with women by a specialist.

Progestogen-Only Injection – Depot Medroxyprogesterone Acetate

Depot medroxyprogesterone acetate (DMPA) has a useful place in contraceptive choice, and when administered at the recommended dosing interval (13 weeks), it has a failure rate of approximately 0.2%. It suppresses the ovaries, preventing ovulation and resulting in amenorrhoea for a significant number of users. It can also be useful for the treatment of endometriosis. Due to its effect on oestrogen levels, it reduces bone mineral density and therefore is not suitable for young teenagers whose bone mass is not fully developed. Acne, decreased libido, mood swings, headache, hot flushes and vaginitis have been reported with the use of DMPA. It seems plausible that oestrogen suppression might account for this. There is evidence of weight gain, particularly in younger women with BMI ≥30, and it can cause delayed return to fertility – up to 1 year.

Traditionally, DMPA is administered by intramuscular (IM) injection every 3 months; however, there is a subcutaneous administration preparation (SC DMPA), which women can self-administer with the correct training. SC DMPA is the same as the IM preparation in relation to dose interval, efficacy, contraindications, risks and side effects, although injection site reaction is more common. The gluteal muscle is the preferred site for IM administration, but it can be administered into the deltoid muscle of the upper arm, particularly in women with deep adipose tissue when standard-length needles may not reach the gluteal muscle layer. SC DMPA is injected into the abdomen or anterior thigh.

Progestogen-Only Pill

Few medical conditions restrict the use of the progestogen-only pill (POP). It is the mainstay of oral contraception when combined methods are contraindicated. The traditional POP has been limited in its use because of its relatively poor efficacy and the requirement to take it within a 3-hour window each day. Traditional POPs thicken the cervical mucus, inhibiting sperm transport. The desogestrel (DSG) POP also inhibits ovulation and allows a 12-hour window for pill taking and thus is likely to have greater efficacy. The pregnancy rate is 0.3% to 0.9%, and women should be advised that regular pill taking every day is required to improve efficacy and to take the pill at a time of day that will best suit them. If a woman vomits within 2 hours of pill taking, another pill should be taken as soon as possible. If a pill is missed, additional precautions are required until 48 hours after pill taking has been resumed.

Women may be given up to a 12-month supply of POPs at their first and follow-up visits and can continue until the age of 55 years, when natural loss of fertility can be assumed for most women. Changes in bleeding patterns associated with the POP are common, and mood changes have been reported in women using the POP, although there is no evidence of a causal association with mood changes or depression.

Combined Hormonal Contraception

Combined hormonal contraception (CHC) contains two hormones, progestogen and ethinylestradiol (EE), giving effective contraception and considerable noncontraceptive benefits. There are three types of CHC: combined oral contraception (COC), combined transdermal patch (CTP) and combined vaginal ring (CVC). They all have the same contraindications and largely the same side effects, which include breakthrough bleeding, acne, headache and mood change. The mode of action is threefold: inhibition of ovulation, reduced sperm transport and a thinning of the endometrial lining to make it less receptive to implantation. If used perfectly, the pregnancy rate is 0.3%.

Despite its popularity, CHC is the most complex of the methods and has the greatest number of contraindications, as well as different doses and types of progestogen to consider. Women with any category 3 or 4 UKMEC contraindications elicited during assessment (see Table 15.4) should be advised that CHC is not a suitable method. CHC is associated with an increased risk of venous thromboembolism (VTE), including deep vein thrombosis and pulmonary and cerebral emboli, and a slightly increased risk of breast and cervical cancer (>5 years use), which reduces with time after stopping.

Because of the increased risk of VTE, advice about ensuring mobility and hydration during long-haul air travel (6 hours or more) and advice to change to a different method if trekking to high altitudes (above 4500 m) for more than a week should be given. Similarly, women having major planned surgery or an expected long period of immobility should be advised to switch methods. CHC is contraindicated at less than 3 weeks postpartum or if breastfeeding.

CHC can be started up to and including day 5 of a normal menstrual cycle without the need for additional contraceptive protection. It can also be 'quick started' at any other time (with additional contraceptive precautions for 7 days) if it is reasonably certain that the woman is not pregnant. Women should be given information about both standard and tailored CHC regimens. This means choosing the length and frequency of the hormone-free interval (HFI). A 12-month supply can be given at initiation and continuation. Annual review is recommended and should include reassessment of medical eligibility (including blood pressure and BMI measurement), method adherence and side effects (Table 15.5).

The noncontraceptive health benefits of CHC are associated with reducing heavy, painful menstrual bleeding (HMB). CHC can improve acne and may be beneficial for women with premenstrual syndrome (PMS) and in the management of polycystic ovary syndrome and can reduce the risk of recurrence of endometriosis. It is also associated with a significant reduction in the risk of endometrial, ovarian and bowel cancer that increases with the duration of CHC use and persists for many years after stopping.

Sterilisation

A detailed discussion of vasectomy and female sterilisation is beyond the scope of this chapter because they are undertaken in specialist settings. GPNs should, however, be aware of these methods and their high efficacy (0.5% for female procedures and 0.15% for vasectomy). Vasectomy is now undertaken using minimally invasive techniques, usually in an outpatient setting, and for women, hysteroscopic tubal occlusion now provides an acceptable alternative to laparoscopic sterilisation. The FSRH has produced a guidance document that is designed for those who undertake and refer for male and female sterilisation procedures (see Box 15.3).

Fertility Awareness Methods (Natural Family Planning)

Detail on how to use fertility awareness methods is not included in this chapter because of the high failure rates associated with their use (typically 24%). Women who are keen to use these methods can be directed to online resources provided by Fertility UK (https://www.fertilityuk.org/).

Emergency Contraception

Emergency contraception (EC) provides women with a means of reducing the risk of the conception of an unintended pregnancy following UPSI. Oral EC methods do not provide contraceptive coverage for subsequent UPSI occurring in this or future cycles, and women will need to use contraception or abstain from sex to avoid further risk of pregnancy. In the UK, oral methods are free and widely available from NHS providers and in some cases from community pharmacies free of charge.

TABLE 15.5
Standard and Tailored Regimens for Use of Combined Hormonal Contraception (CHC)

Type of regimen	Period of CHC Use	Hormone-Free Interval (HFI) Standard Use
Standard use	21 days (21 active pills or 1 ring, or 3 patches)	7 days
Tailored use		
Shortened HFI	21 days (21 active pills or 1 ring, or 3 patches)	4 days
Extended use (tricycling)	9 weeks (3 × 21 active pills or 3 rings, or 9 patches used consecutively)	4 or 7 days
Flexible extended use	Continuous use (≥21 days) of active pills, patches or rings until breakthrough bleeding occurs for 3–4 days	4 days
Continuous use	Continuous use of active pills, patches or rings	None

From Faculty of Sexual and Reproductive Health, Clinical Effectiveness Unit, (2019) Clinical Guidance, Intrauterine Contraception. Reproduced under licence from FSRH. Copyright © Faculty of Sexual and Reproductive Healthcare.

There are three methods of EC – copper IUD (CU-IUD), oral ulipristal acetate (UPA-EC) and levonorgestrel (LNG-EC). A judicial review in 2002 (Munby, 2002) concluded that pregnancy begins at implantation. None of the EC methods noted disrupts *established* implantation. CU-IUD has a toxic effect on sperm and ova, thereby potentially preventing fertilisation. However, if fertilisation does occur, the endometrial inflammatory reaction caused by the copper prevents implantation. The earliest implantation possible is 6 days post-ovulation. A CU-IUD can be inserted in good faith up to 5 days after the predicted ovulation date (e.g., until day 19 of a regular, 28-day cycle).

Oral methods act by delaying ovulation for at least 5 days, until sperm from the UPSI are no longer viable (UPA-EC works even after the start of the luteinising surge). Neither has been demonstrated to be effective when administered after ovulation, suggesting no significant effect on implantation. After taking oral EC, if a woman then ovulates later in the cycle, she will be at risk of pregnancy from further UPSI. If she has had other UPSI earlier in the same cycle, it is safe to take oral EC, and if oral EC has been taken once or more in a cycle, the same type of oral EC can be offered again for subsequent UPSI within the same cycle.

The choice of EC will depend on the woman's preference, her risk of pregnancy, which is highest just before ovulation, and the time elapsed since UPSI. To assess when ovulation might take place, knowing the time of UPSI and the usual pattern of menses is essential. With a very regular cycle, ovulation can be predicted by counting 14 days back from the expected date of onset of menstruation (day 14 in a 28-day cycle, day 16 in a 30-day cycle). Being precise about efficacy with EC is very difficult (FSRH, 2017 [amended 2020]), but the CU-IUD is the most effective method and should always be discussed. It needs to be inserted by a trained fitter within the legal timeframe, so access may be an issue. It is a more invasive method, but once fitted, it gives between 5 and 10 years of ongoing effective contraception with no risk of drug interaction or major side effects.

UPA-EC has been demonstrated to be more effective than LNG-EC from 0 to 120 hours after UPSI and so should be considered the first-line option if the risk of pregnancy is high. From 96 to 120 hours, it is the only effective oral option. However, UPA-EC may not be the most suitable method in certain situations. Most notably, if progestogen has been taken in the preceding 120 hours, or if quick start contraception, within 5 days of EC, has been advised to reduce risk from further UPSI, then efficacy could be reduced. It is not suitable for use by women who have severe asthma controlled by oral glucocorticoids, and breastfeeding women should discard breast milk for 1 week after taking UPA-EC.

LNG-EC has fewer contraindications; however, it must be taken within 72 hours of UPSI, with its efficacy reducing over time (greatest in first 12 hours post-UPSI). Effectiveness also may be reduced in women weighing >70 kg or with a BMI >26, where a double dose of LNG -EC is advised or, preferably, an alternative method.

FEMALE GENITAL MUTILATION

In the provision of SRH, GPNs may encounter women, particularly from some African and Asian backgrounds, who have subjected to FGM. FGM is the collective term that describes the nonmedical cultural practice of cutting of female genitalia, which the WHO (2018) has classified into four types, from a small cut to the clitoral hood to destructive removal of all the external genitalia.

FGM is a gender-based violent violation of human rights that has received worldwide condemnation. FGM is illegal within the UK, irrespective of national or residential status (Female Genital Mutilation Act 2003 England, Wales and Northern Ireland; Prohibition of Female Genital Mutilation (Scotland) Act 2005). FGM can take place at any point between infancy and adulthood, and with reference to the abuse of children, its illegality is recognised within UK safeguarding frameworks.

The health implications for women who have been subjected to FGM are stark and wide-ranging, with death as an immediate risk as a result of haemorrhage and septicaemia. Long term, the impact is associated with pain, infections, abscess and fistula formation, repeated genitourinary infections, period problems and obstetric complications. This is often accompanied by lifelong poor mental health and poor sexual wellbeing.

Consequently, whether in the context of providing SRH or otherwise, GPNs have an important role in supporting these women who have been affected by FGM in meeting their holistic health needs. They also have a crucial a role in the safeguarding of infants, girls and women who may be at potential risk of this abuse. Where the GPN suspects a child may be at risk, the legal and professional implications are apparent in initiating immediate contact with safeguarding leads. Similarly, for situations where the patient discloses to the practice nurse that FGM has occurred or there is suspicion by the GPN that FGM has taken place, this requires mandatory legal reporting (Department of Health (DOH), 2017). To support practice nurses appropriately responding to the challenge of FGM, a number of resources and e-learning materials are available (see Box 15.4 for resources).

TRANSGENDER HEALTHCARE

Transgender is a blanket term for people whose experienced or expressed gender is different from the sex assigned to them at birth and includes trans, nonbinary and other gender non-conforming people. The World Professional Association for Transgender Health (WPATH, 2012, p. 4) asserts that this is a 'common and culturally diverse human phenomenon that should not be judged as inherently pathological or negative'.

There is a lack of reliable evidence on the number of transgender people living in the UK because of a lack of data and different approaches to defining gender identity, making health service planning difficult. It is clear that numbers have been considerably underestimated. In England, gender identity clinics (GICs) have seen a 240% overall increase in referrals over 5 years (Torjesen, 2018). Within NHS Health Scotland, it was estimated that approximately 200 adults would present for treatment per annum; the actual number is approximately 900.

Gender incongruence is a persistent incongruence between a person's experienced gender and their assigned sex at birth, which often leads to a desire to 'transition', to live and be accepted as a person of the experienced gender. Distress associated with this is known as *gender dysphoria*. Hormonal treatment, surgery or other healthcare services are used to make the person's body align, as much as desired and to the extent possible, with the experienced gender. Health professionals can help individuals affirm their gender identity, explore how they wish to express their identity and support individualised treatment options for alleviating gender dysphoria.

BOX 15.4
FEMALE GENITAL MUTILATION (FGM) RESOURCES

Scottish Government	Responding to Female Genital Mutilation in Scotland: Multiagency guidance 2017: https://www.gov.scot/binaries/content/documents/govscot/publications/advice-and-guidance/2017/11/responding-female-genital-mutilation-fgm-scotland-multi-agency-guidance-978-1-78851-364-7/documents/00528145-pdf/00528145-pdf/govscot%3Adocument/00528145.pdf
UK Government	Gov. UK. Female Genital Mutilation Resource Pack 2020: https://www.gov.uk/government/publications/female-genital-mutilation-resource-pack/female-genital-mutilation-resource-pack
UK Government	Gov.UK. Female Genital Mutilation Mandatory Reporting Duty: https://assets.publishing.service.gov.uk/government/uploads/system/uploads/attachment_data/file/525405/FGM_mandatory_reporting_map_A.pdf
Health Education England	FGM E-Learning to improve awareness and understanding of female genital mutilation: https://www.e-lfh.org.uk/programmes/female-genital-mutilation/
Royal College of General Practitioners	Female genital mutilation – online learning: https://www.rcpch.ac.uk/resources/female-genital-mutilation-online-learning

Specialist Gender Identity Services and the Role of General Practice

General practice is most often the first point of contact with the healthcare system for individuals questioning their gender, and healthcare professionals play a vital role in ensuring these patients are treated with respect and sensitivity and that they receive the care they need. Consequently, asking people which pronouns they prefer validates and shows respect and empathy. It is not uncommon to feel anxious about using the right personal pronouns. Gender-neutral pronouns (*they/them/their*) are often preferred and are grammatically correct, but if in doubt, just ask trans-identifying people which pronouns they prefer. Try to avoid using 'sir', 'madam', 'lady' and 'gentleman'; instead, use 'person' or 'individual'. If you think you have made a mistake, you can simply acknowledge the error, apologise, give the person a chance to respond if they want to and move on.

The General Medical Council (GMC) advises that doctors should promptly refer patients requesting treatment for gender dysphoria and has issued guidance on the role of general practitioners (GPs) in the management of people waiting to be seen in GICs. However, the structure of services varies throughout the UK, and there may be a significant wait for a first appointment at GICs. The ability of GPs and GPNs to provide this care depends on the necessary investment in gender services and training. The Royal College of Physicians, with the support of NHS England, is developing an interprofessional postgraduate certificate and diploma (PGCert/Dip) in Gender Identity Healthcare Practice for GPs and other regulated healthcare professionals who wish to deepen their skills and expertise in gender identity and gender variance. The Royal College of General Practitioners (RCGP) has also developed an e-learning module that aims to expand the understanding of gender variance for a wider audience in primary care.

GPs may be asked by patients to prescribe bridging hormones, and they should only consider prescribing with the advice of an experienced gender specialist to mitigate the risk of self-harm or suicide if the patient is already self-medicating from an unregulated source. GICs support GPs and offer clinics where individuals have an opportunity to explore their gender identity and consider appropriate treatment options. Assessment is a collaborative process, usually conducted over several appointments, designed to support the person to explore their gender identity and consider approaches to transition.

A variety of therapeutic options can be considered for individuals with gender dysphoria:

- Peer-support resources or community organisations, which can provide avenues for social support and advocacy for families and friends
- Changes in gender expression and role (which may involve living part time or full time in their experienced gender role)
- Changes in name and gender marker on identity documents

Therapies
- Speech therapy
- Hair removal (electrolysis, laser, or waxing)
- Provision of wigs
- Breast binding or padding, genital tucking or penile prostheses, padding of hips or buttocks
- Psychotherapy may be helpful but is not essential. It can help to address the negative impact of gender dysphoria and stigma and to improve body image and promote resilience and confidence.

Treatments
- Hormone treatment to feminise or masculinise the body and give relief from physical reminders of assigned gender (e.g., menstruation, facial hair growth)
- Surgery to change primary and/or secondary sex characteristics (e.g., breasts/chest, external and/or internal genitalia, facial features, body contouring)
- Genital reassignment surgery requires the person to live for 12 months in their experienced gender and to be proposed for surgery by two clinicians.

GICs refer for therapies, and if someone is interested in hormone treatment, they will support the person to make an informed decision and will supervise the person's treatment until it is stable, at which point they *may* be discharged to the GP with advice about appropriate monitoring. For many people, their medical transition will last for several years, and progress, especially with hormone treatment, can be slow. GICs will help individuals assess their clinical response and make appropriate adjustments to treatment.

BOX 15.5
GENDER RESOURCES

Royal College of General Practitioners	e-learning continuing professional development (CPD) module on gender variance (this is accessible by all health professionals on registration): https://london.ac.uk/courses/gender-identity-healthcare
Royal College of Psychiatrists	Good practice guidelines for the assessment and treatment of adults with gender dysphoria, College Report CR181: https://www.rcpsych.ac.uk/docs/default-source/improving-care/better-mh-policy/college-reports/cr181-good-practice-guidelines-for-the-assessment-and-treatment-of-adults-with-gender-dysphoria.pdf?sfvrsn=84743f94_4
General Medical Council	Guidance for doctors treating transgender patients: https://www.gmc-uk.org/ethical-guidance/ethical-hub/trans-healthcare
Medical and Dental Defence Union (MDDUS)	Link to MDDUS page on treating transgender patients: https://www.mddus.com/resources/publications-library/gpst/gpst-issue-13/transgender-healthcare
British Association of Gender Identity Specialists	'Promote excellence in clinical practice, clinical research, training and education in the field of healthcare for transgender and gender non-conforming people': https://www.bagis.co.uk/
National Gender Identity Clinical Network for Scotland	A full range of information about services, policy, standards, resources, prescribing guidelines, FAQs and data: https://www.ngicns.scot.nhs.uk/

For the GPN, this type of scenario may involve a young person disclosing that they hold concerns about their gender identity. Whilst this may be unfamiliar territory for the GPN, a key issue is not to panic and consider that the patient may not have told many people and is signalling trust in communicating such information. A good starting point is to ask what name and pronoun they prefer, what support they are looking for and who else they have confided in. Accept what they say about their gender, and bear in mind that for many young people, their identity development will be evolving. Counselling and support services can offer support to them and their parents. If they mention mental health difficulties, consider referral to local child and adolescent mental health services. If they want to pursue specialist NHS advice, follow the referral pathway for your area. There are a number of useful training and guideline resources for gender in Box 15.5.

SUMMARY

SRH is a complex, diverse and evolving area of practice requiring a high degree of sensitivity and self-awareness. Practice nurses are embedded in front-line service provision and are likely to encounter a range of presentations and expressions of sexuality and sexual behaviours, which may present challenges to personal beliefs. This chapter provides a practical overview and information on common and significant SRH topics relevant to routine practice. It takes time to develop the knowledge and skill set crucial to screening, treatment and management of the wide variety of SRH conditions; however, modular courses and support, including referral, from specialist services mean that practice nurses can work with confidence to provide holistic, person-centred care, wholly within their scope of practice (NMC, 2018).

ACKNOWLEDGEMENTS

Thanks to Dr. Dan Clutterbuck, clinical lead, Lothian Sexual and Reproductive Health Service, for his support in producing this chapter.

REFERENCES

British Association for Sexual Health and HIV. (2018). *BASHH Clinical Effectiveness Group, update on treatment of* Chlamydia trachomatis *(CT) infection.* https://www.bashhguidelines.org/media/1191/update-on-the-treatment-of-chlamydia-trachomatis-infection-final-16-9-18.pdf

British National Formulary. (2020). *Routine immunisation schedule.* https://bnf.nice.org.uk/treatment-summary/immunisation-schedule.html

Cameron, S. T., Craig A., Sim, J., Gallimore, A., Cowan, S., Dundas, K., Heller, R., Milne, D., & Lakha, F. (2017). Feasibility and accessibility of introducing routine contraceptive counselling and provision of contraception after delivery: The APPLES pilot evaluation. *British Journal of Obstetrics and Gynaecology, 124*(13), 2009–2015.

Clutterbuck, D. (2018). Pelvic infections and sexually transmitted infections. In B. Magowan, P. Owen, & A. Thomson (Eds.), *Clinical obstetrics and gynaecology* (4th ed., pp. 155–166). Elsevier.

Cooper, M., & Cameron, S. T. (2018). Successful implementation of postpartum intrauterine contraception in Edinburgh and framework for wider dissemination. *International Journal of Gynecology and Obstetrics, 143*(Suppl. 1), 56–61.

Faculty of Sexual and Reproductive Health. (2016). *UK medical eligibility criteria for contraceptive use (UKMEC) (updated 2019).* https://www.fsrh.org/ukmec/

Faculty of Sexual and Reproductive Health, Clinical Effectiveness Unit. (2019). *Clinical guidance, intrauterine contraception.*

Faculty of Sexual and Reproductive Health FSRH Guideline Emergency Contraception March 2017 (amended 2020). https://www.fsrh.org/documents/ceu-clinical-guidance-emergency-contraception-march-2017/

Female Genital Mutilations Act 2003 (England, Wales, Northern Ireland). https://www.legislation.gov.uk/ukpga/2003/31/introduction?view=extent

Gupta, N., Gilleece, Y., & Orkin, C. (2020). Implementing U=U in clinical practice: Results of a British HIV Association members survey. *Sexually Transmitted Infection Monthly.* Advance online publication. https://dx.doi.org/10.1136/sextrans20-054462

Health Education England. (2017). *The general practice nursing workforce development plan.* http://www.hee.nhs.uk

Munby, J. (2002). Judicial review of the Prescription-Only Medicines (Human Use) Amendment (No. 3) Order 2000 (SI 2000/3231) (2002).

NHS Education for Scotland. (2013). *Standards for education providers: Cervical cytology in clinical practice.* https://www.nes.scot.nhs.uk/media/14945/Standards%20for%20Cervical%20Cytology_interactive.pdf

Nursing and Midwifery Council. (2018). *The code: Professional standards of practice and behaviour for nurses, midwives and nursing associates.* www.nmc.org.uk/globalassets/sitedocuments/nmc-publications/nmc-code.pdf

Pope, L. (2020). Contraception, sexual problems and sexually transmitted infections. In A. Staten & P. Staten (Eds.), *Practical general practice guidelines for effective clinical management* (7th ed., pp. 247–277). Elsevier.

Prohibition of Female Genital Mutilation (Scotland) Act 2005. https://www.legislation.gov.uk/asp/2005/8/contents

Public Health Agency. (2016). *Northern Ireland standards for nurse and midwife education providers: Cervical screening sample taking.*

Public Health England. (2018). *HPV vaccination programmes for men who have sex with men (MSM). Clinical and operational guidance* (PHE Publications Gateway Number 2017892).

Public Health England. (2019). *Cervical screening campaign.* https://campaignresources.phe.gov.uk/resources/campaigns/85-cervical-screening-campaign/overview

Public Health England. (2020). *Cervical sample taker training guidance: Education pathway.* https://www.gov.uk/government/publications/cervical-screening-cervical-sample-taker-training/training-for-cervical-sample-takers-education-pathway

Royal College of Nursing. (2016). *Genital examination in women. A resource for skills and assessment.*

Scottish Government. (2017). *Chief Medical Officer Directorate, letter, introduction of HPV vaccination programme for men who have sex with men (MSM).*

Torjesen, I. (2018). Trans health needs more and better services: Increasing capacity, expertise, and integration. *British Medical Journal, 362,* Article 3371.

World Health Organisation. (2018). *Care of girls and women living with female genital mutilation: A clinical handbook.* https://www.who.int/teams/sexual-and-reproductive-health-and-research/areas-of-work/female-genital-mutilation/types-of-female-genital-mutilation

World Health Organisation. (2019). *Sexually transmitted infections (STIs).* https://www.who.int/en/news-room/fact-sheets/detail/sexually-transmitted-infections-(stis)

World Professional Association for Transgender Health. (2012). *Standards of care for the health of transgender, transsexual and gender non-conforming people. Version 7.* https://www.wpath.org/publications/soc

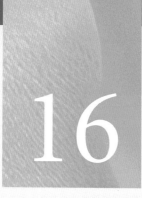

16

THE PRACTICE NURSE'S ROLE IN SUPPORTING PEOPLE WITH LEARNING DISABILITIES

ALAN R. MIDDLETON

INTRODUCTION

This chapter explores the role of the general practice nurse (GPN) in supporting and contributing to the care and treatment of people with learning disabilities. The challenges and opportunities in providing care for this subgroup of the practice population will be highlighted, and the inauspicious gaps in service provision will be identified for consideration. With this in mind, the chapter will help develop the GPN's knowledge and understanding in the care and treatment of people with learning disabilities and the differing patterns of health and illness that they experience. A brief overview of the historical care and treatment of people with learning disabilities is provided, inclusive of policy and legislation, which will help convey the journey that services have undergone in the past few decades to arrive at the current delivery within healthcare and social care partnerships across the UK.

SETTING THE CONTEMPORARY SCENE

Within the UK, there are 1.5 million people with learning disabilities (Office for National Statistics, 2019), with Mencap (2018) estimating that 2.16% of adults and 2.5% of children in the UK are believed to have a learning disability. The specific definition of *learning disability* is one that is open to interpretation and debate, which has resulted in the term *learning difficulty* often being used interchangeably, and indeed many individuals with learning disabilities and advocacy groups prefer this term. The most recognised

terms are used within healthcare policies to delineate a significant lifelong condition beginning in childhood, significant impairment of global intelligence (but not a specific learning difficulty such as dyslexia) and significant impairment of adaptive/social functioning. All three features must be present, albeit they may manifest in varying degrees for learning disabilities to occur, be these mild, moderate, severe or profound. Also noteworthy is that a learning disability is often, but not always, associated with sensory impairments, physical disabilities, communication difficulties and mental health problems. An important point to consider when undertaking research into the health needs of people with learning disabilities is that as well as the terms *learning difficulty* and *developmental disability,* the outdated and less acceptable terminology of *mental handicap* and *mental retardation* can still elicit relevant findings. Fortunately, the term *intellectual disability* (ID) has become the accepted international terminology of choice (Truesdale & Brown, 2017).

Along with these changes in terminology, there have also been advances in approaches to caring for people with learning disabilities, with a shift from the traditional medical model to one that incorporates social constructionism theory. Nunkoosing (2011) clarifies this as interactions that are socially focused on the individual, their relationships and interactions and not the condition (learning disability) itself. This discussion is expanded to include how language can affect how someone is perceived and indeed the care and treatment they receive; this means 'always putting the person first, not the condition' and thus framing this as *people with learning disabilities,* not *the learning-disabled person.*

Clearly advocated in caring for people with learning disabilities are person-centred approaches, and whilst these have been advanced within learning disability services, there remains significant scope for improvement (National Institute for Health Research, 2020). The key concept in care provision is the application of values-based approaches, which aim to maximise the quality of life for the individual based not only on their needs but also their aspirations to lead an enjoyable and healthy life. This clearly infers the use of person-centred planning, which was classically defined by the Department of Health (DOH, 2001) as follows:

Planning should start with the individual (not with services), and take account of their wishes and aspirations. Person-centred planning is a mechanism for reflecting the needs and preferences of a person with a learning disability and covers such issues as housing, education, employment and leisure.

To support practitioners in this crucial role, in 2019 the Social Care Institute for Excellence (SCIE) and National Institute for Health and Care Excellence (NICE) jointly produced *Person-Centred Future Planning: A Quick Guide for Practitioners Supporting People Growing Older With Learning Disabilities* (see Resources section at the end of this chapter).

Significant progress has occurred in developing person-centred care within nursing and healthcare practice based on the development of models, such as the person-centred practice framework by McCormack and McCance (2016). However, the work of O'Brien (1989) has been a seminal influence on how person-centred care and planning has developed, which establishes the five valued experiences that help people with learning disabilities live good lives (Fig. 16.1), which, succinctly, entails:

- **Sharing ordinary spaces:** Experiencing the value that comes from the ability to access and share typical social spaces with others.
- **Making choices:** Experiencing the value that comes from not limiting the ability of people with disabilities to find meaning and make their own meaningful choices.
- **Making contributions:** Experiencing the value that comes from exploiting the potential to widen social interaction and the opportunity to gain employment.
- **Growing in relationships:** Experiencing the value that comes from people with learning disabilities expanding and diversifying in forming relationships and networks.
- **Dignity of valued roles:** Experiencing the value that comes from experiencing respect from others for the person they are rather than being known for their intellectual disabilities.

Further detailed within this model are the five correlated service accomplishments that services could strive towards to help people have more of the valued experience. These accomplishments seek to guide and structure care and service provision, with each accomplishment capturing essential components of the human experience that present limitations for people with learning disabilities in participating as part of the community. In detailing their application, and although considered somewhat dated, Brown and Benson's (1994) articulation of these 'accomplishments' in the context of person-centred planning are still contemporaneous:

- **Community presence:** The right to take part in community life and to live and spend leisure time with other members of the community.
- **Relationships:** The right to experience valued relationships with non-disabled people.
- **Choice:** The right to make choices, both large and small, in one's life. These include choices about where to live and with whom to live.
- **Competence:** The right to learn new skills and participate in meaningful activities with whatever assistance is required.
- **Respect:** The right to be valued and not treated as a second-class citizen.

Relating these principles to the primary healthcare setting is entirely appropriate, and the GPN occupies a pivotal role in promoting an inclusive agenda within this environment. In supporting equality and independence, many individuals with a learning disability are, as part of communities, of course, accessing primary care and therefore the services of the GPN. Within the general practice setting, some individuals may have been identified within the practice population

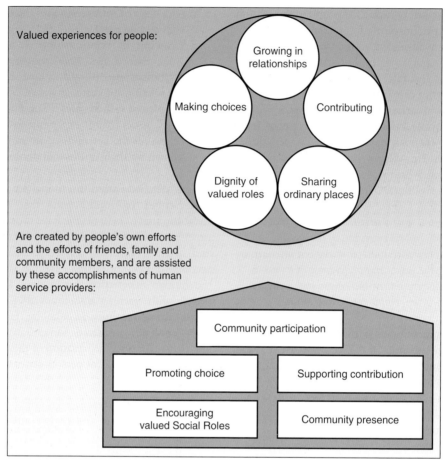

Fig. 16.1 ■ Five valued experiences and essential service accomplishments. (From O'Brien, J. (1989). *What's worth working for? Leadership for better quality human services.* Responsive Systems Associates. https://inclusion.com/site/wp-content/uploads/2017/12/Whats-Worth-Working-For.pdf)

and have the *International Classification of Mental and Behavioural Disorders* (ICD-10; World Health Organisation (WHO), 1992) classification included in their medical records. This classification describes four degrees of learning disability and uses the intelligent quotient (IQ) criteria of mild (IQ 50–69), moderate (IQ 35–49), severe (IQ 20–34) and profound (IQ less than 19). It is worth noting that IQ is not used in contemporary definitions but instead allows consideration of the differing needs across the spectrum of learning disabilities, from minimum support needs to relying totally on others. So within this, there is an opportunity to think about the care provided for people with learning disabilities, raising awareness

of their differing needs, how the practice is responding and looking at where adjustments can be made. The GPN is well placed to champion this agenda within the general practice setting to ensure the care and treatment of people with learning disabilities continues to evolve, as well as to recognise the challenges faced in delivering appropriate healthcare.

ADVANCING THE HEALTHCARE AND SOCIAL CARE LANDSCAPE

In the past two decades, there have been significant changes in the approaches to the care and treatment of people with learning disabilities, which have positively influenced the support individuals and their families receive across healthcare, social care, education and housing. The direction in which healthcare and social care and treatment services has evolved has been informed by the Health and Social Care Act 2012 and additional national directives, for example, the Public Bodies (Joint Working) (Scotland) Act 2014. These legislative drivers indicated the need to address, or indeed readdress, and review the issues around good joint working where there is a focus on integrated practice when delivering services for people with learning disabilities. Intrinsically, key services must evolve and develop to meet local needs and be driven forward at the ground level, which in turn will assist in the improvement of services and optimise the lives of people with learning disabilities.

Having awareness of how the integrated agenda influences the provision of care and treatment will enable the GPN to actively support people with learning disabilities and their families. This includes having a clear understanding of the professional groups involved in service delivery and their specific roles and responsibilities. There are many good examples of joint working relationships already occurring in practice, especially where there are complex and diverse healthcare and social care needs necessitating a multidisciplinary/agency approach.

Influential changes regarding services for children and young people have been advanced via government policies, such as 'Every Child Matters' (ECM) within England and Wales (launched in 2003 and remains current; Gov.UK, 2003) and 'Getting It Right for Every Child' (GIRFEC; Scottish Government, 2006 (updated 2017)) in Scotland, which have changed the focus for children and young people with learning disabilities to one of inclusion within mainstream children's services. The change in thinking within the integrated agenda for children's services focuses on the child first, regardless of disability or health issues, and concentrates on helping every child achieve their potential.

Recent policy direction regarding strengthening of the services available to people with learning disabilities and their families has been unequivocally outlined within the key publications *Valuing People Now* (HM Government, 2009), *The Keys to Life* (Scottish Government, 2013) and the Welsh Government's

(2018) *Learning Disability: Improving Lives* Programme; Northern Ireland has yet to update current policy direction. The positive influences of these policy directives have permitted the implementation of a shift in the balance of funding and care for people with learning disabilities and given a voice to this previously marginalised population. This can be seen in the inclusion of the health needs of people with learning disabilities in current policy, such as the National Health Service (NHS) Long Term Plan (NHS England, 2019), which notes one of its key clinical priority areas as addressing the health needs of people with learning disabilities.

With the shift in the direction of care, people with learning disabilities should, where possible, have the same level of access to general practice and primary care services as anyone else (NICE, 2018). However, it is well documented that people with learning disabilities experience numerous barriers in accessing healthcare services (Truesdale & Brown, 2017), and whilst the reasons for this are multifactorial, involving limited knowledge of both service user and provider, communication barriers and health literacy (Public Health England (PHE), 2015), the consequence is inappropriate healthcare assessment and management. This is particularly noteworthy in respect to some long-term conditions, which are more prevalent in people with learning disabilities in comparison to people who do not have learning disabilities (Kinnear et al., 2018). This disproportionate risk of increased morbidity and early mortality is a clear indicator of health inequalities for people with learning disabilities (Parkin et al., 2020).

Despite direction from the UK governments, professional literature and the legal requirements of the Equality Act 2010, healthcare services for people with learning disabilities continue to ineffectively meet their needs (Parkin et al., 2020). This is further evidenced within a raft of reports on preventing avoidable deaths of people with learning disabilities, with one of the most sobering being *Death by Indifference: 74 Deaths and Counting* (Mencap, 2012). In response, Mencap launched 'Treat Me Well' (Mencap, 2017), an ongoing campaign aiming to change how the NHS provides care and treatment for people with a learning disability. Although the main focus of the campaign centres on challenging the inequalities that exist within hospital care and treatment, the workable changes are focused on ensuring that people with learning disabilities routinely get the care and treatment they need and the equal access to healthcare they are entitled to, the ethos of which is transferable to the primary care setting. With a focus on anticipatory care and treatment, reactive acute hospital admission could be avoided for many people with learning disabilities.

Challenging the health inequalities faced by people with learning disabilities remains a contemporary issue and a persistent challenge (Bollard et al., 2018). Against this backdrop, the importance of primary care and the role of GPNs should not be underestimated as recognised 'gatekeepers' and advocates for people entering healthcare and signposting to other services and support systems. Reviewing the aforementioned policies and professional literature will contribute to ensuring the GPN's skills and knowledge are current (Royal College of Nursing (RCN), 2017) and that they practice within the established legal frameworks in delivering health services that are fit for purpose for people with learning disabilities.

LEGISLATION AND SAFEGUARDING – UK PERSPECTIVES

A crucial aspect of healthcare provision is the legal framework that underpins the safe and effective care and treatment of people with learning disabilities. Legal frameworks recognise the current limitations in practice in assessing capacity or, indeed, the issues arising in adult support and protection of people with learning disabilities. As a complex issue, Jenkins and Middleton (2018) discuss the safeguarding of adults with learning disabilities by exploring professionals' knowledge and skill deficits, which often prevail in working in healthcare and social care settings, which, if addressed, would ensure that the rights of people with learning disabilities are upheld.

The UK's constituent governments stipulate the respective legislative acts in caring for people with learning disabilities across the four home countries; for example, within Scotland, the main legal framework that the GPN would work within is the Adults With Incapacity (Scotland) Act 2000, which references the capacity to consent to treatment within Part 5,

Section 47. This details that a Section 47 certificate must be completed by a doctor or other authorised healthcare professional to provide nonemergency treatment to an adult who lacks the capacity to give or refuse consent. Crucially, this should be completed following an assessment of capacity and thus provide evidence that the treatment complies with the principles of the act and any associated code of practice. In England and Wales, the Mental Capacity Act 2005 (MCA) applies, and within Northern Ireland, the Mental Capacity (NI) Act 2016 applies. There are also wider legislative frameworks that practitioners need to have a working knowledge of when supporting people with learning disabilities, although the following is not an exhaustive list; it will also vary according to specific national application:

- Mental Health Act 1983, amended in 2007
- Mental Health (Care and Treatment) (Scotland) Act 2003
- Care Act 2014
- Adult Support and Protection (Scotland) Act 2007

However, it is important to remember when working within legal frameworks that people with learning disabilities have a wide spectrum of abilities and disabilities. Consequently, many individuals will have the capacity to make choices about their own lives with complete independence, whilst people with more severe or profound learning disabilities will require others to make decisions for them. Practitioners should therefore be mindful that although the person with learning disabilities will have a range of abilities, they may be considered vulnerable for different reasons or, indeed, not at all. Jenkins and Davies (2011) discuss the risks that may increase a person with learning disabilities demonstrating vulnerability. These issues are multifaceted and take consideration of not just the individual's learning disability, physical health and mental health but also the socioeconomic factors that influence their health and wellbeing. This correlates with the Health Equalities Framework (HEF; UK Learning Disability Nurse Consultant Network, 2013), which is an outcomes-based approach addressing the determinants of health inequalities for people with learning disabilities, discussed later in this chapter. However, it is worth keeping in mind that the particular issues concerning vulnerability for a person with learning disabilities are not static and will fluctuate and change over time. Many individuals with learning disabilities, and others receiving additional supportive interventions, are able to develop personal strategies to guard against vulnerability and so protect themselves from harm. However, practitioners also need to consider suitable risk assessments not only to protect individuals but also to enable people to achieve their potential.

Any discussion on the legal capacity of individuals and vulnerability must also be set against the stark reality that people with learning disabilities may be at risk of abuse (O'Malley et al., 2020). As such, practitioners must be alert to the possibility that individuals accessing care and treatment may evidence abuse, be this physical, psychological or sexual. Abuse needs to be acknowledged, believed and responded to when supporting individuals with a learning disability.

Having considered the legislative framework and aspects of safeguarding from a UK perspective, the next section will discuss the differing pattern of health that people with learning disabilities experience.

ASSESSING HEALTH NEEDS: IMPLICATIONS FOR PRIMARY CARE

People with learning disabilities experience a different pattern of mortality and morbidity in comparison to the general population (Truesdale & Brown, 2017). They have a lower life expectancy and higher rates of premature death; men with learning disabilities die 13 years younger, and women with learning disabilities die 20 years younger. Mortality rates are 3 times higher than those of the general population and are higher still for people with severe and profound learning disabilities. Preventable and premature causes of death are associated with higher rates of aspiration pneumonia, respiratory diseases, cardiovascular diseases and seizures. People with learning disabilities are also prone to particular types of cancer, heart disease and stroke, with these being amongst the main causes of mortality (Truesdale & Brown, 2017). Whilst these outcomes are concerning, they are compounded by the fact that people with learning disabilities have poorer access to healthcare services, public health interventions and health initiatives, which, furthermore,

are not designed to meet their complex and diverse needs (Truesdale & Brown, 2017). This resonates with the inverse care law – that is, people with learning disabilities are more in need of health services but are less likely to receive them.

In recognising that large numbers of people with learning disabilities will have unrecognised and therefore unmet health needs, a key issue for the GPN is to ensure that the care and treatment being delivered to people with learning disabilities with their practice population is specific and appropriate and, importantly, that preventative measures and models of supporting anticipatory care are being utilised. The recent publication of NHS Health Scotland's *People With Learning Disabilities in Scotland: 2017 Health Needs Assessment Update Report* (Truesdale & Brown, 2017) represents a key resource in the planning and delivery of care. As an update of an earlier landmark publication, this report verifies that many of the health issues that people with learning disabilities experience could be prevented or at least recognised early through appropriate health needs assessment, screening and early treatment interventions. For the GPN, this publication represents a valuable resource in raising awareness of prevalent health issues, which people with learning disabilities may be at risk of, but also in providing evidence-based information on diagnosis and appropriate treatment. This document provides a clear indication of health risks and wider holistic health assessment relative to the following:

- **Health needs assessment:** Taking the opportunity to consider communication; sensory impairment; visual impairment and hearing, accident prevention, mobility, balance and co-ordination, foot care, physical activity and any life events and trauma. Other aspects of assessment include nutrition and oral and dental health, with particular attention to bone health (as a result of pharmacology), as well as haematological disorders and infections. Pharmacotherapy (polypharmacy) should be explored, and where necessary, the advice of the pharmacologist should be sought, particularly when assessing drug histories and complex interactions.
- **Risk of physical health conditions:** Cardiovascular disease, particularly types of cancers and

respiratory disorders, are indicated as some of the highest causes of death. The incidence of epilepsy is significantly higher for people with learning disabilities, and this increases with the severity of the learning disability. Gastrointestinal disorders such as *Helicobacter pylori*, gastric infection and gastro-oesophageal reflux disorder (GORD) and constipation may occur. The incidence of constipation increases with the severity of the person's learning disability, which, if undiagnosed and untreated, can have significant consequences and implications for health and even premature death. In 2016, PHE published *Making Reasonable Adjustments for People With Learning Disabilities in the Management of Constipation*. There is also the additional online resource Self-Care Forum (n.d.), available from Easy Read guides.

■ **Sexuality and sexual health:** Assumptions should be avoided to ensure individuals do not miss out on receiving important support, guidance and services, which includes cervical screening (PHE, 2019).

■ **Mental ill-health:** People with learning disabilities are up to 50% more likely to experience mental health issues than the general population, which often go undiagnosed and poorly treated. Dementia also has a higher incidence and earlier onset for people with Down's syndrome. Many individuals will require specific psychological interventions and support to assist in behaviour changes and in addressing behaviours that may be perceived as challenging, as well as help with sleep disorders. Some individuals with learning disabilities who offend will require the specific support of forensic care services.

■ **Healthy lifestyles, health improvement and health-promotion activities:** Consideration needs to be given to how campaigns for the general population need to be adapted to ensure that the key messages are received in ways that are meaningful, such as simplifying and editing messages to specific focused points.

■ Noteworthy is that the life expectancy for people with a learning disability correlates with developments in preconceptual care and better accessibility to healthcare and social care services.

This highlights the prevention of fetal alcohol spectrum disorder (FASD), affecting 3.2% of babies born in the UK (Scottish Intercollegiate Guidelines Network, 2019), which, with the right preventative advice and early interventions, could make a difference to individuals' lives.

Finally, another useful resource published by PHE (online) is the Learning Disability Profiles, which provide key data sets on the health status of people with learning disabilities and details of care provided and information that can usefully inform decisions about the care and treatment of people with learning disabilities. This resource includes summaries of specific health inequalities experienced by people with learning disabilities, inclusive of the current evidence base on prevalence and risk factors, the potential impact on people with learning disabilities, healthcare and treatment measures, social determinants of health, signposting to links and other additional resources (see Resources section).

In considering the aforementioned health needs of people with learning disabilities, the GPN is well placed to search out, initiate and manage care in relation to unmet health needs. However, a crucial part of this care entails facilitating effective communication to enable the GPN to address individual health needs.

Facilitating Effective Communication

As highlighted earlier, one of the main issues that affects the lives of people with learning disabilities is communication. Consequently, reasonable adjustments must be made to ensure that individuals have appropriate mechanisms, strategies or support structures to ensure that they are included in all conversations and that, where possible, informed choice and consent is facilitated (Bunning, 2011).

Some individuals with a learning disability, who have limited or indeed no speech, may use Makaton to communicate. Makaton is a unique language that combines symbols, signs and speech to aid and develop communication skills (The Makaton Charity, 2020). Also, the use of 'Easy Read' formats is a key resource in aiding communication and for individuals to receive key health messages. Good examples that have applicability in primary care are those used for cervical screening and, additionally, the guide produced by Bowel

Cancer UK (2017): *Easy Read for the Bowel Health and the Bowel Screening Test in Scotland*.

Hospital passports have also been utilised across the UK to support communication in the care and treatment of people with learning disabilities in both acute and primary care settings. The aim of this single document is that it should relate to the individual and be available during consultations between the individual with learning disabilities and healthcare staff. The passport aims to provide clear information on 'things you must know about me', 'things that are important to me' and 'my likes and dislikes'. However, as Northway et al. (2017) highlight, there is no clear standard format or national approach to using communication passports within the UK, leading to inconsistency in use. The passports do, however, have a strong part to play in the healthcare of people with learning disabilities and continue to be developed by NHS boards/trusts, third-sector charitable and voluntary organisations, families and learning disabilities health services. Lunsky (2018) and Northway et al. (2017) strongly petition on the need for a consistent approach that considers not just the medical information but also the personal. The focus should be on making reasonable adjustments and for capacity to be considered within the appropriate legal framework(s).

Communication processes also involve carers, family and informal paid support workers in the context of appropriate legislation. However, the individual with learning disabilities needs to be at the centre of any care and treatment decisions. This will be explored in the next section, which will look at ways to assist in consultations and the assessment process.

Consultation Skills and Approaches

A key consideration for the GPN is that individuals with a learning disability often suffer significant anxiety when coming into contact with unfamiliar people and environments, which may impede the provision of appropriate care and treatment. So there may need to be flexibility in the scheduling of appointments that would be best for the individual as well as the length of the appointment. Sensitivity is also needed in the provision and staging of treatment because clinical interventions may not be appropriate as part of a first visit to the practice and may require the support of others to help facilitate the process. There have been a

number of changes in the approach to the assessment of people with learning disabilities by registered learning disability nurses, with models of nursing being reviewed and considered with current evidence-based practice. Moulster et al. (2019) have established an eclectic framework for learning disability nursing practice that has been recognised as a significant asset to the learning disability nurse's toolkit as a validated assessment tool that uses person-centred approaches in conjunction with current evidence-based practice.

Although there are specific and specialist assessments that can be used in the diagnosis and treatment of the health needs of people with learning disabilities, as discussed previously, the GPN has an important role to undertake in this process. The GPN is a vital link for people with learning disabilities in supporting their primary healthcare needs and, in turn, signposting to other services as required. Research by Truesdale and Brown (2017) recognises the pivotal role that primary healthcare has in addressing and maintaining the health needs of people with learning disabilities and has established a clear rationale for annual health checks to be undertaken for every individual on the GP register. In the delivery of anticipatory care, annual health checks not only contribute to the early detection and treatment of specific health conditions (National Institute for Health Research, 2020) but also allows for monitoring of long-term conditions. NHS England provides excellent guidance and tools for conducting annual health checks for people with learning disabilities (see Resources section). The Royal College of General Practitioners (RCGP) has also created the *Health Checks for People With Learning Disabilities Toolkit* (RCGP 2020). Aimed at general practitioners (GPs), GPNs and the primary administration team, the toolkit has collated guidance and resources to effectively undertake annual health checks for people with a learning disability.

The HEF, as previously mentioned, is an outcomes framework based on the determinants of health inequalities. Although this framework is intended for specialist learning disability services to set out and evaluate outcomes with and for people with learning disabilities, it is also useful for the GPN in having an overview of the factors affecting the health and wellbeing of this population. The framework can, in fact, be useful to a range of services to measure their effectiveness in tackling health inequalities for people with learning disabilities. Additionally, the framework can be used, with the input of families and carers, to set out person-centred outcomes and measure progress, which can be particularly useful when individuals may lack capacity and rely on others to improve and maintain their health and wellbeing. Another excellent resource for people with learning disabilities, produced by Macmillan Cancer Support (2018), is *7 Steps to Equal Health Care: Your Guide to Getting Good Health Care If You Have a Learning Disability*, which is structured as follows:

1. Imagine being me.
2. Find out who and what matters to me.
3. Listen to me.
4. Give me the information that I need, in the way that I need it.
5. Think about where we are.
6. Work with others who are in my life.
7. Giving treatment seems too difficult? Think again.

Having established that the mortality and morbidity of people with learning disabilities differ from that of the general population (Truesdale & Brown, 2017), the GPN's role in early detection, management and ongoing promotion is vital. With the appropriate knowledge base, the GPN can begin to consider what may be 'different' for people with learning disabilities and, in doing so, 'make a difference' in providing essential and equitable care. This will include the recognition of morbidities and, indeed, multiple morbidities, and where diagnostic overshadowing (i.e., not seeing beyond the diagnosis) can affect a clear and accurate diagnosis. The GPN will also have to consider, where appropriate, the health needs of any family/carers who support people with learning disabilities, whose role may be lifelong, and the impact this may have on their health and wellbeing.

In the context of consultations with people with learning disabilities, the GPN is required to be mindful of conversations that may, as previously discussed, indicate concerns regarding the safeguarding of vulnerable adults. Consequently, the GPN may, in the context of duty of care (Nursing and Midwifery Council (NMC), 2018), need to consider when it is appropriate to raise and escalate safeguarding concerns.

Although the GPN has a key role to play in addressing the healthcare needs of people with learning disabilities, it is also important to have an awareness of the services that are available locally. This will enable the GPN to network to seek additional support and guidance or indeed make referrals to specific learning disability services. The next section of this chapter will provide an overview of some of the services available, discussed within the context of the evolving healthcare and social care arena.

NETWORKING HEALTHCARE AND SOCIAL CARE SERVICES FOR PEOPLE WITH LEARNING DISABILITIES

The political landscape was discussed earlier in this chapter, and concerted efforts are also being made in the development and integration of healthcare and social care services across the UK. This has been implemented to varying degrees, with many areas via the creation of health and social care partnerships, whose aim is to create services that provide access to appropriate healthcare and social care and treatment by having a multiple-agency approach.

The registered learning disability nurse remains the only healthcare and social care professional to receive specific educational preparation in the care and treatment of people with learning disabilities. The role of learning disability nurses, many of whom work within community teams, is explored as part of *Strengthening the Commitment: The Report of the UK Modernising Learning Disabilities Nursing Review* (Scottish Government, 2012). Community teams are multidisciplinary and, in some cases, multiagency, including social work/social care professionals. The medical provision within learning disability services is usually provided by a consultant psychiatrist. Allied health professionals working within the team/services will include psychologists, physiotherapists, occupational therapists, speech and language therapists and dieticians, with some teams inclusive of art, music and drama therapists. Across the NHS, some areas have seen the introduction of acute and primary care liaison nursing roles to help facilitate the care journey for people with learning disabilities (MacArthur et al., 2015). Additionally, in-patient facilities exist for assessment and treatment as well as within mental health services, with many children and young people accessing child and adolescent mental health services (CAMHS). Having an awareness of the range and types of services available within the locality will enable the GPN to signpost individuals, families and carers to appropriate support services. With earlier sections having discussed some of the services available, the final section will provide a brief summary of the chapter, draw some conclusions and discuss implications for practice.

SUMMARY

In exploring the role implications for the GPN in the care and treatment of people with learning disabilities in the context of primary care, a clear picture emerges of how the GPN can make a significant difference in shifting the healthcare imbalance that can still occur for people with learning disabilities in the UK. Utilising the existing and emerging evidence base that identifies the additional and unmet health needs of people with learning disabilities gives substance to the GPN role to improve healthcare outcomes for this population. Additionally, having a greater understanding of specific legislation and vulnerability can ensure that people with learning disabilities receive appropriate care and protection. This also ensures that nursing practice remains legal and professional registration and that integrity is not compromised (NMC, 2018).

Working with individuals and carers, both family and paid, can maximise the best outcomes for people with learning disabilities, but GPNs must also recognise where the individual's voice can and should be heard. Taking on the role of 'gatekeeper' and 'navigator' within the primary care setting will ultimately lead to better signposting for the person with learning disabilities to appropriate services. For services that may be in mainstream general health services or, indeed, referral to specialist learning disability services, the GPN should have an understanding of the differing requirements and use this to guide and support people with learning disabilities.

Through building on communication skills and making reasonable adjustments as required, the GPN can improve the consultation process for people with learning disabilities accessing their care and treatment. Taking time to understand the situation and accommodate adaptations will not only benefit the individual but also the smooth operation of the GPN/primary care service.

Where the GPN is able to facilitate access to appropriate supports, the individual's journey into healthcare can be a less stressful experience. This may be a primary care liaison nurse, an acute liaison nurse, or a referral to the local learning disability community team. Having knowledge and understanding of the possible networks and specialist services where support may be available will enhance the role the GPN has in improving the health of people with learning disabilities.

RESOURCES

Social Care Institute for Excellence/National Institute for Health and Care Excellence: https://www.scie.org.uk/person-centred-care/care-planning/learning-disabilities

Public Health England – Learning Disability Profiles: https://fingertips.phe.org.uk/profile/learning-disabilities

NHS England – Annual Health Checks: https://www.england.nhs.uk/learning-disabilities/improving-health/annual-health-checks/

Royal College of General Practitioners – Learning Disabilities Toolkit: https://www.rcgp.org.uk/clinical-and-research/resources/toolkits/health-check-toolkit.aspx

REFERENCES

Adult Support and Protection (Scotland) Act 2007. http://www.legislation.gov.uk/asp/2007/10/contents

Adults With Incapacity (Scotland) Act 2000. http://www.legislation.gov.uk/asp/2000/4/pdfs/asp_20000004_en.pdf

Bollard, M., McLeod, E., & Dolan, C. (2018). Exploring the impact of health inequalities on the health of adults with intellectual disability from their perspective. *Disability and Society, 33*(6), 831–848.

Bowel Cancer UK. (2017). *Easy read for the bowel health and the bowel screening test in Scotland.* https://bowelcanceroruk.s3.amazonaws.com/Publications/BowelHealthAndTheBowelScreeningTestInScotland.pdf

Brown, H., & Benson, S. (1994). *A practical guide to working with people with learning disabilities* (2nd ed). Hawker.

Bunning, K. (2011). Let me speak – Facilitating communication. In H. Atherton & D. Crickmore (Eds.), *Learning disabilities: Toward inclusion* (6th ed., pp. 91–112). Churchill Livingstone Elsevier.

Care Act 2014. http://www.legislation.gov.uk/ukpga/2014/23/contents/enacted

Department of Health. (2001). *Valuing people: A new strategy for learning disability for the 21st century* (Cm 5086).

Gov.UK. (2003). *Every child matters.* https://www.gov.uk/government/publications/every-child-matters

Health and Social Care Act 2012. https://www.legislation.gov.uk/ukpga/2012/7/contents/enacted

HM Government. (2019). *Valuing people now: A new three-year strategy for people with learning disabilities: Making it happen for everyone.* https://webarchive.nationalarchives.gov.uk/20130105064234/http://www.dh.gov.uk/prod_consum_dh/groups/dh_digitalassets/documents/digitalasset/dh_093375.pdf

Jenkins, R., & Davies, R. (2011). Safeguarding people with learning disabilities. *Learning Disability Practice, 14*(1), 32–39.

Jenkins, R., & Middleton, A. (2018). Safeguarding adults with learning disabilities. In G. MacIntyre, A. Stewart, & P. McCusker (Eds.), *Safeguarding adults: Key themes and issues* (pp. 132–151). Macmillan Education.

Kinnear, D., Morrison, J., Allan, L., Henderson, A., Smiley, E., & Cooper, S-A. (2018). Prevalence of physical conditions and multimorbidity in a cohort of adults with intellectual disabilities with and without Down syndrome: Cross-sectional study. *BMJ Open, 2018*(8), Article e018292. https://bmjopen.bmj.com/content/bmjopen/8/2/e018292.full.pdf

Lunsky, Y. (2018). Hospital passports require standardisation to improve patient safety and person-centred care for those with intellectual disability. *Evidence-Based Nursing, 21*(2), 56–56.

MacArthur, J., Brown, M., McKechanie, A., Mack, S., Hayes, M., & Fletcher, J. (2015). Making reasonable and achievable adjustments: The contributions of learning disability liaison nurses in 'Getting it right' for people with learning disabilities receiving general hospitals care. *Journal of Advanced Nursing, 71*(7), 1552–1563.

Macmillan Cancer Support. (2018). *7 steps to equal health care: Your guide to getting good health care if you have a learning disability.* https://www.macmillan.org.uk/_images/enable-scotland-7-steps_tcm9-326880.pdf

McCormack, B., & McCance, T. (Eds.). (2016). *Person-centred practice in nursing and health care: Theory and practice* (2nd ed.). Wiley-Blackwell.

Mencap. (2012). *Death by indifference: 74 deaths and counting.* https://www.mencap.org.uk/sites/default/files/2016-08/Death%20by%20Indifference%20-%2074%20deaths%20and%20counting.pdf

Mencap. (2017). *Treat me well: Simple adjustments make a big difference: A campaign to transform how the NHS treats people with a learning disability.* https://www.mencap.org.uk/sites/default/files/2018-07/2017.005.01%20Campaign%20report%20digital.pdf

Mencap. (2018). *How common is learning disability in the UK?* https://www.mencap.org.uk/learning-disability-explained/research-and-statistics/how-common-learning-disability

Mental Capacity Act 2005. http://www.legislation.gov.uk/ukpga/2005/9/contents

Mental Capacity Act (Northern Ireland) 2016. https://www.legislation.gov.uk/nia/2016/18/contents/enacted

Mental Health (Care and Treatment) (Scotland) Act (2003). http://www.legislation.gov.uk/asp/2003/13/contents

Mental Health Act 1983 (amended in 2007). http://www.legislation.gov.uk/ukpga/2007/12/contents

Moulster, G., Lorizzo, J., Ames, S., & Kernohan, J. (2019). *The Moulster and Griffiths learning disability nursing model – A framework for practice.* Kingsley.

National Institute for Health and Care Excellence. (2018). *Care and support of people growing older with learning disabilities* (NICE Guideline NG96). https://www.nice.org.uk/guidance/ng96/chapter/Recommendations

National Institute for Health Research. (2020). *Better health and care for all; better care and services for people with learning disabilities.* https://content.nihr.ac.uk/nihrdc/themedreview-04326-BCAHFA/Better-Health_Care-For-FINALWEB.pdf

NHS England. (2019). *NHS long term plan.* https://www.longtermplan.nhs.uk/

Nursing and Midwifery Council. (2018). *The code: Professional standards of practice and behaviour for nurses, midwives and nursing associates.* https://www.nmc.org.uk/globalassets/sitedocuments/nmc-publications/nmc-code.pdf

Northway, R., Rees, S., Davies, M., & Williams, S. (2017). Hospital passports, patient safety and person-centred care: A review of documents currently used for people with intellectual disabilities in the UK. *Journal of Clinical Nursing, 26*(23–24), 5160–5168.

Nunkoosing, K. (2011). The social construction of learning disability. In H. Atherton & D. Crickmore (Eds.), *Learning disabilities: Toward inclusion* (6th ed., pp. 3–16). Churchill Livingstone Elsevier.

Office for National Statistics. (2019). *Dataset: Estimates of the population for the UK, England and Wales, Scotland and Northern Ireland.* https://www.ons.gov.uk/peoplepopulationandcommunity/populationandmigration/populationestimates/datasets/populationestimatesforukenglandandwalesscotlandandnorthernireland

O'Brien, J. (1989). *What's worth working for? Leadership for better quality human services.* Responsive Systems Associates. https://inclusion.com/site/wp-content/uploads/2017/12/Whats-Worth-Working-For.pdf

O'Malley, G., Irwin, L., & Guerin, S. (2020). Supporting people with intellectual disability who have experienced abuse: Clinical psychologists' perspectives. *Journal of Policy and Practice in Intellectual Disabilities, 17*(1), 59–69.

Parkin, E., Kennedy, S., Long, R., Hubble, S., & Powell, S. (2020). *Learning disability – Policy and services.* https://commonslibrary.parliament.uk/research-briefings/sn07058/

Public Bodies (Joint Working) (Scotland) Act 2014. http://www.legislation.gov.uk/asp/2014/9/contents/enacted

Public Health England. (2015). *Local action on health inequalities: Improving health literacy to reduce health inequalities.* http://www.healthliteracyplace.org.uk/media/1239/hl-and-hi-ucl.pdf

Public Health England. (2016). *Making reasonable adjustments for people with learning disabilities in the management of constipation.* https://www.ndti.org.uk/uploads/files/Constipation_RA_report_final.pdf

Public Health England. (2019). *Having a smear test. An easy guide about a health test for women aged 25 to 64.* https://assets.publishing.service.gov.uk/government/uploads/system/uploads/attachment_data/file/790791/CSP05_an_easy_guide_to_cervical_screening.pdf

Royal College of Nursing. (2017). *Dignity in health care for people with learning disabilities.* http://oxleas.nhs.uk/site-media/cms-downloads/RCN_Dignity_in_healthcare.pdf

Scottish Government. (2006). *Getting it right for every child 2006, updated 2017.* https://www.gov.scot/policies/girfec/

Scottish Government. (2012). *Strengthening the commitment: The report of the UK Modernising Learning Disabilities Nursing Review.* https://www.gov.scot/publications/strengthening-commitment-report-uk-modernising-learning-disabilities-nursing-review/

Scottish Government. (2013). *The keys to life: Improving quality of life for people with learning disabilities.* https://www.gov.scot/publications/keys-life-improving-quality-life-people-learning-disabilities/

Scottish Intercollegiate Guidelines Network. (2019, January). *Children and young people exposed prenatally to alcohol* (SIGN Publication No. 156). https://www.sign.ac.uk/assets/sign156.pdf

Self-Care Forum. (n.d.). *Fact Sheet No. 5: Constipation.* http://www.easy-read-online.co.uk/media/50962/constipation-lo-res-_v3pages.pdf

The Equality Act 2010. http://www.legislation.gov.uk/ukpga/2010/15/contents

The Makaton Charity. (2020). *About Makaton.* https://www.makaton.org/aboutMakaton/

Truesdale, M., & Brown, M. (2017). *People with learning disabilities in Scotland: 2017 health needs assessment update report.* NHS Health Scotland.

UK Learning Disability Nurse Consultant Network. (2013). *The Health Equalities Framework (HEF): An outcomes based approach on the determinants of health inequalities.* https://www.ndti.org.uk/assets/files/The_Health_Equality_Framework_final_word.pdf

Welsh Government. (2018). *Learning disability: Improving lives programme.* https://gov.wales/sites/default/files/publications/2019-03/learning-disability-improving-lives-programme-june-2018.pdf

World Health Organisation. (1992). *The ICD-10 Classification of Mental and Behavioural Disorders: Clinical descriptions and diagnostic guidelines.* https://www.who.int/classifications/icd/en/bluebook.pdf

17

MANAGING WOUNDS IN PRIMARY CARE

EDWIN TAPIWA CHAMANGA

INTRODUCTION

Wound management in general practice remains a challenge, with continuous contractual changes at the local and national levels to healthcare delivery, variations in wound care classifications (simple wounds and complex wounds) and variations in practitioners' knowledge and skill in wound management. The latter two are further influenced by the practitioner's previous role, access to education and the sharing of wound care practice between healthcare assistants and practice nurses. As a result of such challenges, wound care and wound assessments are poorly conducted, negatively affecting patient outcomes (Guest et al., 2015) and resulting in prolonged healing times and chronic wounds. This chapter seeks to explore wound assessment, management and factors that may affect wound healing in primary care.

Most patients in primary care will at some point experience a wound, and this may be as innocuous as an injection site. In most cases, such small wounds heal with no complications, except in situations where the site is infected or deteriorating. It is common for patients within the general practice setting to present with leg ulcers, pressure ulcers, neuropathic ulcers, diabetic foot ulcers, surgical wounds, cancerous wounds, lacerations, burns and scalds, bites and sinuses. The general management of such wounds is determined by the presenting characteristics of the wound bed at the time of assessment. The characteristics encountered influence the practitioner's decision-making in terms of wound dressing choice and the option to refer for specialist input.

Wound management does not occur in isolation. An effective wound management plan assesses the patient holistically. In general practice in the UK, practices use different electronic systems and wound assessment tools. For generalisation purposes, a version of the Generic Wound Assessment Minimum Dataset by Coleman et al. (2017) will be used as a guide to holistic wound assessment in this chapter. The dataset forms the basic information that should be collated as part of wound assessment whilst acknowledging intrinsic and extrinsic factors that may affect the wound-healing process.

NORMAL WOUND-HEALING PROCESS

Wound healing is a complex and dynamic process by which the skin repairs itself. It is characterised by a series of events that occur from the time of the injury to the point of wound healing, classified as four phases: *haemostasis, inflammation, proliferation,* and *remodelling.* In clinical practice, these phases often overlap, and some wounds become stuck in one phase, predominantly the inflammatory phase, which can lead to the development of a chronic wound. Table 17.1 outlines the phases of the normal wound-healing process and what happens at each stage.

Haemostatic Phase

The first phase of the normal wound-healing process involves haemostasis. This begins as the blood vessels constrict (vasoconstriction), the platelets aggregate and a clot is formed to prevent excess blood loss (Wilkinson

TABLE 17.1				
Normal Wound-Healing Process				
Phase	Time Frame	Cells Involved	Function	Cellular and Biophysical Events
Haemostasis	Immediate	Platelets (also called *thrombocytes* and involved in blood clotting)	Clotting	Vascular constriction Platelet aggregation, degranulation and fibrin formation (thrombus)
Inflammation	Day 1–4	Monocytes Lymphocytes Neutrophils Macrophages	Phagocytosis (ingestion of bacteria)	Neutrophil infiltration, monocyte infiltration and differentiation of macrophages Lymphocyte infiltration
Proliferation	Day 4–21	Macrophages Lymphocytes Angiocytes Neutrophils Fibroblasts Keratinocytes	Re-establishment of skin function Wound bed filling Wound closure	Re-epithelialisation Angiogenesis (growth of new capillaries) Collagen synthesis
Remodelling	Day 21–year 2	Fibrocytes	Develop tensile strength	Collagen remodelling Vascular maturation and regression

Adapted from Stacey, M. (2016). *Why don't wounds heal?* http://www.woundsinternational.com

& Hardman, 2020). This phase is commonly associated with surgical or traumatic wounds where bleeding is observed; it does not occur with burns or pressure ulcers because they do not present in this phase.

Inflammatory Phase

Inflammation is predominantly characterised by the presence of neutrophils and macrophages in the wound bed and surrounding tissue, which combat any invading harmful microorganisms or foreign materials (Harper et al., 2014). As the wound progresses through the phases of the healing process, neutrophils reduce in number and are replaced by macrophages, which can ingest bacteria and alter the body's immune function, to fight infection. As stated previously, in relation to burns and pressure ulcers, they present in the late inflammatory phase, despite the wound bed biochemistry being the same.

Proliferation Phase

In the proliferation phase, new granulation tissue is formed, which comprises microscopic blood vessels and elements that form the extracellular matrix (ECM), for example, polysaccharides and elastin and collagen proteins. The ECM surrounds and supports cells in the body's tissues and is the main component of the dermal skin. Fresh granulation tissue has a moist, beefy appearance and begins to fill the wound bed from the base upward to the skin level, where epithelialisation will occur in the next phase of wound healing (Meyers & Hudson, 2013). The growth of fresh granulation tissue is supported by angiogenesis, the formation of new blood capillaries.

Remodelling Phase

Remodelling is the final phase of wound healing, in which the collagen content of the wound changes to become smoother and new epithelial cells adjacent to the wound migrate across the wound surface (Leoni et al., 2015). Cells that were required to repair the wound are removed by apoptosis (programmed cell death). The remodelling phase involves closure of the wound edges. It should be noted that following total wound closure, the tissue on the healed wound site will retain 70% to 80% of the tensile strength of the original tissue.

HOLISTIC WOUND ASSESSMENT

There is a wealth of literature on the importance of undertaking a comprehensive patient assessment for those presenting with wounds (Benbow, 2016; Ousey & Cook, 2012). Wound assessments must be holistic, evolving and able to facilitate differential diagnosis to identify any causative or contributing factors that could potentially delay or prevent wound healing. Primary care patients can present with complex wounds as a result of multiple comorbidities because of increased longevity and advances in medicine. Practitioners must consider the social, family and emotional needs of the patient because wounds can lead to frustration for both patients and their families. Frustration increases the release of cortisol, an anti-inflammatory that will adversely affect the second phase of the wound-healing process. This frustration may also negatively affect the patient's quality of life, leading to social isolation, depression and anxiety. Primary care practitioners need to assess patients' community support networks and resources for both families and patients.

Wound History

The primary care practitioner must ascertain a full history of the wound, including factors that may have led to wound development or deterioration, such as infection or poor sitting posture as a result of immobility. This is essential for all types of wounds, including pressure ulcers, because there is a need for risk reduction/elimination of pressure to enhance wound healing. Also, this influences the focus of treatment, be it wound management or wound healing. Wound management is often associated with wounds that cannot be healed – for example, those with an untreatable underlying pathology, such as cancerous lesions. As a result, the care of these wounds becomes palliative by focusing on symptom relief, be it malodour, pain or exudate management. In primary care, this category consists mainly of fungating tumours, chronic pressure ulcers and any lesions where tissue repair or regeneration cannot be achieved, such as arterial ulcers (Rogers, 2015). In contrast, wound healing aims at encouraging tissue repair and regeneration in wounds that can be healed, mainly superficial traumatic wounds, acute wounds and chronic wounds without any complications.

Wound Types

Primary care practitioners must be able to clearly identify the cause of the wound because this influences

the treatment plan. Failure to accurately diagnose the underlying cause can delay the wound-healing process (Cook, 2012). Wounds managed in primary care may be acute or chronic wounds, healing by either primary or secondary intention. Acute wounds normally progress through the normal wound-healing trajectory because they are a result of surgery and trauma and usually have a short healing time frame as the wound edges are brought together (primary intention wound closure). However, chronic wounds could also be acute wounds that have not followed the normal healing pattern as a result of infection or other physical or physiological factors, thereby presenting with gaping edges as a result of loss of skin (secondary intention wound closure). These wounds typically result in longer healing time and increased levels of exudate as a result of prolonged inflammation.

It is the primary care practitioner's responsibility to provide an accurate diagnosis, clear treatment plan, rationale for dressing choice and therapy. If the patient presents with multiple wounds, each wound must be assessed individually and documented separately with an individualised care plan (Ousey & Cook, 2012).

Wound Location

Wound location may provide insight into its aetiology and assist in the implementation of an effective care plan. For example, pressure ulceration should be suspected where excessive prolonged sitting, reduced repositioning and immobility are present if the wound overlies bony areas. Alternatively, pressure ulcers can be evident around the insertion site of intervention tubes, such as the nostrils for nasogastric tubes. This could also be a result of the body rejecting foreign material — for example, where patients present with sinuses and nonhealing surgical wounds as a result of the body rejecting the foreign body (e.g., surgical mesh/nondissolvable sutures). Care must be taken to establish what structures lie beneath the wound:

- A wound over a capsule joint, such as the knee, could leak synovial fluid, which can be mistaken for wound exudate.
- Areas with exposed bone, such as diabetic foot ulcers, heel pressure ulcers or sacral pressure ulcers, must be carefully treated to eliminate the risk of osteomyelitis.

- Where an organ is exposed or the depth of a sinus is unknown, negative-pressure machines (advanced wound therapies) may be inappropriate.
- Where an exposed tendon or ligament is present, this needs to be kept moist because there is a high risk of drying, which ultimately results in death of the exposed tendon or ligament (Lie et al., 2019).

Wound Dimensions

Wound measurement forms part of the assessment process. However, measurement is effective when only recorded as wound volume (length from head to toe, width from side to side and depth). The measurement of wound size will help inform whether the wound is increasing or decreasing in volume. It is important when measuring the wound that cavities, sinuses, undermining, tracts, fistula and/or tunnelling are measured with a measuring probe. Anecdotal evidence suggests these can be documented using a clock system to elaborate an area of wound tunnelling – for example, a 5-cm tunnelling between 2 o'clock and 5 o'clock. Although this is not exact, it enables consistent measurement and documentation to be completed easily in primary care. Examples of wound tunnelling and tunnelling measurement are shown in Figs. 17.1, 17.2 and 17.3.

Wound Bed Condition

Wound bed condition varies, and wounds can be classified according to tissue type at any given time. For example, a wound bed can be necrotic, sloughy, granulating and epithelializing. A healthy granulation tissue is red in colour and granular in appearance; this is a positive indicator of healing and a good blood supply. In some cases, the wound bed may be invisible, covered with necrotic tissue or slough tissue. Such tissue impedes healing and will require debridement (Ousey & Cook, 2012). As part of the wound bed assessment, the primary care practitioner must consider whether the tissue easily bleeds and whether there is any swelling, cellulitis, malodour or collection of pus, which can be clinical indicators of wound infection. However, wound infection may also present as shown in Fig. 17.4.

Exudate

Exudate is essential for the wound-healing process. It encourages cellular migration on the wound bed

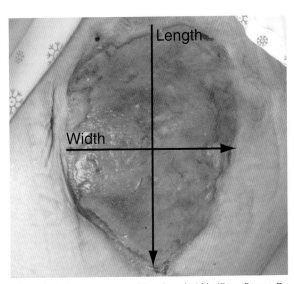

Fig. 17.1 ■ Measuring wound length and width. (From Bryant, R., & Nix, D. (2016). *Acute and chronic wounds: Current management concepts* (5th ed.). Elsevier.)

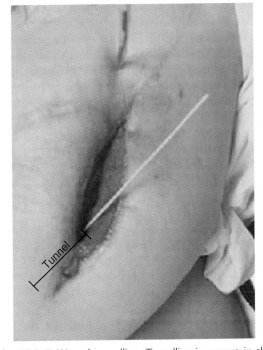

Fig. 17.2 ■ Wound tunnelling. Tunnelling is present in this abdominal wound at the 7 o'clock position and measures 2 cm in length. *Tunnel* and *sinus tract* are often used interchangeably. (From Bryant, R., & Nix, D. (2016). *Acute and chronic wounds: Current management concepts* (5th ed.). Elsevier.)

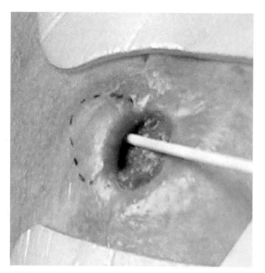

Fig. 17.3 ■ Undermining extends 2 cm from 7 to 11 o'clock. (From Bryant, R., & Nix, D. (2016). *Acute and chronic wounds: Current management concepts* (5th ed.). Elsevier.)

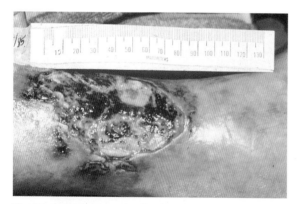

Fig. 17.4 ■ After 1 week of hydrocolloids and compression therapy, autolysis has occurred, and venous ulcer has the presence of granulation tissue. Amount of slough and eschar is reduced; remaining eschar is softened. (From Bryant, R., & Nix, D. (2016). *Acute and chronic wounds: Current management concepts* (5th ed.). Elsevier.)

(World Union of Wound Healing Societies (WU-WHS), 2019). Most of the wound exudate properties are essential for the wound-healing process, except for metabolic waste products. However, it is important that wound exudate is well managed because it can lead to either periwound maceration as a result of

moisture damaging the epidermis or excoriation when the skin pH creates a chemical reaction with wound exudate. Although wound exudate varies throughout the wound-healing process, its volume and consistency should be recorded.

The measurement and documentation of exudate have not been standardised in primary care. For example, exudate has been classified as lightly, moderately, or heavily exuding, and it has always been assumed that nurses can differentiate between these terms. Such terminology has also included subjective terms, such as the following:

- High/Excessive/+++
- Medium/moderate/++
- Low/minimal/+

This can make clinical communication/documentation and dressing choices difficult and subjective, which may lead to poor management of exudate and delay wound healing. It may be beneficial to use terms and descriptors as detailed in Table 17.2.

TABLE 17.2
Exudate Classification Chart

Term	Descriptor
Dry	No visible moisture
	Not an ideal wound-healing environment
	Surrounding skin may be dry, flaky and hyperkeratotic (exceptions are dry stable plaques in patients with inoperable ischaemia/peripheral arterial disease; may need experienced/expert assessment)
Moist	An ideal wound environment
	Primary dressing may have absorbed low amount of exudate
	Wound bed could appear glossy
	Surrounding skin may be intact and hydrated
Wet	Primary dressing may have absorbed large amounts of exudate
	Potential for periwound maceration
Saturated	Primary dressing may be saturated, and leakage is visible on the secondary dressing

Adapted from World Union of Wound Healing Societies. (2019). *Wound exudate: Effective assessment and management.* http://www.woundsinternational.com

Referrals

In primary care, as part of holistic wound assessment and management, some patients may need the involvement of a multidisciplinary team. Therefore referrals must be made to other services, and multidisciplinary teamwork must be established, with clear channels of communication, to improve patient outcomes. For example, in complicated diabetic foot ulcers, where a patient presents with a history of peripheral vascular disease, poor glycaemic control, neuropathy, loss of adipose tissue, renal disease and multiple infections, there is a need to involve the vascular team, diabetic podiatry, diabetic nurse specialists and endocrinologist. Where patients present with autoimmune ulcers, they may require the involvement of a rheumatologist or a dermatologist.

Condition of Wound Edges and Surrounding Skin

A thorough assessment of the periwound area can facilitate a holistic assessment by providing the primary care practitioner with information about the effectiveness of current therapy and aetiology. For example, arterial ulcers usually are well demarcated, with steep sides, whereas venous ulcers are defined by sloped and demarcated edges (Todhunter, 2019). Evidence of maceration of the surrounding skin can be an indicator of poor exudate management by the current dressing product. High levels of exudate can encourage bacterial growth, leading to infection, and slow down wound healing because the epithelium is unable to migrate across the new granulating tissue.

Pain

Wounds can cause continuous or intermittent pain. Intermittent pain is usually experienced during dressing changes or at repositioning. In such instances, the primary care practitioner will need to advise the patient to take analgesia before their appointment. For example, paracetamol can be taken 20 to 30 minutes before a dressing change. Poorly managed pain can negatively affect the wound-healing process and quality of life because high levels of cortisol (stress hormone) are released as a way of addressing homeostasis. This inhibits the inflammatory process, which is essential for wound healing. Continuous pain can be related to the inflammation phase, tissue excoriation, nerve damage, stress/anxiety, the site of the wound, ischemia, neuropathy, oedema or infection. A pain diary using a validated pain assessment scale will enable the prescribing of appropriate pain management therapy (Benbow, 2016). The assessment scale will also enable pain evaluation instead of the descriptors that are sometimes used in clinical practice, such as +, ++ or +++. In some cases, wound pain management involves the use of adjunctive therapies, such as amitriptyline (Joint Formulary Committee, 2021). In other situations, a patient may need a referral to the pain management team.

Neuropathy

Most practitioners are more familiar with sensory neuropathy, which is the most often documented type of neuropathy. It is a result of neurological deficit that results in patients losing sensation. In most cases, it is considered a complication of diabetes mellitus or excessive consumption of alcohol (alcoholic neuropathy). It is usually assessed in primary care with the use of a 10-g monofilament. In the absence of a monofilament, practitioners can conduct an Ipswich Touch Test (Volmer-Thole & Lobmann, 2016). Sensory neuropathy can lead to a patient developing a wound without realising it. For example, patients have presented with foreign objects (glass and needles) in their feet without knowing how these objects entered their skin.

The second most common type of neuropathy seen in primary care is autonomic neuropathy. This is a direct result of the lack of the ability to produce sweat to keep the skin moist. As a result, patients present with 'cracked heels' known as *fissures,* and these are commonly managed by the application of urea-based creams. The urea in the cream draws moisture from the dermis, thereby rehydrating the skin and addressing the dryness.

The third and final type of neuropathy is motor neuropathy. This is common in patients presenting with altered gait, which could be a direct result of removed bones or fixed ankles leading to toe muscular atrophy, and in most cases, patients present with shrivelled toes, known as 'picnic sausages'. In the presence of a wound, this may negatively affect the provision of nutrients and blood circulation to the area. For more information on feet neuropathy, please refer to Volmer-Thole and Lobmann (2016).

Wound Deterioration and Chronicity

Despite the efforts made by primary care practitioners, wounds often stall and become chronic. Chronic wounds are often stuck in one of the wound-healing phases, often the inflammatory phase, and fail to progress to the next phase. This is evidenced by exudate from chronic wounds presenting with elevated levels of protease as a result of higher levels of inflammatory molecules (WUWHS, 2019). There are multiple risk factors for wound chronicity, which are both intrinsic and extrinsic. The primary care practitioner must consider and discuss these factors with the patient.

INTRINSIC FACTORS

Age

Ageing results in changes to the structure and function of the skin that may impair the rate and quality of the wound-healing process. For example, the skin of older adults is more fragile, thinner, less elastic and drier than that of younger adults, with new cells being generated slowly. In addition, the fatty content of the subcutaneous tissue, which protects against infections and trauma, decreases in older adults. The major challenges associated with longevity are that patients present with multiple comorbidities and polypharmacy, which negatively affect the wound-healing process.

Stress

Haynes and Holloway (2019) reported that stress disrupts the neuroendocrine immune equilibrium, which causes a significant delay in wound healing by prolonging the inflammation phase. A prolonged inflammatory phase results in a higher bacterial count and increases the incidence of infection, which disrupts wound closure and the healing process. Stress can also lead to anxiety, depression, suboptimal sleeping patterns, inadequate nutrition, reduced exercise and increased susceptibility to alcohol consumption, cigarette smoking and drug use, all of which have a negative effect on wound healing.

Diabetes Mellitus

Patients with a diagnosis of diabetes are at risk of presenting with multiple comorbidities, including suboptimal wound healing and chronic ulceration as a result

of microvascular and macrovascular complications (Okonkwo & DiPietro, 2017). Although the diagnosis of diabetes does not automatically mean that a patient's wound will become chronic, patients with suboptimally controlled blood glucose levels are at high risk of developing chronic wounds because of hypoxia, dysfunction in the role of fibroblasts and epidermal cells, and impaired angiogenesis and neovascularisation (the natural formation of new blood vessels).

Nutrition

Adequate nutritional intake is essential to enable wound healing because some patients lose large volumes of protein through wound exudate, and patients with wounds have a higher metabolic rate compared with those who do not have wounds (Guo & DiPietro, 2010). There are several aspects of nutrition that influence the wound-healing process. For example, vitamin K and calcium are essential for the formation of fibrin clots during the haemostasis phase. Vitamin K is responsible for enzyme activation of prothrombin VII, IX and X clotting factors, which enables fibrin formation, of which calcium is essential for binding clotting factors to membranes at the site of injury (Sherman & Barkley, 2011). Protein deficiency can impair capillary formation, cell proliferation and wound remodelling, as well as reducing the efficiency of the immune system, thereby increasing the risk of infection (Gould et al., 2015). Other essential nutrients for wound healing include vitamins A, B and C and zinc, iron and copper. A referral to the dietetics service for assessment may be required if a person with a wound is suspected of having a suboptimal nutritional intake. Obesity and being underweight also have a negative effect on the wound-healing process. Patients who are obese are at risk of compromised wound healing resulting from inadequate blood supply to the adipose tissue or protein malnutrition, whereas patients who are underweight may lack the oxygen and nutritional stores required for wound healing.

EXTRINSIC FACTORS

Medicines

Some medicines, such as cytotoxic drugs, interfere with cell migration on the wound bed and may cause neutropenia, leaving the wound bed susceptible to infection. The use of antiplatelet agents, long-term corticosteroids and anti-inflammatory drugs suppresses the body's usual inflammation process or disrupts the clotting mechanism, thereby disrupting the wound-healing process through vasoconstriction (Maver et al., 2015). Because of prolonged vasoconstriction in the wound bed, the healing process becomes disrupted, with an inadequate number of macrophages reaching the wound to facilitate the inflammation process. This could potentially lead to a chronic wound caused by a lack of growth factors or disruption from infection.

Alcohol Consumption

Excessive alcohol consumption has been found to negatively affect the wound-healing process. It increases the incidence of infection by suppressing the release of pro-inflammatory enzymes (Tønnesen et al., 2012). Primary care practitioners must include questions on alcohol consumption as part of ongoing patient assessment because alcohol consumption patterns may change in relation to wound outcomes.

Smoking

Smoking reduces the oxygen-carrying capacity of red blood cells, thereby inducing wound chronicity because the lack of oxygenated blood inhibits angiogenesis on the wound bed (Meyers & Hudson, 2013). It is associated with delayed wound healing, wound infection and wound dehiscence (breaking down of postsurgical wounds, as shown in Fig. 17.5), despite research indicating that topical application of nicotine in low doses improves healing by the formation of new blood capillaries (Kean, 2010). However, tar from cigarette smoking causes vasoconstriction, which reduces blood flow to the skin. This results in tissue ischaemia; reduced proliferation of red blood cells, fibroblasts and macrophages; and impaired wound healing.

Infection

One of the functions of the skin is to provide protection to internal organs from external microorganisms. Once the skin is injured, the underlying tissue can become contaminated. It is essential that any contaminating microorganisms are removed or reduced so that the inflammation phase of the wound-healing

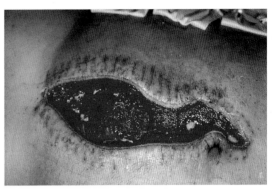

Fig. 17.5 ■ Full-thickness abdominal wound healing by secondary intention with healthy (red, cobblestone) granulation tissue and attached wound edges. (From Bryant, R., & Nix, D. (2016). *Acute and chronic wounds: Current management concepts* (5th ed.). Elsevier.)

process is not prolonged (Gould et al., 2015). The major function of neutrophils is to remove foreign material, bacteria and nonfunctional tissue that may be present on the wound bed. Phagocytosis occurs when neutrophils identify the chemical signals displayed by microorganisms and ingest them (Harper et al., 2014).

Temperature

It is essential that wound bed temperature is maintained at body temperature, between 36°C and 38°C. Delayed healing has been noted in cases where temperatures have been observed to be below the core body temperature or above 42°C (Lloyd-Jones, 2012). A drop in temperature leads to vasoconstriction, which results in a disruption of blood flow to the wound bed. An increase in temperature risks vasodilation, which may lead to an uncontrollable leaking of vital nutrients on the wound bed. This means a temperature drop in the wound as a result of cleansing solution or exposure to air can take up to 40 minutes before the temperature returns to normal and up to 3 hours for the cell-division process to be re-established (Beam et al., 2016).

WOUND MANAGEMENT

Wound Bed Preparation

Wound bed preparation is considered crucial to accelerate wound healing or to enhance the effectiveness of interventions designed to heal chronic wounds (Frykberg & Banks, 2015). Wound bed preparation involves identifying and eliminating factors that may hinder the wound-healing process, such as nonviable tissue in the wound bed or increased levels of exudate. This facilitates wound healing and provides an effective means of chronic wound management by promoting an understanding of the barriers to healing, providing a systematic approach, and enhancing the effects of advanced therapies. Wound bed assessment can be summarised using the TIME framework (Dowsett et al., 2015), which consists of four components:

- T – tissue. Is the tissue viable or nonviable? Is removal (debridement) of nonviable tissue, for example, necrotic tissue and eschar, necessary to encourage wound healing?
- I – infection or inflammation. Are there any visible clinical signs of infection that need to be addressed to encourage the wound-healing process? These signs might include heat, redness, pain, swelling and odour.
- M – moisture balance. Is the wound environment moist enough to support the principle of moist wound healing?
- E – edges of the wound and epithelialisation. Are the wound edges nonadvancing or undermining (deep tissue damage around the wound margin)? What are the characteristics of the wound edges? Are they thick and nonadvancing (callus)? If so, they may require debridement.

The TIME framework provides primary care nurses with a systematic approach to selecting appropriate wound interventions and should be implemented as part of a holistic assessment of any wound. The TIME framework can also identify appropriate wound bed objectives, which can often change during the wound-healing process, for example:

- Debride – to remove the nonviable tissue to encourage granulation.
- Hydrate – to moisten the wound bed to encourage moist wound healing or debridement.
- Protect – to keep the tissue in the wound bed free from trauma and contamination.
- Manage pain – to ensure that the patient is comfortable.

- Manage exudate – to encourage a moist environment and protect the periwound skin.
- Encourage granulation – to support the formation of new capillaries.
- Aid epithelialisation – to encourage total wound closure by ensuring that epithelial cells cover the wound bed and are not being damaged.
- Reduce bacterial bioburden – to minimise the risk of infection.

One of the main principles of wound healing is moist wound healing, a concept first posited by Winter in 1962, which states that the wound bed must be kept moist using conventional dressings to encourage wound healing. Although this principle was initially based on managing acute wounds, it has also been proven to be effective in managing chronic wounds. Wound bed preparation has largely superseded Winter's (1962) work. Ensuring that the wound is adequately hydrated is one of the cornerstones of modern wound care and an essential element of the TIME framework. Wound healing in moist wounds is 2 to 3 times faster than healing in dry wounds.

SELECTING AN APPROPRIATE WOUND DRESSING

The dressing-selection process is influenced by the objective of the wound bed, as stated previously. Each dressing type has its own unique properties, and the primary care practitioner and patient should consult to choose the appropriate dressing to be used on the wound. The most common types of dressings include passive dressings, interactive dressings and occlusive dressings, as listed in Table 17.3.

CHALLENGES IN PRIMARY CARE

Overgranulation

One of the major challenges faced in primary care when treating wounds healing by secondary intention is overgranulation. This is when the wound bed tissue 'overgrows' beyond the surface of the wound, also referred to as *hypergranulation, exuberant granulation, hyperplasia of granulation, hypertrophic granulation* or *'proud' flesh* (Stephen-Haynes & Hampton, 2010); some examples are shown in Fig. 17.6. The exact

TABLE 17.3
Types of Dressings and Their Properties

Dressing Type	Dressing Examples	Dressing Properties
Passive dressings	Foams	For low-exudation and epithelialising wounds
	Films	Provide protection by covering the wound
	Silicone	Provide protection against dehydration
Interactive dressings	Alginates	For clean granulating wounds
	Hydrocolloids	Actively interact with the wound surface by either filling space to encourage granulation or resting on top of nonviable tissue to encourage wound debridement
	Hydrofibres	
	Hydrogels	Promote an optimal environment for wound healing
	Semipermeable films	Provide protection against dehydration
		Many, but not all, interactive dressings are semi-impermeable to moisture, which promotes moisture balance
	Some foams	
Occlusive dressings	Hydrocolloids	Completely seal off the wound from the external environment
		Occlusive

Adapted from Sussman, G. (2014). Ulcer dressings and management. *Australian Family Physician, 43*(9), 588–592.

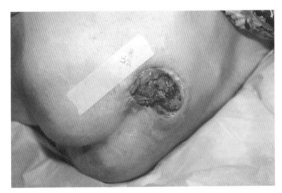

Fig. 17.6 ■ Stage III pressure ulcer with excess granulation tissue. (From Bryant, R., & Nix, D. (2016). *Acute and chronic wounds: Current management concepts* (5th ed.). Elsevier.)

causes of overgranulation are unknown, and it can be challenging to manage because it will delay the wound-healing process or increase exudate volume. Different options are being used in clinical practice to manage overgranulation (Table 17.4). Malignance (disrupted cell division that leads to cell mutation) may also lead to overgranulation, and it is best practice to investigate the aetiology of persistent overgranulating tissue with dermatological examinations (Dabiri et al., 2016). Although Table 17.4 lists different procedures

carried out across the UK to manage overgranulating wounds, primary care practitioners should always practice within their own sphere of competence and local guidelines.

LEG ULCERS

The term *leg ulcer* is not a diagnosis; instead, it is an indicator that a patient has a wound that is located between the knee and the ankle. Consequently, this is not a diagnostic term because leg ulcers are defined by the nature of their origin, and this determines the care plan and treatment approach. There are three main common types of leg ulcers: venous leg ulcers, arterial leg ulcers and mixed-aetiology leg ulcers. It is the duty of the primary care nurse to differentiate between the origins on initial assessment and on an ongoing basis to maintain an optimal appropriate treatment for the patient's condition because the three categories of leg ulceration are treated or managed differently. It is therefore essential that the practice nurse has the evidence-based knowledge and skills to effectively assess and competently manage leg ulceration.

Venous Leg Ulcers

Venous leg ulcers are open lesions between the knee and the ankle joint (the gaiter area). They tend to occur

TABLE 17.4

Treatment for Overgranulation

Treatment Option	Objective of Treatment	Evidence Base
Application of foam dressing	To flatten and absorb moisture	Carter, 2003; WUWHS, 2019
Change from an occlusive to a nonocclusive dressing	To reduce moisture	Carter, 2003
Use of antimicrobials	To reduce bacteria	Leak, 2002; Lloyd-Jones, 2006
Topical corticosteroid	Reduces the cell division and production of granulation tissue	Carter, 2003; WUWHS, 2019
Silver nitrate pencil	Only if all else has been ineffective	Borkowski, 2005
Foam and silver	Has antimicrobial effect and provides compression because of the foam	Lloyd-Jones, 2006
Surgical excision	Undertaken in theatre as very last resort	

WUWHS, World Union of Wound Healing Societies.
Adapted from Stephen-Haynes, J., & Hampton, S. (2010). *Achieving effective outcomes in patients with overgranulation*. Wound Care Alliance UK. https://www.wcauk.org/uploads/files/documents/resources/educational-booklets/booklet_overgranulation.pdf

on both the lateral and medial aspects of the leg and occur in the presence of venous insufficiency. They are also known as *varicose* or *stasis ulcers*, which are usually superficial, with poorly defined wound margins and a granulating wound bed, and exhibit moderate to high exudate. They are a common, recurring condition, with an estimated prevalence of 730,000 in the UK (Guest et al., 2015), which increases with the aging process and is highest in those between the ages of 60 and 80 (Atkin, 2019). They occur in people from all socioeconomic backgrounds; however, evidence indicates that they take longer to heal, with a higher recurrence rate, in people from lower socioeconomic backgrounds (Scottish Intercollegiate Guidelines Network, 2010), with a recurrence risk of between 26% and 69% in 12 months (Nelson & Bell-Syer, 2014).

There are multiple theories attributed to venous leg ulceration aetiology, such as the fibrin cuff theory, the white cell entrapment theory and the growth factor 'trap' theory. In addition, patients with venous leg ulcers also present with physical signs of venous insufficiency or skin changes, which must be documented on assessment as part of good clinical practice and care planning. Risk factors to the development of venous ulcers must also be identified and addressed or minimised. Evidence-based treatment for venous leg ulcers is compression bandaging (Team et al., 2019), and with advances in research and technology, there are different devices, such as bandages, compression

stockings and compression wraps, at the primary care nurse's disposal to offer compression therapy to a patient with venous leg ulcers.

Arterial Leg Ulcers

Arterial leg ulcers occur as a result of poor arterial blood flow, resulting in some parts of the leg lacking the provision of essential nutrients and oxygenation. These ulcers are often deeper and rounded, with clearly defined edges. In most cases, patients with arterial leg ulcers may already have a diagnosis of atherosclerosis (narrowing of the arteries as a result of plaque) or peripheral vascular disease (Todhunter, 2019). Because the arterial blood flow is inhibited, patients experience pain in the lower limb on exertion because the blood flow cannot meet the demand to the active area, thus causing hypoxia in the muscle nearest to the affected area. Pain can also be experienced at night, during rest or on leg elevation, and this is often addressed once the leg is put in a dependent position because the oxygenated blood will find it easier to flow through the narrowing part of the arteries.

The poor blood flow in the limb, if left untreated, will eventually lead to tissue death in areas close to the affected artery, which in turn will present with a rapid ulcer development and deep destruction of tissue. There are risk factors associated with arterial leg ulceration, which are smoking, obesity, hyperlipidaemia, hypertension and diabetes (European Society of Cardiology,

2018). All patients with suspected/possible arterial problems are referred to the vascular team for further assessments and care planning as a matter of urgency.

Mixed-Aetiology Leg Ulcers

Approximately 10% to 20% of leg ulcers are of mixed aetiology, exhibiting a mixture of signs of venous and arterial disease. The term *mixed aetiology* is commonly associated with venous leg ulcers with a concomitant arterial occlusive disease (Harding et al., 2015). These ulcers are often managed by compression therapy, but in some cases, this may include the involvement of the vascular team, depending on the severity of the arterial insufficiency.

SUMMARY

Wound assessment and evaluation are an ongoing, dynamic process that must identify changes that occur during the wound-healing/management process. As a result, this influences the plan of care to meet the needs of both the wound bed and the patient. It is essential that all care plans and changes are well documented to enhance wound management that is supported by effective communication. It is essential that primary care practitioners can identify their limitations and make necessary referrals to respective departments or therapists to improve wound healing and patient outcomes.

REFERENCES

Atkin, L. (2019). Venous leg ulcer prevention 1: Identifying patients who are at risk. *Nursing Times, 115*(6), 24–28.

Beam, J. W., Buckley, B., Holcomb, W. R., & Ciocca, M. (2016). National Athletic Trainers' Association position statement: Management of acute skin trauma. *Journal of Athletic Training, 51*(12), 1053–1070.

Benbow, M. (2016). Best practice in wound assessment. *Nursing Standard, 30*(27), 40–47.

Borkowski, S. (2005). G tube care: managing hypergranulation tissue. *Nursing, 35*(8), 24.

Carter, K. (2003). Treating and managing pilonidal sinus disease. *Journal of Community Nursing, 17*(7), 28–33.

Coleman, S., Nelson, E. A., Vowden, P., et al. (2017). Development of a generic wound care assessment minimum data set. *Journal of Tissue Viability, 26*(4), 226–240.

Cook, L. (2012). Wound assessment: The missing link. *British Journal of Nursing, 21*(20), 4–6.

Dabiri, G., Damstetter, E., & Phillips, T. (2016). Choosing a wound dressing based on common wound characteristics. *Advanced Wound Care, 5*(1), 32–41.

Dowsett, C., Nylokke, M., & Harding, K. (2015). *Taking wound assessment beyond the edge.* http://www.woundsinternational.com

European Society of Cardiology. (2018). 2017 ESC guidelines on the diagnosis and treatment of peripheral arterial diseases, in collaboration with the European Society for Vascular Surgery (ESVS). *European Heart Journal, 39,* 763–821.

Frykberg, R. G., & Banks, J. C. (2015). Challenges in the treatment of chronic wounds. *Advances in Wound Care, 4*(9), 560–582.

Gould, L., Adabir, P., Brem, H., et al. (2015). Chronic wound repair and healing in older adults: current status and future research. *Wound Repair and Regeneration, 23*(1), 1–13.

Guest, J. F., Ayoub, N., McIlwraith, T., et al. (2015). Health economic burden that wounds impose on the National Health Service in the UK. *BMJ Open, 5*(12). https://bmjopen.bmj.com/content/bmjopen/5/12/e009283.full.pdf

Guo, S., & Dipietro, L. A. (2010). Factors affecting wound healing. *Journal of Dental Research, 89,* 219–229.

Harding, K., et al. (2015). *Simplifying venous leg ulcer management.* Consensus recommendations. http://www.woundsinternational.com

Harper, D., Young, A., & McNaught, C. (2014). The physiology of wound healing. *Surgery, 32*(9), 445–450.

Haynes, S., & Holloway, S. (2019). Theories of stress and coping and how they relate to individuals with venous leg ulceration. *British Journal of Healthcare Management, 25*(5). https://www.magonlinelibrary.com/doi/full/10.12968/bjhc.2019.25.5.187

Joint Formulary Committee. (2021). *British National Formulary.* http://www.medicinescomplete.com

Kean, J. (2010). The effects of smoking on the wound healing process. *Journal of Wound Care, 19*(1), 5–8.

Leak, K. (2002). PEG site infections: A novel use for Actisorb Silver 220 (562kb). *British Journal of Community Nursing, 7*(6), 321–325.

Lei, J., Sun, L., Li, P., Zhu, C., Lin, Z., MacKey, V., Coy, D., & He, Q. (2019). The wound dressings and their applications. Wound healing and management. *Health Science Journal, 13*(4), 662. https://www.hsj.gr/medicine/the-wound-dressings-and-their-applications-in-wound-healing-and-management.php?aid=24605

Leoni, G., Neumann, A., Sumagin, R., et al. (2015). Wound repair: Role of immune-epithelial interactions. *Mucosal Immunology, 8*(5), 959–968.

Lloyd-Jones, M. (2006). Treating overgranulation with a silver hydrofibre dressing. *Wound Essentials, 1,* 116–118.

Lloyd-Jones, M. (2012). Wound cleansing: Is it necessary, or just a ritual? *British Journal of Healthcare Assistants, 6*(6), 269–273.

Maver, T., Maver, U., Kleinschek, K. S., Smrke, D. M., & Kreft, S. (2015). A review of herbal medicines in wound healing. *International Journal of Dermatology, 54,* 740–751.

Meyers, L., & Hudson, S. L. (2013). *Wound care: Getting to the depth of the tissue.* http://www.nursece.com/pdfs/720_WoundCare.pdf

Nelson, E. A., & Bell-Syer, S. E. (2014). Compression for preventing recurrence of venous ulcers. *Cochrane Database of Systematic Reviews, 2014*(9), Article CD002303.

Okonkwo, U. A., & DiPietro, L. A. (2017). Diabetes and wound angiogenesis. *International Journal of Molecular Sciences, 18*(1419), 1–15.

Ousey, K., & Cook, L. (2012). Wound assessment: Made easy. *Wounds UK, 8*(2), 1–4.

Rogers, G. (2015). Palliative wound care: Part 1. *Wound Care Advisor, 4*(1), 25–27.

Scottish Intercollegiate Guidelines Network. (2010). *Management of chronic venous leg ulcers. A national clinical guideline.* http://www.sign.ac.uk/pdf/sign120.pdf

Sherman, A. R., & Barkley, M. (2011). Nutrition and wound healing. *Journal of Wound Care, 20*(8), 357–367.

Stephen-Haynes, J., & Hampton, S. (2010). *Achieving effective outcomes in patients with overgranulation.* Wound Care Alliance UK. https://www.wcauk.org/uploads/files/documents/resources/educational-booklets/booklet_overgranulation.pdf

Team, V., Chandler, P. G., & Weller, C. D. (2019). Adjuvant therapies in venous leg ulcer management: A scoping review. *International Journal of Tissue Repair and Regeneration, 27*(5), 562–590.

Todhunter, J. (2019). Detecting and treating peripheral arterial disease in primary care. *Journal of Community Nursing, 33*(4), 35–41.

Tønnesen, H., Pedersen, S., Lavrsen, M., et al. (2012). Reduced wound healing capacity in alcohol abusers-reversibility after withdrawal. *Research and Best Practice, 2*(3), 89–92.

Volmer-Thole, M., & Lobmann, R. (2016). Neuropathy and diabetic foot syndrome. *International Journal of Molecular Science, 17*(917), 1–11.

Wilkinson, H. N., & Hardman, M. J. (2020). Wound healing: Cellular mechanisms and pathological outcomes. *Open Biology, 10,* 200223. https://royalsocietypublishing.org/doi/pdf/10.1098/rsob.200223

Winter, G. D. (1962). Formation of the scab and the rate of epithelialization of superficial wounds in the skin of the young domestic pig. *Nature, 193,* 293–294.

World Union of Wound Healing Societies. (2019). *Wound exudate: Effective assessment and management.* http://www.woundsinternational.com

18 MANAGING DERMATOLOGICAL CONDITIONS IN PRIMARY CARE

KIRSTY ARMSTRONG

INTRODUCTION

The knowledge and understanding of how to assess and manage dermatological conditions is a fundamental part of the skill set of the general practice nurse (GPN). However, this represents a complex area of practice because dermatological conditions, whilst primarily involving the skin, can often require consideration of other body systems. Consequently, dermatological presentations can demonstrate wide and varied aetiology in that they can present as stand-alone conditions, such as molluscum contagiosum, or form part of a more complex set of conditions, for example, psoriasis and psoriatic arthropathy. Moreover, the emergence of a skin rash may also be indicative of the acute phase of a communicable infection, such as measles or varicella (chickenpox), which have potentially serious sequelae, such as encephalitis in the case of measles or severe bacterial skin sepsis in the case of varicella (UK Sepsis Trust, 2016). As a frontline practitioner, the GPN's knowledge of the potential 'red flags' associated with making a dermatological diagnosis is a critical part of safe and effective care. Therefore any cursory temptation to dismiss an abnormal skin presentation as 'just a rash' must be avoided because this may be indicative of significant clinical risk.

As the body's largest organ, the skin performs numerous complex functions in protecting and maintaining health and wellbeing. This includes being the tactile window to the world in transmitting, via sensory receptors located within the skin, sensations such as touch, temperature, pain, pressure and movement. For the GPN, fundamental knowledge of skin anatomy, physiology and systemic diseases that may affect this system, along with the use of relevant diagnostic tools, is necessary to ensure accurate assessment, management and treatment.

SKIN PHYSIOLOGY AND ANATOMY

Physiologically, skin functions include regulation of pressure and touch sensation, maintaining temperature by controlling heat/cold and water loss and, critically, providing a protective barrier against bacteria and other pathogenic organisms (Hess, 2011). When the skin loses its integrity, infection is more likely, so maintaining soft, supple skin is vital, and the homeostatic function of the skin is essential for health and wellbeing. Consequently, if large areas of blistering, erythema (redness) or exudate develop, this may affect temperature control and increase the risk of dehydration and heat loss, allowing the patient to become cold or potentially hypothermic.

Skin thickness varies on bodily regions, being only 2 mm thick in some areas. In many patients with pre-existing comorbidities, such as diabetes or autoimmune diseases, or patients prescribed particular types of medications (e.g., steroids), the skin will become progressively thinner and thus more friable and particularly prone to traumatic tears, infection and bruising, which can be difficult to manage clinically.

As a body system, the skin comprises two key layers, the epidermis and the dermis (Fig. 18.1), the former being the protective layer that contains melanin and the latter containing nerve endings, sweat glands, hair

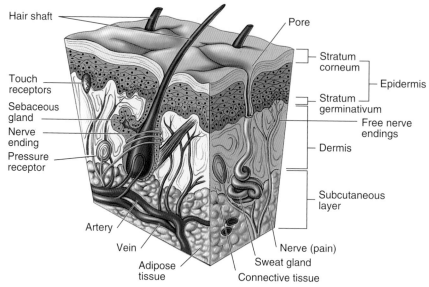

Hair shaft

Pore

Touch receptors

Sebaceous gland

Nerve ending

Pressure receptor

Stratum corneum

Epidermis

Stratum germinativum

Free nerve endings

Dermis

Subcutaneous layer

Artery

Vein

Adipose tissue

Nerve (pain)

Sweat gland

Connective tissue

Fig. 18.1 ■ Dermis cross-section of the skin. (From Larson, L. W. (2018). *Surgical implantation of cardiac rhythm devices* (1st ed.). Elsevier.)

follicles and oil glands. Collagen, within the dermis layer, provides structure and support for the skin.

MANAGING THE DERMATOLOGY CONSULTATION

In managing the consultation, the GPN requires the ability to undertake a comprehensive history and physical examination and develop a management plan, irrespective of the presentation appearing acute or unclear and the potential need for onward referral to the general practitioner (GP). Acknowledging that patients presenting with dermatological conditions will have anxieties means the GPN must utilise excellent communication skills, which include active listening.

The use of active listening skills is a crucial part of clinical decision-making processes in gathering vital clinical cues, particularly when the diagnosis may be unclear, and these skills are critical in avoiding misdiagnosis, which may lead to inappropriate management, including erroneous discharge from the service. The need to obtain an accurate and comprehensive history as part of holistic assessment for any

presenting complaint cannot be overstated (Armstrong 2019). Practical guidance on evidence-based history taking approaches is provided within Chapter 6 and with specific reference to dermatological conditions within Table 18.1 as detailed below.

ASSESSMENT AND MANAGEMENT OF DERMATOLOGICAL LESIONS AND RASHES

Examination and Assessment of the Skin

Despite the commonality of rashes and lesions being localised to certain areas of the skin, the skin in its entirety, plus the hair/scalp and nails, must be assessed. The aetiology of skin disease can include nail disorders, such as psoriasis (nail pitting), and if seborrhoeic dermatitis or fungal infections are present, these can affect the scalp, resulting in tinea capitis (*tinea* meaning 'fungal').

Clinically, rashes can be classified according to the colour, distribution, type of lesion and arrangement; for instance, the shingles rash is generally observed as pale blisters, linear in their presentation, vesicular (blistered) and unilateral (one side of the torso),

TABLE 18.1

Structured History Taking and Assessment of Dermatological Presentations

History taking	Site	Location
		Where first started (e.g., eczema typically starts in flexures)
	Onset	How long has the skin rash or lesion been present
		Any changes in the rash or lesion
		Is this a recurrence or seasonal presentation
	Character	Experiencing pain, swelling, tenderness, itching, burning sensation
		Exudate or bleeding from the rash or lesion
	Radiate	If experiencing pain, does it radiate anywhere?
	Associated features	General health status: currently well; exclude fever, malaise, joint pain, and unexplained weight loss
	Exacerbating factors	Does any thing make it worse, (e.g., heat, cold)?
		Does anything make it better, (e.g., heat, cold, medication, such as antihistamines or topical application)?
	Past medical history	Any underlying disease or condition?
		Allergies: medication, foods, other products or triggers
	Drug history	Currently taking any medications (prescribed, or over the counter)
	Family history	Close relatives living with a skin conditions (e.g., eczema), familial history of skin disease
	Social history	Occupation
		Recent recreational activities(e.g., hill walking)
		Recent travel, if so, where and type of excursion
		Use of sun beds
		Recent contacts with persons experiencing a skin infection (e.g., impetigo)
Physical Assessment	Skin, nails, hair, and scalp	**Observe and examine:**
		Condition and appearance and establish moisture, dryness, temperature, colour
	Site(s) of rash or lesion	**Observation:**
		Distribution and pattern; unilateral or bilateral in character
		Discrete appearance of rash, determine character of individual lesions (e.g., pustule, macule, papule, vesicle nodule, wheal, plaque)
		Shape (noting symmetry), colour (noting pigmentation), and border definition
		Evidence of blistering, scaling, bleeding, excoriation, and crusting
		Examination:
		Size of palpable and nonpalpable lesions (measure)
		Palpate to establish texture, thickness, tenderness, warmth, mobility, friable, and if blanches on palpation

whereas varicella (chickenpox) (Fig. 18.2) tends to have lesions that are varying shades of red, which may initially exhibit a scattered pattern on the torso and then spread to the limbs. These lesions are vesicular but sometimes become pustular and occur in isolation (singular).

The rash associated with measles infection is typically described as maculopapular, representing a combination of macules and papules, where the macule (Fig. 18.3) is flat and the papule is raised, so measles will contain both types of lesions. The pattern exhibited by the measles rash is scattered, and patients may also present with Koplik's spots, which occur within the mouth (have the appearance of grains of salt clinging to the mucous membranes); patients may also exhibit conjunctivitis.

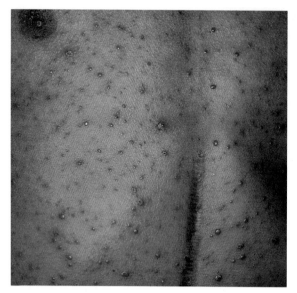

Fig. 18.2 ■ Varicella (chickenpox). (Courtesy Robert Hartman, MD. In Bolognia, J. L., Schaffer, J. V., & Cerroni, L. (2018). *Dermatology* (Vol. 2, 4th ed.). Elsevier).

Differentiating between dermatological conditions and observing the different types of lesions can help the GPN to distinguish between chronic and acute conditions. Extremely widespread itchy rashes that are accompanied or preceded by a fever are often indicative of a viral or bacterial aetiology, whereas lesions that have been present for some time and have not changed in their presentation can be indicative of a more chronic problem, for example, psoriasis. When undertaking the examination of a skin rash, it is important to palpate the rash and confirm if the rash pattern is scattered, linear, coalescing (joining up with other lesions), scaly or widespread. Also, determine whether singular lesions are apparent or whether any of the lesions are discoid or oval-shaped.

Examination and assessment of skin presentations require a structured and systematic approach to aid the diagnostic process and inform decision-making regarding ongoing treatment, management and, where indicated, onward referral (Narayan, 2017; Watson & Lawton, 2018). Table 18.1 provides a guide to undertaking a structured approach to history taking and assessment of dermatological problems to ensure an accurate diagnosis and facilitate onward referral.

TREATING COMMON SKIN COMPLAINTS

Emollient preparations are commonly used in the treatment of a variety of skin conditions. Steroid creams can be useful in treating areas of thickened skin, as in psoriasis, although vitamin D analogues are sometimes preferred. In scaly, hard, lichenified eczema, that is, noninfected thickened areas, topical steroid cream can help in returning the skin to its original integrity. Steroid ointments can be used for drier skin rather than creams, but emollients should always be applied before applying steroid cream. This enables softening and moisturising of the skin and will also promote absorption and allow a smaller amount to be used.

The medicinal strengths of steroid creams are described as mild, moderate, potent and high potency (Dinwoodie et al., 2020), and these are effective in reducing itching. Despite their ubiquitous use, they should only be used for a short duration, that is, a few days, as opposed to prolonged use over a period of weeks because skin thinning can occur. Commencing treatment with mild, rather than potent, creams (Joint Formulary Committee, 2014) is preferable because the strength can be increased as necessary. A potent cream may, however, be considered if the presenting complaint is severe or when the problem affects the palms or soles of the feet, but this is generally only initiated by a dermatology specialist. Potent creams may help in keeping the condition under control, at which point milder creams can be reintroduced. A mild preparation should always be used on the face. Finally, ointment or creams should be considered for dry skin because this will help with moisturising and aid the absorption of steroid creams.

Emollients are essential in the treatment and management of most dry skin conditions, particularly eczema and dermatitis. When used appropriately, before the application of steroid creams, they can potentiate absorption. When applied to varicose eczema, they promote venous return and can reduce

PRIMARY LESIONS-MORPHOLOGICAL TERMS

Term	Clinical features	Clinical example	Clinical disorders
Nodule	• Palpable, circumscribed • Larger volume than papule, usually >1 cm in diameter • Involves the dermis and/or the subcutis • Greatest portion may be beneath the skin surface or exophytic	Epidermoid cyst	• Epidermoid and tricholemmal cysts • Lipomas • Metastases • Neurofibromas • Panniculitis, e.g. erythema nodosum • Lymphoma cutis
Wheal	• Transient elevation of the skin due to dermal edema • Often pale centrally with an erythematous rim	Acute annular urticaria	Urticaria
Vesicle	• Elevated, circumscribed • <1 cm in diameter • Filled with fluid – clear, serous, or hemorrhagic • May become pustular, umbilicated or an erosion	Herpes zoster	• Herpes simplex • Varicella or zoster • Dermatitis herpetiformis • Dyshidrotic eczema
Bulla	• Elevated, circumscribed • >1 cm In diameter • Filled with fluid – clear, serous, or hemorrhagic • May become an erosion	Bullous pemphigoid	• Friction blister • Bullous pemphigoid • Linear IgA bullous dermatosis • Bullous fixed drug eruption • Coma bullae • Edema bullae
Pustule	• Elevated, circumscribed • Usually <1 cm in diameter • From its onset, filled with purulent fluid	Folliculitis	*Follicularly centered* • Folliculitis • Acne vulgaris *Non-follicularly centered* • Pustular psoriasis • Acute generalized exanthematous pustulosis • Subcorneal pustular dermatosis

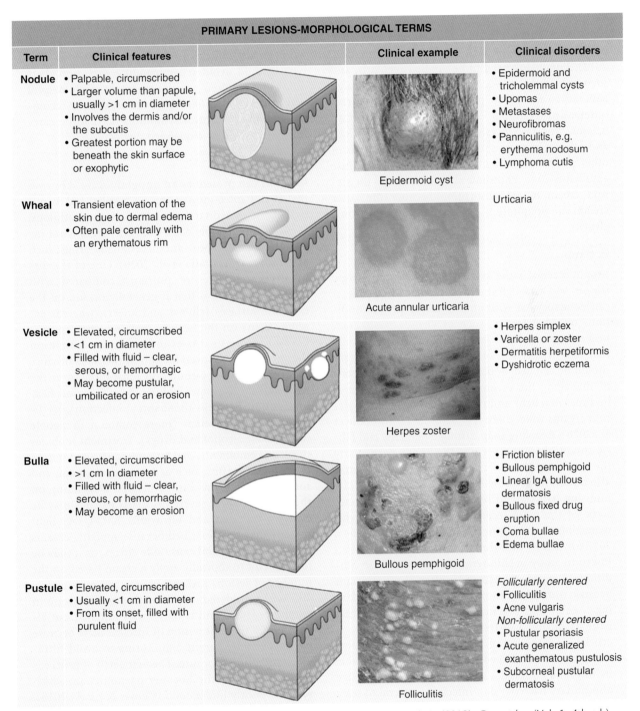

Fig. 18.3 ■ Types of skin lesions. (From Bolognia, J. L., Schaffer, J. V., & Cerroni, L. (2018). *Dermatology* (Vol. 1, 4th ed.). Elsevier.).

bacterial load (using an emollient with an antibacterial agent). This bacterial load is often increased in patients with eczema (UK Medicines Information, 2012). Emollients need to be applied regularly, and soap substitutes are also recommended, although aqueous cream as a soap substitute is no longer recommended (National Eczema Society, 2014). If an eczema-type rash persists, the patient's nails, hair and other skin areas should be assessed for signs of other pathology. Patients should be advised to use emollients 20 to 30 minutes before applying the steroid cream to aid absorption because the latter creams are lipophilic (i.e., fatty based) (Armstrong, 2014).

Eczema

Atopic eczema is the skin's response to an allergic trigger, and although the cause is often idiopathic, it can be associated with atopy (allergy prone condition) or other causes, such as viruses, soap, cold, heat or even as a result of ingesting something orally that may trigger a response. If known, the trigger should be avoided, and treatment generally consists of managing the eczema with emollients when it becomes dry, itchy and inflamed and using mild steroid creams when there is a 'flare-up' (Dinwoodie et al., 2020). Avoiding soap, strong detergents and fabric conditioners and keeping the home, particularly the bedroom area, as trigger-free as possible may also be helpful (National Eczema Society, 2014). Minimising bathing and bleach baths (very weak) are some of the more recent suggestions to help with managing the condition (National Eczema Society, 2017). A history of asthma and/or hay fever is often linked to atopy in children, so managing these conditions alongside the eczema is often also important because it may help in minimising symptoms. Having a calm and practical approach to supporting patients during a distressing flare-up of eczema is crucial, as is the use of topical treatments. Patients may also be prescribed antihistamines to subdue itching, and antibiotics may be indicated to manage a secondary bacterial skin infection; referral to see a specialist may become necessary if the condition is severely affecting the person's life. Iatrogenic eczema, or dermatitis, generally means there is a trigger, but its source is unknown, and trialling different creams and environments may be helpful. The GPN should avoid recommending exclusion diets for young children because these are rarely helpful and lead to nutritional deficiencies; dietary recommendations to control symptoms need to be carefully supervised by a qualified dietician.

Psoriasis

Psoriasis can present as an unsightly scaly skin rash that is not infectious; it can be familial but is not necessarily hereditary. In terms of the aetiology, some of the possible causes include stress, viral infections, alcohol abuse and occasionally drugs, such as lithium (Dinwoodie et al., 2020). One of the distinguishing features of psoriasis, compared with other skin rashes, is that it generally occurs on the extensor surfaces (elbows and knees), whereas eczema occurs on the flexural surfaces; rarely seen is flexural psoriasis. Assessment of the condition should include an examination of the nails because these may exhibit pitting and separation from the nailbed. Psoriasis types include chronic plaque, flexural, guttate (6 weeks after a throat infection), erythrodermic and pustular (more common in people who misuse alcohol and drugs). Treatment includes the use of emollients, coal tar ointments and vitamin D analogue creams, such as calcipotriol cream, and some steroid creams can be helpful. Depending on the severity, where several psoriasis patches may be evident, psoralen and ultraviolet A (PUVA) light therapy may be prescribed because applying creams may be excessive and cause side effects, or it may be too difficult to topically apply a cream based on the number of lesions present. PUVA therapy is generally not considered first-line treatment except in guttate psoriasis and is only rarely initiated but always under the supervision of specialist care because patients require careful monitoring to avoid ultraviolet radiation exposure. The first patch of psoriasis can be caused by the Koebner phenomenon, which remains poorly understood (Kumar & Clark, 2018), but evidence indicates that it can occur following trauma to the skin.

Fungal Infections (Tinea) and Angular Cheilitis

Fungal infections of the skin are also known as *tinea,* specifically, *tinea cruris* (groin), *tinea capitis* (head) and *tinea corporis* (body). When tinea manifests within the nails (unguium), this should be treated with caution because this may be indicative of serious systemic disease, such as immunosuppression, or the development of long-term conditions, such as diabetes or peripheral vascular disease. Even mild nail infections should be investigated and treated to prevent comorbidity. Intertrigo (Fig. 18.4) is a rash that can occur in the folds of the skin and may develop to host a fungal infection, and this may become exacerbated in hot weather or in obese patients with multiple skin folds.

This type of fungal infection can be caused by *Candida albicans,* and the treatment normally prescribed is clotrimazole cream. However, depending on the location/site of the infection and severity, ketoconazole or miconazole cream or oral antifungal medication (which needs to be prescribed with caution in elderly people because of possible renal or hepatic toxicity from failing kidneys or poor hepatic function associated with aging) may be necessary. Topical antifungal creams that have steroid components should be avoided because these may make the tinea 'incognito'; that is, it may become difficult to ascertain effectiveness and aetiology because the steroid cream will markedly change the appearance of the rash. Dermatophyte infections (yeast spores rather than a fungus) include rashes such as seborrhoeic dermatitis and pityriasis rosea. Treatment of these conditions may start with a common *Candida* treatment such as clotrimazole, but a lack of resolution may sometimes necessitate the introduction of additional medication (such as oral therapy). This may include antibiotics such as lymecycline orally or topical treatments such as an imidazole cream.

Angular cheilitis can be a result of *Candida* occurring in the mouth. This can result in painful fissure-like cracks in the corners of the mouth. Treatment for this type of fungal infection is straightforward using oral nystatin; however, the GPN needs to be mindful that this presentation may be symptomatic

of diabetes, poorly fitting dentures, immunosuppression through disease or treatment and malnutrition, so the causative factor requires investigation (Primary Care Dermatology Society, 2019a).

Rashes and Viral Exanthems

The treatment and management of rashes triggered by a viral infection initially warrant an assessment of the severity of the underlying condition. Consequently, those patients who present with clinical symptoms of a stiff neck, high fever and confusion with a non-blanching purpuric (haemorrhagic) rash indicating meningococcal infection need immediate transfer, with support, to acute care. Treatment of vesicular rashes, such as recurrent herpes simplex (appears similar to shingles rash but is linear in presentation and recurrent), can be treated with antiviral medication. The treatment of shingles, genital herpes (can be caused by herpes simplex virus 2) and other blistering types of rashes is dependent on the age and health status of the patient, whether this is a first episode or recurrent, the disability caused by the rash and the effectiveness of the treatments available.

Molluscum contagiosum (MC) presents with unsightly, fluid-filled blisters/lesions (with an umbilicated centre) that have a scattered pattern, and when large crops occur, they can be accompanied by a viral-type illness. This is generally a self-limiting infection, occurring any time from the age of 18 months up to 10 years, but normally, it does not last longer than a year. The GPN will undoubtedly encounter situations involving dealing with anxious parents who will require support and information about the trajectory of this infection. Treatment options involve freezing with cryotherapy, but this may cause scarring and is painful. Enquiry regarding homeopathic remedies may be sought; however, the evidence base for this approach is unconfirmed. Parents – and children, where age permits – should be advised of the chance of their child infecting others, and in terms of resolution, this entails waiting for the body to develop immunity; these actions are all essential tools in the management of MC. The treatment of warts and verrucae is similar, although it is more common to use cryotherapy to

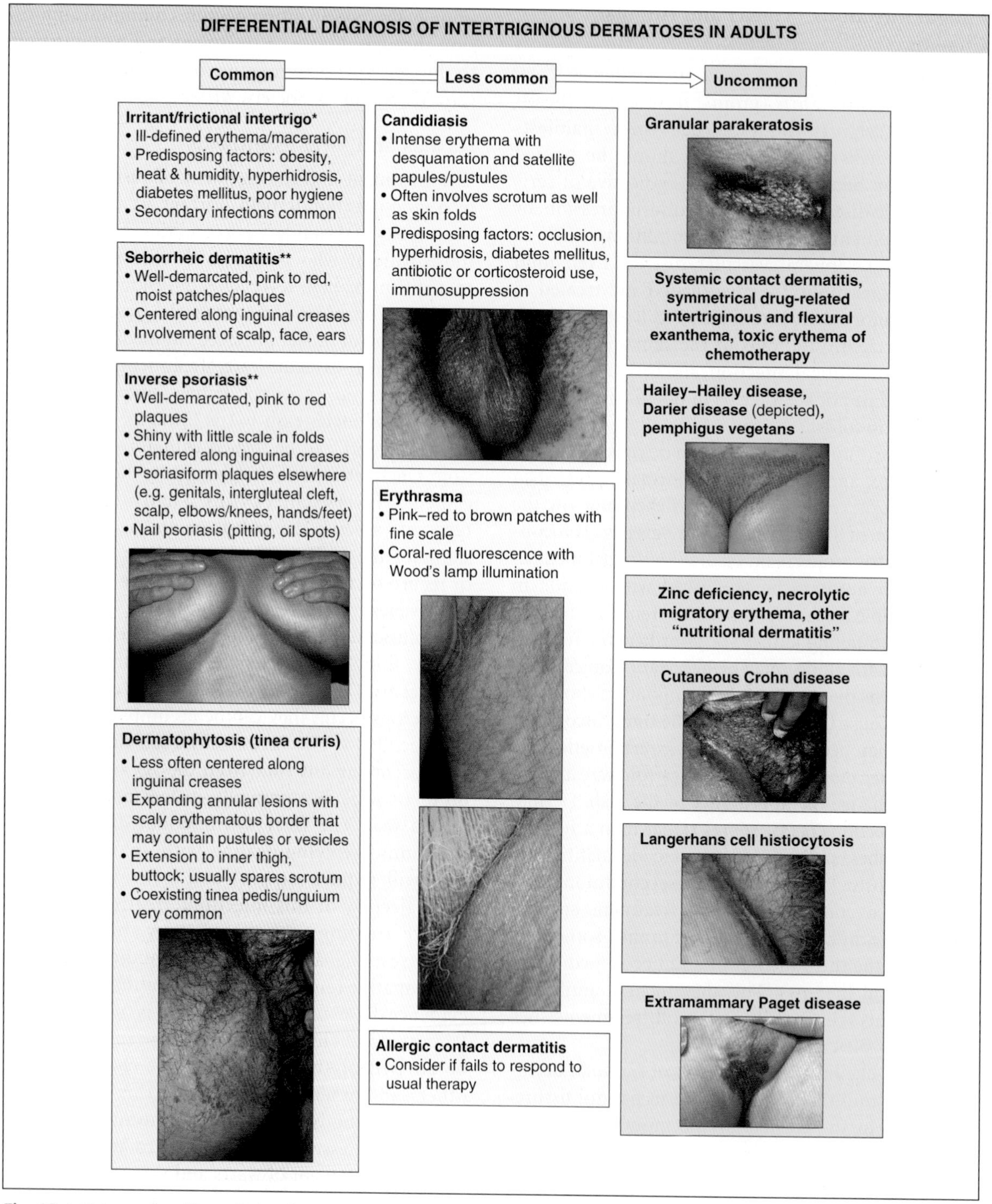

DIFFERENTIAL DIAGNOSIS OF INTERTRIGINOUS DERMATOSES IN ADULTS

Common ————————————→ Less common ————————————⇢ Uncommon

Irritant/frictional intertrigo*
- Ill-defined erythema/maceration
- Predisposing factors: obesity, heat & humidity, hyperhidrosis, diabetes mellitus, poor hygiene
- Secondary infections common

Seborrheic dermatitis**
- Well-demarcated, pink to red, moist patches/plaques
- Centered along inguinal creases
- Involvement of scalp, face, ears

Inverse psoriasis**
- Well-demarcated, pink to red plaques
- Shiny with little scale in folds
- Centered along inguinal creases
- Psoriasiform plaques elsewhere (e.g. genitals, intergluteal cleft, scalp, elbows/knees, hands/feet)
- Nail psoriasis (pitting, oil spots)

Dermatophytosis (tinea cruris)
- Less often centered along inguinal creases
- Expanding annular lesions with scaly erythematous border that may contain pustules or vesicles
- Extension to inner thigh, buttock; usually spares scrotum
- Coexisting tinea pedis/unguium very common

Candidiasis
- Intense erythema with desquamation and satellite papules/pustules
- Often involves scrotum as well as skin folds
- Predisposing factors: occlusion, hyperhidrosis, diabetes mellitus, antibiotic or corticosteroid use, immunosuppression

Erythrasma
- Pink–red to brown patches with fine scale
- Coral-red fluorescence with Wood's lamp illumination

Allergic contact dermatitis
- Consider if fails to respond to usual therapy

Granular parakeratosis

Systemic contact dermatitis, symmetrical drug-related intertriginous and flexural exanthema, toxic erythema of chemotherapy

Hailey–Hailey disease, Darier disease (depicted), **pemphigus vegetans**

Zinc deficiency, necrolytic migratory erythema, other "nutritional dermatitis"

Cutaneous Crohn disease

Langerhans cell histiocytosis

Extramammary Paget disease

Fig. 18.4 ■ Intertrigo. (From Bolognia, J. L., Schaffer, J. V., & Cerroni, L. (2018). *Dermatology* (Vol. 1, 4th ed.). Elsevier).

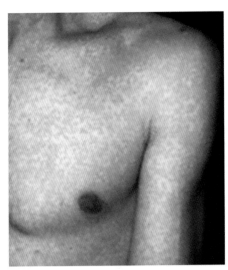

Fig. 18.5 ▪ Viral rash from dermis. (From Perry, S. E., Hockenberry, M. J., Lowdermilk, D. L., Wilson, D., Alden, K. R., & Cashion, M. C. (2018). *Maternal child nursing care* (6th ed.). Elsevier.)

freeze warts. Warts are caused by HPV (Primary Care Dermatology Society, 2019b), and therefore, essential enquiry by the GPN entails asking patients about their vaccination history against viral disease, such as HPV vaccination, possible contacts and other vaccination history, to aid clinical decision-making and, where necessary, onward referral. A detailed discussion on HPV and the management of genital warts can be found in Chapter 15.

The GPN also needs to be aware that some viral rashes can be harmful in pregnancy, such as slapped cheek in naïve patients and rubella in nonvaccinated pregnant patients (Public Health England, 2019) (Fig. 18.5 and Box 18.1). In this scenario, the GPN should seek immediate advice from the GP.

Bites and Stings

Patients presenting to the GPN with insect bites and stings is a common seasonal occurrence. Bites tend to induce an inflammatory reaction; hence, the standard treatment involves the use of antihistamines, drowsy and nondrowsy preparations, which can be used together to facilitate the reduction of swelling

---

BOX 18.1
EXANTHEMS CAUSED BY VIRAL ILLNESSES

1. Vesicular – such as those caused by herpes simplex and varicella zoster
2. Maculopapular, for instance, measles because there are some raised lesions (i.e., papular) and some flat (i.e., macular)
3. Purpuric rashes as in rubella and meningococcal disease
4. Warty as in molluscum contagiosum and human papilloma virus (warts and verrucae)

---

and reduce the localised cellulitis. Occasionally oral steroids may be indicated if the reaction is severe, and prompt review and/or referral may be needed and must be timely. A critical aspect in the immediate management of bites and stings is to exclude the minor bites from those that require urgent attention, that is, those that involve an allergy to bee stings or other flying insect bites/stings and trigger an anaphylactic reaction necessitating the administration of adrenaline via an injector (Sheikh 2020). In line with updated guidance from the National Institute for Health and Care Excellence (NICE) (2020), part of the GPN's role may also entail teaching parents and patients how to use an adrenaline injector, which includes ensuring the pen is 'in date' and checking that the dose is correct for the adult or child. Post-injector use includes cardiac monitoring (generally in a pre-hospital environment or possibly within the emergency department); this must be emphasised to parents and children.

Wasp stings can be treated with vinegar (acetic acid), and jellyfish stings can be managed with a urea-based cream or hot water. Tick bites need careful attention in adhering to evidence-based guidance, such as that provided by the National Institute for Health and Care Excellence (NICE), which may indicate the need for further follow-up to exclude Lyme disease. It is therefore imperative that patients who present with an area of erythema migrans (creeping redness) with a target-shaped lesion should be assessed for the possibility of Lyme disease (Fig. 18.6). Moreover, irrespective of patients being able to provide a history of

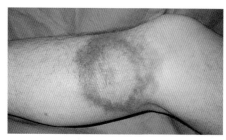

Fig. 18.6 ■ Lyme disease rash. (From Ball, J., Dains, J., Flynn, J., Solomon, B., & Stewart, R. (2019). *Seidel's guide to physical examination* (9th ed.). Elsevier, 2019.)

tick bite, symptoms of myalgia, fatigue or fever and antibiotic treatment should be considered with this type of rash presentation and immediate referral made to the GP. Reactions to mosquito bites or flying insects should be assessed in the light of the severity of the reaction, the effectiveness of antihistamines, pre-existing comorbidity and detailed history of recent travel to an area of insect-borne disease (see Chapter 19).

With insect or tick bites, a detailed history of the recent whereabouts/activities undertaken by the patient is essential. For instance, in European forested areas, consider Lyme disease (as discussed earlier), or if the patient has been in areas of endemic insect-borne disease, such as malaria, consider the additional likelihood of this or other insect-borne disease, such as Dengue or Chikungunya fever (see Chapter 19). Heat rashes are intensely uncomfortable for patients, and their immediate treatment involves keeping cool, taking antihistamines and/or using refrigerated, nonoily calamine lotion to reduce the length of time the rash may be present. If this is nonresolving, timely review is essential to rule out red flags.

Urticaria and Allergies

Urticaria of the skin, emerging as red raised bumps/wheals as a reaction to known or unknown allergens, is concerning, and there is often the uncertainty that this may lead to an anaphylactic reaction. Seeing patients promptly, treating with both nondrowsy and drowsy antihistamines, assessing for the trigger allergens and remaining open-minded to causation are essential skills in the management of urticaria.

Follow-up care may involve referral for patch testing and/or serological screening via radioallergosorbent (RAST) testing for immunoglobulin E (IgE) antibodies. Advice about future management is essential, especially if this has entailed an emergency situation, and lifestyle advice about allergens may need to be discussed. Should this involve food allergies, any discussion concerning exclusion diets must be formally assessed and reviewed by a qualified dietician.

Dermatitis – Occupational, Hobby Related, Iatrogenic

Occupational dermatitis, such as that caused by allergy to frequent hand washing or strong grease-removing products, can prove difficult to manage. Avoiding the causative trigger and using gloves and non–soap-based products, with regular application of emollients, may be helpful in assisting patients in managing this condition.

Biologics

Pharmacological immunomodulators, which aim to ameliorate the body's immune response, such as infliximab and other related medications, are being used more frequently in treating a wide range of autoimmune diseases and conditions. These medications may be used to replace more traditional treatments, such as methotrexate, although the latter still has its place. In relation to dermatological conditions, immunomodulators can be an effective alternative when other medications and topical creams have been unsuccessful. Patients taking biologic treatments and those on high-dose oral steroids may be immunocompromised, and specialist clinician management via secondary care is necessary. However, whilst a specialist clinician may initiate treatment of this type of medication, the GPN may be asked to monitor the patient for signs of infection or problems that arise from the patient being immunocompromised.

Skin Infections – Cellulitis, Impetigo and Sepsis

Cellulitis is an acute bacterial infection of the skin, most likely to occur as a result of infiltration by *Streptococcus pyogenes* or *Staphylococcus aureus*

(Dinwoodie et al., 2020). More superficial skin infections are termed *erysipelas,* usually caused by group A beta-hemolytics streptococci or *S. aureus,* and can be treated with topical antibacterial cream such as fusidic acid twice daily, if the patient does not have any accompanying 'red flag' symptoms. These include fever, feeling shivery or a rapidly spreading area of erythema (Oh et al., 2014). Should this manifest, the patient may require oral or intravenous antibiotics.

Skin infections can also occur in postoperative wounds, ulcers, blisters and insect bites, and first-line treatment should involve topical antibiotic therapy initially. Impetigo (infection of small, cracked areas with *S. aureus*) and boils/furuncles are also best treated with topical antibiotic therapy, unless the problem is spreading or the patient is systemically unwell, in which case, oral therapy may be indicated. Flucloxacillin or co-amoxiclav is a suitable antibiotic for skin infections, with erythromycin being the alternative for those patients who are allergic to penicillin. The GPN needs to be diligent in considering if patients who present within population subgroups (those with pre-existing comorbidity) are more at risk of severe risk or skin sepsis. In these cases, the patients may need immediate specialist referral (UK Sepsis Trust, 2016).

Impetigo can be caused by the common skin commensal *S. aureus* and is more common in children, particularly those with pre-existing skin conditions, such as eczema, where skin integrity has compromised and there are increased levels of the bacteria on the skin (Dinwoodie et al., 2020). The honey-coloured crust seen in many presentations is pathognomonic (indicative) of impetigo, and first-line treatment should be topical antibiotics for small areas in immunocompetent individuals. Treatment may also involve the use of oral antibiotics in the immunocompromised patient or where there are widespread and/or spreading lesions. Advice to the patient should detail that the condition is highly infectious, and lesions should be covered where possible, with careful personal hygiene used at home, such as not sharing baths, towels and flannels.

Impetigo may be a precursor to systemic sepsis, particularly for people who are immunocompromised.

Consequently, the GPN has a critical role in providing safety-netting advice to parents or patients who present with this skin condition. They need to seek immediate medical advice if the rash spreads alarmingly, if fever persists, despite antipyretics, or in the case of a child or elder, there is oliguria and/or they become confused (UK Sepsis Trust, 2016).

Infestations

Scabies, head lice, fleas and pubic lice (crabs) should always be considered for extremely itchy rashes that have a recent and sudden onset (although scabies can occur up to 6 weeks after contact). Detailed history taking is important, involving specific probing of recent and previous events/activities/travel, and the clinical examination should include, in relation to scabies, the webs of the fingers and under the nails for scabies burrows. Examination for head lice includes inspection for small sacs clinging to the hair shafts (head lice) and both arthropods (insects) and eggs in the pubic hair (pubic lice or 'crabs'). Fleas may be the likely culprit in an itchy rash for patients with a history of homelessness or neglect (National Health Service (NHS), 2018), and fleas are often seen within items of clothing in the hems. In assessing all skin problems, the practitioner should inspect the hair/scalp, all of the skin and the nails of the hands and the feet, not just the patch of skin that the patient proffers. Attention to the original cause of the problem should also be addressed, be this homelessness, neglect or lack of education on the causative factor (NHS, 2018).

Erythema Nodosum and Lichen Planus

Erythema nodosum (Fig. 18.7) is an erythematous eruption commonly associated with adverse drug reactions or infection (often viral) and is characterised by inflammatory nodules that are usually tender, multiple, and bilateral. These nodules/lesions are located predominantly on the shins but less commonly on the thighs and forearms. They undergo characteristic colour changes, ending in temporary bruise-like areas (Kumar & Clark, 2018). This condition usually subsides in 3 to 6 weeks without scarring or atrophy and is self-limiting.

Long-term treatment may involve the use of oral steroids, which can predispose patients to skin thinning,

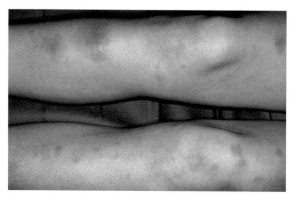

Fig. 18.7 ■ Erythema nodosum. (Courtesy Louis A. Fragola, Jr., MD. In Bolognia, J. L., Schaffer, J. V., & Cerroni, L. (2018). *Dermatology* (Vol. 1, 4th ed.). Elsevier.).

BOX 18.2

SYSTEMIC CONDITIONS RELATED TO SKIN PROBLEMS AND RASHES

- Fever and malaise – consider herpes, erythema nodosum or roseola (measles).
- Red, sticky eyes – consider rosacea and Kawasaki's disease.
- Upper respiratory infection and/ or viral – think of erythema nodosum or a viral rash.
- Asthma or episodic cough – these may accompany atopic dermatitis.
- Varicosities and/or pedal oedema – these may be noted with stasis dermatitis.
- Arthritis and joint stiffness – psoriasis may be the long-term syndrome.

and in the long term, osteoporosis is among the potential side effects if medication is taken orally. It is essential for the practice nurse to ensure there are no underlying causes for this condition. In contrast, lichen planus (Fig. 18.8), a separate condition, is an inflammatory, intensely itchy disease of the skin and mucous membranes that can be generalised or localised. It is characterised by distinctive purple, flat-topped papules, sometimes silvery in colour, generally on the trunk of the body and the flexor surfaces, but it can also be seen in the mucous membranes. It can also be very itchy and is generally treated with emollients and steroid creams. In erythema nodosum with lichen planus, the lesions may be discrete or merging to form plaques, and generally, the cause is unknown

but presents as a very itchy, silvery rash. As noted in Fig. 18.7, the hard, blistering lines should be differentiated from sudden-onset blisters, which are mostly fluid filled. Some systemic conditions seen alongside and related to skin problems and rashes can be found in Box 18.2.

SKIN LESIONS OR RASHES OF IMMEDIATE OR INTERMEDIATE CLINICAL CONCERN

Syndromes related to skin conditions may include rosacea, psoriasis and rashes in those patients who are immunocompromised and may need more prompt attention. When assessing patients who present with

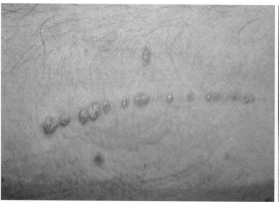

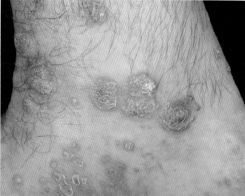

Fig. 18.8 ■ Lichen planus.

lesions (spots on the skin) or rashes, always consider that they may be malignant or suspicious, especially if these are in sun-exposed areas. The mnemonic ABCDE can be a useful tool (NICE, 2016; Skin Cancer Foundation, 2014). This can be helpful in aiding decision-making regarding onward referral to GP or specialist services. If in doubt, seek advice on the need for referral. The guidance in Table 18.2 may be helpful in differentiating between lesions. See also Fig. 18.9 and Box 18.3.

Managing Risk in Dermatological Presentations

There are numerous physiological and pathophysiological factors that can affect the condition of the skin, including age, being immunocompetent and pharmacological treatment, as well as lifestyle and environmental factors (Hess, 2011). Consequently, the GPN must be mindful of population subgroups that may be at increased risk of dermatological ill health.

In older people, epidermal thinning is a normal physiological process; however, minor dermatological conditions that may arise can subsequently become difficult to manage as a result of a variety of intrinsic and extrinsic factors. Furthermore, a decrease in vitamin D production, resulting from a lack of sun exposure, in this population subgroup can result in a loss

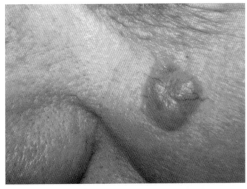

Fig. 18.9 ■ Basal cell carcinoma. (From Bolognia, J. L., Schaffer, J. V., & Cerroni, L. (2018). *Dermatology* (Vol. 1, 4th ed.). Elsevier.).

TABLE 18.2
Different Types of Basal-Cell Carcinoma (BCC)

	Common Location	Features
Nodular	Face	Cystic, pearly, telangiectasia
		May be ulcerated
		Micronodular and microcystic types may infiltrate deeply
Superficial	Upper trunk and shoulders	Erythematous, well-demarcated, scaly plaques, often >20 mm
	Often multiple	Slow growth over months or years
		May be confused with Bowen's disease or inflammatory dermatoses
Morphoeic (or sclerosing or infiltrative)	Midfacial sites	Skin-coloured, waxy, scar-like
		Prone to recurrence after treatment
		May infiltrate cutaneous nerves
Pigmented		Brown, blue or greyish lesion
		Nodular or superficial histology
		May resemble malignant melanoma
Basosquamous		Mixed BCC and squamous-cell carcinoma
		Potentially more aggressive than other forms of BCC

© NICE 2010. *Improving outcomes for people with skin tumours including melanoma (update) – The management of low-risk basal cell carcinomas in the community* (Cancer Service Guideline 8). http://www.nice.org.uk/guidance/csg8. All rights reserved. Subject to Notice of rights. NICE guidance is prepared for the National Health Service in England. All NICE guidance is subject to regular review and may be updated or withdrawn. NICE accepts no responsibility for the use of its content in this publication.

BOX 18.3

ABCDE MNEMONIC TO ASSESS SKIN MOLES

A – Asymmetry – the two halves of the area differ in their shape

B – Border – the edges of the area may be irregular or blurred, and sometimes show notches

C – Colour – this may be uneven. Different shades of black, brown and pink may be seen

D – Diameter – most melanomas are at least 6 mm in diameter

E – Evolution – rapid change in a pre-existing mole

From British Association of Dermatologists (2018). *Melanoma in Situ. Patient Information Leaflet.* https://www.bad.org.uk/shared/get-file.ashx?id=2126&itemtype=document

---

of bone density and decreased muscle strength with a decline in melanocyte activity. As the skin's glandular activity declines, the skin becomes dry and scaly, and thermoregulation is less efficient. Thermal regulation is also affected by a reduced dermal blood supply and may even be affected by poor hair follicle function. The dermis will become less flexible as a result of a decrease in elastic fibres, with the skin becoming wrinkled and beginning to sag. There is also a reduction in the speed with which skin heals and can repel infection. Additionally, elderly patients, especially those living alone, can be at particular risk because they can be vulnerable to poor nutrition, hydration and hygiene, which can significantly affect skin health. Consequently, sensitive, holistic inquiry is necessary to ensure patients are coping at home, hydrated and maintaining a balanced diet because those in this age group tend to be long-suffering and may not recognise a deteriorating skin condition (Armstrong, 2014). An emergent skin condition should be promptly assessed, and in keeping with structured care provision, long-term chronic dermatological conditions must be regularly reviewed and monitored. Where the GPN may doubt the aetiology, diagnosis or associated prognosis of a presenting skin condition, advice should be sought from the GP or a senior nursing colleague.

Babies and young children represent another population subgroup that may frequently present to the GPN with rashes (often viral) or illnesses that affect the skin (Kumar & Clark, 2018). These can include eczema, dry skin, cradle cap and viral exanthem (a rash related to a virus). A fundamental part of the assessment of dermatological presentations involves obtaining a comprehensive history from the parent/guardian/carer and checking clinical records to ascertain the child's immunisation status. The latter should be in accordance with the UK immunisation schedule (Public Health England, 2019) because this information may help to rule out some obvious causes of the rash in relation to communicable disease but cannot, however, completely exclude them from being a causative factor.

As with any assessment, considering the patient holistically is essential because what might appear as a simple rash that blanches and disappears under pressure (i.e., a glass applied to the skin) may still be indicative of a more serious condition. Quality management of dermatological conditions requires a detailed systematic assessment, comprehensive clinical history, evidence-based treatment and appropriate follow-up within an appropriate time frame. Additionally, the GPN's role also entails the diligent assessment and management of any high-risk 'red flag' skin problems that are reported by a patient, such as a rash spreading quickly and existing in conjunction with other physical symptoms such as fever, loss of appetite and/or loss of function. Crucially, symptoms such as visual loss, auditory or renal symptoms, that is, anuria or reduced urine output, can indicate a clinical emergency, necessitating immediate medical intervention. Similarly, an elderly patient who is usually fit and well but suddenly deteriorates and presents with a rash needs timely medical assessment and attention. A good example is pemphigoid, an autoimmune disease presenting with a serious blistering rash that may have rapidly spread, become infected and be accompanied by fever. Once diagnosed, this condition requires treatment with steroids and often antibiotics: topical if localised, oral if widespread or if not responding to local/topical treatment.

Another high-risk group is those patients presenting with a shingles rash that is affecting the facial area, presenting as ophthalmic shingles or herpes zoster

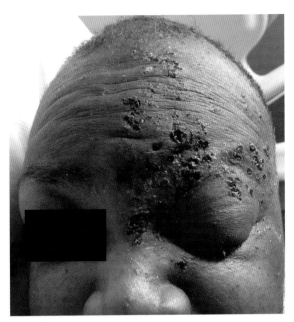

Fig. 18.10 ■ Shingles/herpes zoster.

(Fig. 18.10). This necessitates immediate referral to a specialist clinician within the acute setting because any ear, eye or facial nerve involvement may have serious outcomes. Facial nerve symptoms are hard to resolve once established and may result in Ramsey Hunt syndrome or facial nerve palsy. The definition of *ophthalmic zoster* is a rash in the distribution of the ophthalmic division of the ophthalmic nerve, (Drummond 2020) that is, the forehead to the tip of the nose. There is a risk to the eye, which necessitates urgent referral to an ophthalmologist in addition to systemic management. High-level decision-making to rule out significant clinical risk in the assessment and management of dermatological conditions is based on robust information gathering drawn from the clinical history and systematic physical assessment.

Pregnancy-Related Dermatological Presentations

Itching, rashes and skin discomfort during pregnancy are not uncommon phenomena. However, it is of critical importance that dermatological presentations during pregnancy be comprehensively assessed because they may be indicative of a serious underlying condition, such as biliary or intrahepatic cholestasis, which can result in a stillbirth. Consequently, should pregnant women consult with the GPN for a complaint of the sudden onset of very itchy hands and feet and no rash visible (excluding scratch marks that have been caused by itching), this needs immediate referral to the GP for assessment. These actions reflect evidence-based guidance from Public Health England (2019), which must be followed to ensure appropriate and timely management. In contrast, there are some benign rashes that occur in pregnancy and can be managed with emollients, but as noted, a differential diagnosis is mandatory in this situation, indicating referral to GP.

Acne and Rosacea

Rosacea is a common chronic cutaneous disease primarily affecting the facial skin. It is common in the third and fourth decade of life, peaking at the age of 40 to 50 years. The causes of rosacea are still unidentified. Patients may, however, complain of skin sensitivity to light, sun, weather or alcohol or all of these. Rosacea occurs in stages and may cause ophthalmic problems, most commonly resulting in blepharitis and conjunctivitis. Management is through avoiding triggers and treatment using antibiotics or creams such as azelaic acid. Ophthalmic symptoms should be managed to avoid corneal irritation and ulceration but may necessitate referral to specialist services (Fig. 18.11).

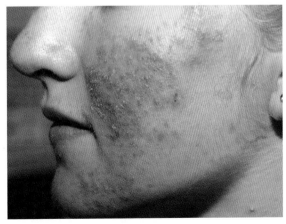

Fig. 18.11 ■ Rosacea. (Courtesy Kalman Watsky, MD. In Bolognia, J. L., Schaffer, J. V., & Cerroni, L. (2018). *Dermatology* (Vol. 1, 4th ed.). Elsevier.)

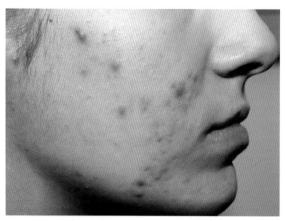

Fig. 18.12 ■ Acne vulgaris. (From Bolognia, J. L., Schaffer, J. V., & Cerroni, L. (2018). *Dermatology* (Vol. 1, 4th ed.). Elsevier.).

Acne (Fig. 18.12) can cause serious body dysmorphia and is initially treated topically in accordance with evidence-based treatment pathways. However, ensure shared decision-making with patients because this may indicate referral to specialist care regarding the use of more potent medication and needs careful monitoring and assessment of side effects.

SUMMARY

As a frontline service, the GPN is likely to be a point of contact for patients who develop dermatological conditions. Observing skin conditions and rashes will help develop confidence and expertise, but expert supervision and auditing practice remain essential. Further, there are multiple clinical resources for the GPN to access, but these must be evidence-based to ensure the delivery of safe and effective quality care (see Resources section at the end of this chapter).

However, given the complexity and the associated morbidity and mortality of skin presentations, the GPN needs to be mindful that because of the sheer number of simple and complex skin conditions, it is not always possible to identify and diagnose the presenting skin condition. If the diagnosis of the dermatological presentation is unclear after a detailed and structured assessment of the patient, checking image databases and seeking advice from GPs and senior colleagues is essential. Safety netting of the patient is a critical requirement in the assessment and management of dermatological presentations, and this includes establishing that the patient is well, physically stable and shows no accompanying systemic reaction. This being the case, then dermatological conditions presenting in primary care can be managed and reviewed as appropriate.

RESOURCES

Dermatology Online Atlas: https://www.dermis.net/doia/
Evidence-based guidelines for assessment, management and treatment of skin conditions:
https://cks.nice.org.uk
https://www.nhs.uk/conditions

REFERENCES

Armstrong, K. (2014). Common skin conditions in the community and primary care. *British Journal of Community Nursing, 19*(10), 482, 484–488.

Armstrong, K. (2019). Taking a patient history as part of a respiratory assessment. *GPN, 5*(8), 40–46.

British Association of Dermatologists (2018). *Melanoma in Situ.* https://www.bad.org.uk/shared/get-file.ashx?id=2126&itemtype=document

Dinwoodie, K., Goyal, A., Nisbett, C., & Colgan, J. (2020). Skin problems. In A. Staten & P. Staten (Eds.), *Practical general practice guidelines for effective clinical management* (7th ed., pp. 381–402). Elsevier.

Drummond, S. (2020). Eye Problems. In A. Staten & P. Staten (Eds.), *Practical general practice guidelines for effective clinical management* (7th ed., pp. 371–380). Elsevier.

Hess, C. T. (2011). *Clinical guide to skin and wound care* (6th ed.). Lippincott Williams & Wilkins.

Joint Formulary Committee. (2014). *British National Formulary.* BMJ Group and Pharmaceutical Press.

Kumar, P., & Clark, M. (2018). *Clinical medicine* (9th ed.). Elsevier Saunders.

Narayan, S. (2017). Dermatological history taking and examination. *Medicine, 45*(6), 352–358.

National Eczema Society. (2014). *Why is aqueous cream bad for eczema? Patient information.* https://eczema.org/information-and-advice/faqs/

National Eczema Society. (2017). *Bleach bathing explained.* https://nationaleczema.org/10-tips-bleach-baths-nea-community/

National Health Service. (2018). *Abuse and neglect of vulnerable adults.* https://www.nhs.uk/conditions/social-care-and-support-guide/help-from-social-services-and-charities/abuse-and-neglect-vulnerable-adults/

National Institute for Health and Care Excellence. (2016). *Skin cancers – Recognition and referral. NICE clinical knowledge summary*. http://cks.nice.org.uk/skin-cancers-recognition-and-referral

National Institute for Health and Care Excellence (2020). Assessment and referral after emergency treatment (CG 134). https://www.nice.org.uk/guidance/cg134/resources/anaphylaxis-assessment-and-referral-after-emergency-treatment-pdf-35109510368965

Oh, C. C., Ko, H. C., Lee, H. Y., Safdar, N., Maki, D. G., & Chlebicki, M. P. (2014). Antibiotic prophylaxis for preventing recurrent cellulitis: A systematic review and meta-analysis. *Journal of Infection, 69*(1), 26–34.

Primary Care Dermatology Society. (2019a). *Angular cheilitis.* http://www.pcds.org.uk/clinical-guidance/angular-chelitis

Primary Care Dermatology Society. (2019b). *Warts.*

Public Health England. (2019). *Guidance on the investigation, diagnosis and management of viral illness, or exposure to viral rash illness, in pregnancy*. https://assets.publishing.service.gov.uk/government/uploads/system/uploads/attachment_data/file/821550/viral_rash_in_pregnancy_guidance.pdf

Sheikh, A. (2020). Allergic problems. In A. Staten & P. Staten (Eds.), *Practical general practice guidelines for effective clinical management* (7th ed., pp. 403–408). Elsevier.

UK Medicines Information. (2012). *Can topical steroids be applied at the same time as emollients?* Medicines Q&As. http://tinyurl.com/k2er3l3

UK Sepsis Trust. (2016). Toolkit: Emergency *Department management of sepsis in adults and young people over 12 years – 2016*. https://sepsistrust.org/wp-content/uploads/2018/06/ED-toolkit-2016-Final-2.pdf

Watson, J., & Lawton, S. (2018). Skin infections. *Primary Health Care, 28*(3), 42–49.

19 TRAVEL HEALTHCARE

JANE CHIODINI

INTRODUCTION

Travel healthcare has been a role of the practice nurse for many years. Protecting the traveller's health in terms of disease prevention is not only important for the individual but also from a public health perspective in terms of preventing the spread of infectious disease on their return home to the UK. In addition, travellers can be at personal risk from other threats, such as road traffic accidents, solar damage, personal safety and security, and need to be advised appropriately based on an individual pre-travel risk assessment. Travel health is a very complex subject and is frequently misunderstood by some working in general practice. The viewpoint that travel is 'just about giving the injections' is not only incorrect but can be detrimental to the care of the traveller and the professional integrity of the healthcare practitioner delivering this care. A general practice is paid for the provision of this additional service. This concept is occasionally ignored, and travel health sometimes takes a lower priority in many settings.

THE PROVISION OF TRAVEL HEALTH IN A PRIMARY CARE SETTING

Whilst the provision of 'vaccinations and immunisations' has been an additional service in a primary care setting since 2004, the newly negotiated general practice contract 2020/21–2023/24 in England has stated that vaccinations and immunisations will become an essential contractual service (NHS England & British Medical Association, 2020). All practices will be expected to offer all routine, pre- and post-exposure vaccinations and National Health Service (NHS) travel vaccinations to the eligible practice population. A named lead for vaccination services will be introduced in all practices, who is responsible for meeting the core standards and requirements of the contract and 'maximising' vaccination opportunities. At the time of writing, the details are not known, but the vaccination payment model will be 'overhauled' to boost vaccination coverage, a change that the contract called the 'most significant in 30 years' (NHS England, 2019). The vaccines that comprise NHS provision for the purpose of travel health protection are hepatitis A, typhoid, cholera and polio (Box 19.1).

In addition to the vaccines provided, the service needs to do the following:

- Provide an initial travel risk assessment.
- Advise on the travel health risks (which would include risk of diseases for the private travel vaccines, which may not be administered within the individual surgery).
- Signpost the traveller to a selection of centres where the private travel vaccines may be provided if the general practice surgery opts not to provide them.
- Provide malaria prevention advice if required within the itinerary.
- Signpost the traveller towards additional reading and advice for individual health risks.
- Provide documentary evidence of vaccine history.

BOX 19.1
TRAVEL-RELATED VACCINES

Travel-Related Vaccines That Must Be Provided to National Health Service (NHS) Patients as an NHS Provision	Travel-Related Vaccines That Must Be Charged for If Provided in an NHS Setting
Hepatitis A (and all vaccines that have a hepatitis A component in them)	Rabies
Typhoid (both injectable and oral presentations)	Yellow fever
Cholera	Japanese encephalitis
Polio (administered for a traveller as Revaxis, which is a combination vaccine of tetanus, polio and diphtheria; therefore all three components are provided by the NHS)	Tick-borne encephalitis
	Meningitis ACWY (for travel purposes)
	Hepatitis B*

*Guidance for hepatitis B indicates that this vaccine may be charged for (British Medical Association, 2018). It is the decision of the individual surgery as to whether or not it will charge the patient if given for the purpose of travel; however, the Medicine Management Committees within Clinical Commissioning Groups (CCGs) often stipulate that it must be charged for.

In Scotland, it was decided to remove the provision of travel healthcare within general practice, and the Vaccine Transformation Programme is currently in progress to decide how the service will be delivered from 2021 (NHS Health Scotland, 2019), but it is expected that the NHS vaccines will still be administered as an NHS provision to travellers.

TRAVEL RISK ASSESSMENT

No travel health consultation should take place without undertaking a travel risk assessment (Royal College of Nursing (RCN), 2018) (Box 19.2). This process will determine the level of risk for the individual traveller with regard to their travel itinerary, combined with their personal health history. No two consultations will be the same, which is one of the elements that make travel health an interesting and dynamic field of practice. Numerous travel risk assessment forms have been developed, and many of them have been transformed into templates used within computer systems within general practice. Examples are listed in the Resources section at the end of this chapter.

The Importance of a Travel Risk Assessment

Travellers generally do not appreciate the rationale for requesting this information, but the detail could affect the outcome. Many resources have written comprehensive explanations of the importance of the questions asked, and general practice nurses (GPNs) are advised to become familiar with these texts (Box 19.3), but the following information provides an initial insight.

Travel risk assessment is based on a number of factors, and the evaluation of the risk assessment will inform the management of the advice subsequently given, vaccines advised and malaria prevention advice required, if it is also a risk in their trip. The key areas to consider are as follows:

- Who is travelling
- Where they are going
- When they are going and for how long
- What they will be doing

Case Study to Demonstrate the Risk Assessment Decisions

A 6-year-old boy is travelling to Turkey to visit relatives for 6 weeks over the summer holiday, staying in the family home in a rural location. He is up to date with his UK vaccination programme but has not travelled outside the UK before, so he has received no travel vaccines. He is fit and well and has no medical problems.

Issues to Consider – An Overview

Age is important, particularly for the young, who are more vulnerable because of a lack of awareness of risk, for example, from road traffic accidents, to safety and security (National Travel Health Network and Centre

BOX 19.2
TRAVEL RISK ASSESSMENT

Traveller-Focussed Questions	Trip-Focussed Questions
Age and gender	Country to be visited and exact location or region – capture all details for a multidestination trip, including time spent at all destinations
Traveller country of origin	Whether travel will be rural or urban
Current health status	Total length of stay for the trip
Previous medical history, including: heart disease; diabetes; anaemia; bleeding or clotting disorders; epilepsy/seizures; gastrointestinal complaints; liver or renal problems; HIV/AIDS; immune system conditions; mental health conditions; neurological illness; respiratory disease; rheumatological conditions; previous surgical operations including thymectomy or splenectomy; splenic disorders; and for women only, pregnancy, planning pregnancy, breastfeeding, female genital mutilation previously performed	Type of travel and accommodation – examples include holiday; business trip; visiting friends and family; expatriate travel; volunteer work; healthcare work; military work; cruise ship travel; safari; adventure; diving; backpacking; school trip; pilgrimage; medical tourism; staying in hotel/hostel/camping
Current medication	Budget for the trip if appropriate
Allergies to food, latex and medication	Mode of travel: air travel, by sea, overland, trucking, etc.
Previous vaccine history	Future travel plans
Tendency to faint with injections	Travel insurance obtained

(NaTHNaC), 2019a). The small child is lower in stature and therefore would be at a higher risk of contact with a rabid dog. This peril may not be appreciated, and therefore the child may fail to report any contact to a responsible adult, resulting in a lack of treatment, which, if rabies were to develop, would be fatal (NaTHNaC, 2019d). In addition, children are at greater risk from diseases transmitted by the faecal-oral route because of poor knowledge or understanding of hygiene. Travel-related diseases can be severe in small children because their immune systems are less well developed, and illnesses such as travellers' diarrhoea, which is the most common non–vaccine-preventable disease in travellers, can be a severe risk if not managed adequately at onset as a result of problems of dehydration in particular. Hepatitis A is a risk in Turkey, and for this child traveller, who would be classified as a 'visiting friends and relatives' (VFR) type of traveller who is living with the locals and will be there for a longer period of time (NaTHNaC, 2019b), there could also be an increased risk for the acquisition of typhoid, so vaccines for both hepatitis A and typhoid should be considered. Tetanus is also a risk,

but if the child is up to date on the UK vaccination schedule, this should be sufficient, but the child's vaccination record would need to be checked, not only for tetanus but also to ensure it includes protection against measles, mumps and rubella (MMR), given the current global concern of measles outbreaks. Turkey is an intermediate to high-risk country for hepatitis B, and this child will not have been included in the national immunisation programme for babies, which started in the UK in 2017. Education regarding transmission risk and prevention would be important, as would possible consideration of vaccination, which may also be influenced by the activities planned on the trip. The risk of acquiring malaria in Turkey is considered to be low, so no chemoprophylactic agents are advised, but awareness of risk, bite prevention precautions and knowledge of symptoms and diagnosis are still important. The parents of this child need to appreciate that all risks increase with a longer duration of stay. Other risks would include altitude, depending on the exact areas the family is visiting, and tick-borne encephalitis, which is known to exist in Turkey (NaTHNaC, 2019e) (see Box 19.3).

BOX 19.3
TRAVEL RISK ASSESSMENT RESOURCES

Royal College of Nursing (2018) Competencies: Travel Health Nursing – Career and Competence Development: https://www.rcn.org.uk/professional-development/publications/pdf-006506 (For the risk assessment/management section, see pages 11–20.)

Centers for Disease Control and Prevention (CDC) – The Yellow Book 2020 (Health Information for International Travel): https://wwwnc.cdc.gov/travel/page/yellowbook-home (See also Chapter 2 – Pre-travel Consultation, found at https://wwwnc.cdc.gov/travel/yellowbook/2020/preparing-international-travelers/the-pretravel-consultation.)

National Travel Health Network and Centre – e-learning course on risk assessment: https://travelhealthpro.org.uk/news/238/e-learning-course-on-risk-assessment

VACCINE-PREVENTABLE RISKS AND THEIR MANAGEMENT

There are a number of vaccine-preventable diseases for which travellers can be at risk. After the provision of clean water, vaccination is the most important public health measure. It is important to ensure travellers are up to date with the national immunisation schedule during the pre-travel consultation. This includes checking the vaccine history and giving any further necessary vaccines required. Influenza and pneumococcal vaccines are also important considerations for travellers, especially those travelling to the southern hemisphere in the UK summer period, when it will be the winter season in that part of the globe, and infections such as flu will be of greater intensity. The recent increase in the risk of measles infection both in the UK and countries abroad makes it particularly important to ensure that travellers have a record of two doses of MMR vaccine and, if not, that they are vaccinated – NHS stock of vaccine can be used for this purpose (Public Health England (PHE), 2017).

The following sections provide brief information about the diseases, what causes them, the vaccines available and additional preventive measures that should be taken. For more extensive knowledge on specific diseases, the reader is advised to refer to *Immunisation Against Infectious Disease* – commonly known as the Green Book (PHE, 2013). NHS Choices also provides comprehensive information.

The NHS Available Vaccines

Hepatitis A is a viral infection transmitted via contaminated food and water. Those at higher risk are VFRs, long-term travellers and those exposed to conditions of poor sanitation. The incubation period averages 28 to 30 days (range of 15 to 50 days), and young children are often asymptomatic. The disease can present with abrupt onset of malaise, anorexia, nausea and fever, followed by jaundice. Fulminant hepatitis is more likely in those with pre-existing liver disease and in older individuals. The overall case fatality rate is low but, again, is greater in older patients and those with pre-existing liver disease (Department of Health and Social Care (DHSC), 2012).

Hepatitis A vaccine is available in paediatric and adult formulations and is very effective in providing protection. There are a number of different brands, but the basic principle is that there are two doses in a course of hepatitis A vaccine, given a minimum of 6 months apart, and then as currently advised, the traveller would be protected for 25 years from the date of receiving the second dose of the course. Prevention of disease, in addition to vaccination, is through food, water and personal hygiene advice in the main. For further information about the many questions relating to hepatitis A vaccine, see http://bit.ly/2RYG437.

Typhoid is a gram-negative bacterial infection, transmitted by the faecal-oral route, through water-borne spread and through human-to-human spread. Those at higher risk include VFRs, young children, long-term travellers and those exposed to conditions of poor sanitation – mainly in Asia, particularly UK visitors going to India, Pakistan and Bangladesh. The incubation period is 7 to 14 days, and the disease can present with fever, chills, headache, malaise, weakness, anorexia, abdominal pain and diarrhoea. Complications found in 10% to 15% of those with illness can lead to intestinal perforation, bacteraemia and meningitis. Chronic carrier status is also feasible in <3% infected persons.

There are currently two vaccines to provide some protection against typhoid, although the available injectable product is a polysaccharide vaccine, which does not evoke a long-term immune response and will not give particularly good protection in all cases. One dose of the injectable vaccine gives up to 3 years of protection, but this will wane as time progresses. The oral typhoid vaccine also does not provide particularly good protection in all recipients. In addition, it is always important for travellers to follow careful food, water and personal hygiene advice.

Cholera is an acute intestinal infection caused by the bacterium *Vibrio cholerae*. It is transmitted by the faecal-oral route, and 90% of cases are mild to moderate, with 10% of cases being very severe and leading to profuse diarrhoea, vomiting, circulatory collapse and shock. The mortality rate can be over 50% in untreated cases unless rapid rehydration therapy is given promptly. Chronic carriage is rare. The organism survives for up to 2 weeks in fresh water and 8 weeks in saltwater. Transmission is normally through infected drinking water, and this disease is usually associated with poverty, poor sanitation and inadequate access to clean drinking water (PHE, 2013). The oral cholera vaccine provides some protection but is variable between individuals, and again, behavioural prevention measures remain very important, addressed through food, water and personal hygiene advice.

At the current time, there is one cholera vaccine available, but a second is due to be launched in the UK in early 2020, which will be a single-dose preparation. In comparison, the current vaccine requires two or three doses in the course, depending on the age of the individual receiving it.

Tetanus, Polio and Diphtheria

Because these vaccines are only available in a combination preparation, they are described here collectively.

Tetanus is caused by bacteria that can survive for a long time outside the body and are usually found in soil or animal manure, so the risk cannot be eliminated. If the bacteria enter the human body through a wound, they multiply and release a toxin that affects the nerves, causing symptoms of the disease, such as muscle stiffness and spasms. Tetanus can be dangerous and even fatal, but because vaccine coverage for tetanus in the UK is good, with the national programme having started in 1961, this is a rare disease affecting those who never received complete vaccination. A tetanus-containing vaccine continues to be given every 10 years to travellers going to risk areas, in case they are unable to obtain treatment in the country they visit.

Polio is a serious viral infection, and although most people will only experience it mildly, to the extent that they have no symptoms, in its severest form, it can cause muscle weakness, atrophy, contractures and deformities and even paralysis. Routine vaccination came into the UK vaccination programme from 1954 onward, and there has not been a naturally acquired case in the UK since 1984 (PHE, 2013). A global eradication programme for polio is under way, but at the present time, the disease remains endemic in three countries, and significant immunisation campaigns are in place using live polio vaccine. The live polio vaccine provides herd immunity as well as individual protection; its use was discontinued in the UK in 2004, in favour of the killed vaccine, because herd immunity was high, and the live vaccine itself can put individuals at risk of disease. A Public Health Emergency of International Concern (PHEIC) programme was initiated by the World Health Organisation (WHO) in 2014 and continues today (Global Polio Eradication Initiative, 2019). It is therefore important to observe the information about polio in each country-specific guidance publication provided by PHE via the NaTHNaC on the website TravelHealthPro and through Health Protection Scotland via TRAVAX. This affects the recommendation for polio-containing vaccine for travellers to certain countries, aiming to stop international spread in the case of travellers.

Diphtheria is an infection caused by the bacterium *Corynebacterium diphtheriae*; it is a highly contagious and potentially fatal infection that can affect the nose and throat and sometimes the skin. It is rare in the UK, but there is a small risk of catching it while travelling in some parts of the world. It is spread by coughs and sneezes or through close contact with someone who is infected but also by sharing items such as cups, cutlery, clothing or bedding with an infected person. Vaccination was introduced to the UK in 1942, and cases in this country are rare.

Because tetanus, polio and diphtheria vaccines are not available as monovalent vaccines in the UK, disease protection can only be administered for travellers in the combination vaccine called *Revaxis*. Five doses of vaccine containing these components are provided in the national programme and then continued routinely every 10 years if travelling to a destination where any of these diseases are a risk. Provision of this protection continues as an NHS provision, but the vaccine must be purchased into the surgery, and the cost is then claimed back from the Prescription Pricing Authority.

The **bacillus Calmette–Guérin (BCG) vaccine** is not part of the national immunisation programme and is only given to small babies in certain circumstances (e.g., born to a parent or grandparent who originates from a country where the annual incidence of tuberculosis is 40:100,000 or greater). BCG can be given for travel purposes in unvaccinated children under 16 years of age who are going to live for more than 3 months in countries where there remains a risk. A tuberculin skin test is required before vaccination for all children from 6 years of age and may be recommended for some younger children. This would not be provided in primary care, and the traveller would often be referred to the local NHS chest clinic. The vaccine is not given to travellers outside this age range, except travelling healthcare workers who may be at risk through their activities at the destination (PHE, 2013).

Privately Available Vaccines

Yellow fever is a virus spread by an infected mosquito bite. It is uncommon in tourist areas but can cause serious, often fatal illness. Outbreaks of disease do sometimes occur, so the country-specific information needs to be read carefully. Yellow fever is only found in parts of Africa, South America, Central America and the Caribbean. The vaccine is licensed from 9 months of age, and one dose now protects for life in most individuals, with a few exceptions identified in the Green Book. The vaccine is given for disease protection, but sometimes it is required because the receiving country has an entry requirement for evidence of protection, which is provided by the vaccine administration being recorded on the International Certificate of Vaccination or Prophylaxis, as required under the International Health Regulations from the WHO. The WHO issues regular updates on these country requirements, with some being advised if travellers are entering from a country that has a risk of disease and others where there is a mandatory requirement. The summary of this requirement will then be found on the NaTHNaC and TRAVAX websites. Yellow fever vaccine can only be administered in a registered yellow fever centre. General Practice surgeries can apply for this option, and if located in England Wales or Northern Ireland, they have to apply through NaTHNaC; in Scotland, they apply through Health Protection Scotland. Training needs to be undertaken every 2 years, and there are a number of regulations that the surgery has to abide by (NaTHNaC, 2016). Serious adverse events identified from yellow fever vaccine are important, particularly in those aged 60 years and over (NaTHNaC, 2019f; Public Health England et al., 2019). This is a complex subject; consequently, GPNs who have limited experience in the provision of travel healthcare should avoid the provision of yellow fever vaccine services until they have competence and developed expertise in general travel health. The RCN competency framework considers yellow fever administration to be a skill of the experienced nurse in travel health (RCN, 2018). However, all practitioners need to understand the risk assessment for yellow fever vaccine to appropriately refer the traveller to a private travel clinic for further advice.

Rabies virus is carried in the saliva of any infected warm-blooded mammal. Although dogs are the most common animals to infect travellers, cats and monkeys are often reported as well. Rabies is spread through a bite, scratch or lick onto broken skin from the infected animal. Rabies is usually fatal. Vaccination is advised for those going to risk areas that will be remote from a reliable source of vaccine for post-exposure treatment. A full course of three doses of rabies vaccine before travel ensures immunity to the rabies virus. If the traveller then has an exposure, they still need to get post-exposure treatment of two further doses of rabies vaccine, but this is more achievable. Those who have no pre-exposure vaccine or an incomplete course, depending on the risk of exposure (i.e., the risk within the country, the type of animal and the severity of the wound), will require a full course of vaccine, which in the UK is four doses (or five doses in an immunocompromised individual), and they may also need to receive rabies-specific immunoglobulin (RIg). This provides antibodies enabling immediate protection, whereas the vaccine will take several days to develop an antibody response. However, there is a global shortage of RIg, which may result in the traveller possibly needing to fly to another country to find it or having to return home early. No traveller who received a full course of rabies vaccine before travel has died from rabies exposure (Warrell, 2012). This information, together with the risk of fake rabies vaccines being found in some countries (NaTHNaC, 2019c), provides compelling reasons for travellers to have a pre-exposure course. However, because of the high cost of vaccine, it is often difficult to persuade travellers to invest in this protection. Whether or not they have vaccine before travel, if they have any animal contact, it is absolutely essential that they know to wash the wound thoroughly with soap and running water for a minimum of 15 minutes, add an antiseptic (something like povidone-iodine is very effective) and then seek immediate medical help. If a general practice does not provide a service for the provision of pre-exposure rabies vaccine administration, it is still essential that the GPN offers post-exposure protection advice, advises the traveller to seek vaccination from a private clinic and documents this information within the patient's record. There are two licenced rabies vaccines at the current time in the UK and two different course schedules: (1) days 0, 7 and 21 to 28 days or (2) days 0, 3, 7 and 365. A booster may be given 1 year or more after the primary course, and current guidance suggests this is sufficient pre-travel protection for life, remembering that the post-exposure treatment must always be applied after a potential risk exposure. The rabies vaccine should be administered via the intramuscular route in the general practice setting (PHE, 2013).

Japanese encephalitis (JE) is caused by a virus spread by mosquitoes but maintained in a life cycle between waterfowl and pigs. Human-to-human transmission is not possible. It is found mainly in rural areas in Southeast Asia, the Pacific Islands and the Far East, so rural areas near pig farms and paddy fields are higher-risk areas. Whilst JE is usually a mild infection, it can be very serious, causing a cerebral infection with severe, life-changing consequences. Bite prevention is essential, with the mosquito being active between dusk and dawn. Whilst this is a rare disease in travellers, the seriousness of the infection is an important factor for travellers at significant risk, especially those going for longer periods of time, travelling or working rurally, going to live in such an area or making frequent trips to a risk area, even if only for short stays each time. Only one vaccine is available for the prevention of this disease in the UK (Ixiaro), which is licenced from 2 months of age, giving doses at days 0 and 28, although there is a licence for a 0- and 7-day schedule in 18- to 64-year-olds. However, the Green Book also says this schedule can be used off-licence for children from 2 months and in the 65-plus age group if there is genuinely no time to complete the standard schedule. The course should ideally be completed at least 1 week before JE virus exposure (PHE, 2013).

Tick-borne encephalitis (TBE) is a viral infection that is usually transmitted through the bite of an infected tick and found in areas that extend from central, eastern and northern Europe across Russia to parts of eastern Asia. TBE is a rare disease in UK travellers, but risk increases if travellers are undertaking activities in woodland or grassland (e.g., when camping or hiking). Illness from the disease is usually mild, although the Asian form can be more severe, with central nervous system problems; it can be fatal in up to 20% of these cases, and long-term neurological sequelae are more common. Prevention includes appropriate clothing (wearing long sleeves, tucking trousers into socks to prevent ticks from getting under any clothing, insect repellents, checking for the presence of ticks at the end of a day out). If any are found, careful removal is required using fine tweezers to ensure that all of the mouthparts are removed.

The vaccine is available in both paediatric and adult formulations. It can be given from 1 year of age, with the course comprising three doses, with a booster at 3-year intervals for those at continued risk (PHE, 2013).

Meningococcal disease is caused by the bacterium *Neisseria meningitidis* – there are six different strains: A, B, C, E, W135 and Y. The most serious forms of the disease are meningitis and septicaemia, which can be life threatening. The disease is spread most commonly via droplet infection, and travellers should practice good hand hygiene and avoid activities that promote the exchange of respiratory secretions, such as sharing drinks and eating utensils. This risk is greater for people who travel to countries where the diseases are common (the four major meningococcal groups abroad are A, C, W135 and Y) and the traveller is mixing in areas that are highly populated, particularly with local people, or for those who are at risk from their occupation. The highest-risk area is the 'meningitis belt' of sub-Saharan Africa, particularly during the dry season, but travellers to the Kingdom of Saudi Arabia (KSA) attending for pilgrimage (Umrah and Hajj) also require vaccination to obtain a visa, which is required by the Saudi Arabian government for entry to the country. Vaccines are available to help provide protection against these diseases. There are two different brands of a conjugate ACWY vaccine in the UK (Menveo and Nimenrix). One dose is required before travel (10 days before entry for those entering KSA), and for travel purposes, it provides 5 years' protection (PHE, 2013).

Hepatitis B virus (HBV) is spread through infected blood, contaminated needles and sexual intercourse. Infection causes inflammation of the liver, which can result in jaundice and occasionally hepatic failure. Around 20% to 25% of individuals with chronic HBV infection worldwide have progressive liver disease, leading to cirrhosis in some patients, who are also at higher risk of developing hepatocellular carcinoma (PHE, 2013). Vaccination should be considered if travellers are visiting high-risk areas for long periods or are at social or occupational risk. There are two vaccine brands (Engerix B and HBVaxPro), both available in adult and paediatric formulations, with a number of different schedules that can be used. The choice depends on various factors, including the importance of adequate protection as soon as possible and the number of vaccines to be given – an important consideration when advising for children or the needle-phobic. Because hepatitis B and other bloodborne infections such as hepatitis C and HIV constitute a risk to travellers, especially if going to areas of the world where the risk is greater and healthcare facilities are less optimal, preventive advice is important, including only accepting adequately screened blood if a transfusion is required, refusing medical procedures with nonsterile equipment, not sharing needles (e.g., tattooing, body piercing, acupuncture and drug abuse) and always practising safe sex, including the use of condoms.

NON–VACCINE-PREVENTABLE RISKS AND APPROPRIATE ADVICE

Insect-Borne Diseases

Yellow fever, JE and tick-borne encephalitis have already been discussed, and vaccination can help in their prevention, but there are other mosquito-borne diseases for which there are currently no vaccines available for travellers – these include malaria, dengue fever, Zika virus, chikungunya, West Nile virus and Rift Valley Fever. Infected mosquitoes will bite day or night, depending on the mosquito type, but in all situations, stringent bite-prevention methods are essential to minimise disease risk. For malaria prevention, the insect repellent commonly recommended is N,N-diethyl-m-toluamide (DEET), up to a 50% concentration. Alternatives are available for those who do not wish to use DEET. Repellents should be applied to any exposed skin at the risk times and reapplied as required, remembering that in a hot and humid country, the traveller may sweat off the repellent more quickly. Repellents and insecticides can be used on cotton clothing. Room protection may be by the use of air-conditioning units, screening over the windows, insect vaporisers (electric or battery operated), knock-down sprays and impregnated mosquito nets. The UK Malaria Guidance document has an excellent section on insect-bite prevention, which should be studied for greater knowledge; see https://www.gov.uk/government/publications/malaria-prevention-guidelines-for-travellers-from-the-uk.

Malaria is a parasitic infection spread by the bite of an infected anopheline mosquito. There is currently no vaccine available that is suitable for use in travellers, and prevention is by awareness of the risks, bite prevention, taking the appropriate antimalarial tablets and being aware of the symptoms of malaria to help identify and treat the disease promptly. Common symptoms are those of a flu-like illness with fever, aching, headache and sometimes diarrhoea or cough, and travellers should be advised to seek urgent medical advice if this happens; they should tell the practitioner they have travelled to a malarious country and ask for a malaria blood test. Malaria is a notifiable disease, and each year, an average of 1500 travellers return to the UK with malaria, of whom about 6 people die. Most cases are caused by the most dangerous human species, *Plasmodium falciparum*, which can, in some circumstances, kill a person within 24 hours of developing the symptoms of malaria. Malaria is both preventable and treatable, but those at greatest risk are VFRs, so it is important that they understand the risk and take advice (PHE, 2019). The GPN is advised to undertake further study on this important topic by reading the UK Malaria Guidelines, and a free e-learning course is available at http://bit.ly/2VyaDLN.

Travellers' Diarrhoea

This is the most common infectious disease in travellers for which there is no vaccine and can be caused by bacteria, parasites or viruses. Prevention relies on the traveller's behaviour, such as taking care regarding what they eat and drink and ensuring they always wash their hands before eating or preparing food. Travellers' diarrhoea is 3 or more looser stools in a 24-hour period, often accompanied by abdominal pain, cramps and vomiting. It usually lasts 2 to 4 days, and whilst it is not a life-threatening illness, it can disrupt travel for several days. Risk is variable in different countries of the world, with high-risk countries generally including North Africa, sub-Saharan Africa, the Indian subcontinent, South East Asia, South America, Mexico and the Middle East. The main danger from the illness is dehydration, and this, if very severe, can kill if it is not treated. Treatment is therefore by rehydration. In severe cases and particularly in young children and the elderly, commercially prepared rehydration solution is extremely useful. Anti-motility drugs may be used for adults but should never be used in children under 4 years of age, and only on prescription for children aged 4 to 12 years. Commonly used oral agents are loperamide and bismuth subsalicylate. None of these should ever be used if the person has a temperature or blood in their stool, and medical help should be sought if the affected person has a fever, has blood in the diarrhoea, has had diarrhoea for more than 48 hours (or 24 hours in children) or becomes confused. In some circumstances, antibiotics are used as a standby treatment for travellers' diarrhoea. Medication advised in anticipation of a traveller being ill whilst away is not usually available from the NHS and needs to be prescribed privately. A clinical knowledge summary (CKS) written by the National Institute for Health and Care Excellence (NICE) is available on this topic at https://cks.nice.org.uk/diarrhoea-prevention-and-advice-for-travellers.

Accidents and Personal Safety

Accidents are leading causes of death in travellers abroad, predominantly road traffic accidents and swimming/water accidents. Travellers can help prevent them by following sensible precautions, such as avoiding alcohol and food before swimming; never diving into water where the depth is uncertain; only swimming in safe water; checking for currents, sharks, jellyfish and other hazards; avoiding alcohol when driving, especially at night; avoiding hiring motorcycles and mopeds and if hiring a car, renting a large one if possible, ensuring the tyres, brakes and seat belts are in good condition; using reliable taxi firms; and knowing where emergency facilities are. The Foreign and Commonwealth Office (FCO) provides excellent information about personal safety and security. The FCO has information for many different types of travel and also advises on travel to specific destinations in times of political unrest and natural disasters. The FCO website has important information at https://www.gov.uk/government/organisations/foreign-commonwealth-office. It is also advisable to raise awareness of insurance coverage with a traveller, to include medical repatriation and if a traveller has any pre-existing medical conditions, that the insurance company is informed of this predeparture.

Other Health Risks

The GPN is advised to review the resources provided to further consider many other risks to which the traveller may be exposed, including diseases such as schistosomiasis, cutaneous larva migrans, and respiratory illnesses such as Middle East respiratory syndrome (MERS) and influenza. The newly discovered coronavirus disease (COVID-19) is a serious and developing situation as this chapter is being finalised, with the WHO declaring it a PHEIC (WHO, 2020). Additionally, other non–infection-related risks, such as altitude sickness, motion sickness, solar damage and air travel advice, and then individual risks for more vulnerable travellers, such as young children and pregnant women, senior travellers, the immunocompromised and others with underlying health conditions, should be reviewed. Female genital mutilation may be identified in a pre-travel consultation, and it is important for the practice nurse to understand the risks to help prevent this from happening, or an LGBTQ traveller may be unaware that such sexual orientation is illegal in the destination they are travelling to.

TRAINING FOR TRAVEL HEALTH

This chapter aimed to provide an overview of travel healthcare, but training is required to develop the requisite knowledge and skills to become a competent practitioner within this field of practice. The RCN guidance suggests a minimum of 15 hours of training initially, which would include mentorship (RCN, 2018). Whilst travel health courses are available, there is no official requirement for practitioners to undertake these, either for the practice of travel medicine or for those training in the subject. However, the GPN, in practising effectively, must, of course, always abide by the Nursing and Midwifery Council (NMC) Code of practice (NMC, 2018). The yellow fever vaccine can only be administered in registered yellow fever centres, and those doing so need to undertake training every 2 years (NaTHNaC, 2016). All those undertaking travel health training should be competent in immunisation and should have completed a generic immunisation training course before studying travel health (PHE, 2018). The Royal College of Physicians and Surgeons of Glasgow has a Faculty of Travel Medicine, and this body's focus is on education and standards in the field (Chiodini et al., 2012). More information can be found in the Resources section.

SUMMARY

Travel health is an important, challenging and wide-ranging area of professional practice but one that GPNs can make valuable contributions to in protecting health and promoting wellbeing. This chapter has provided an introduction to the subject area, and for those GPNs developing and delivering travel health services, further study will be required.

RESOURCES

Essential Guidance for Travel Health Practice

Royal College of Nursing (2018) Competencies: Travel Health Nursing – Career and Competence Development: https://www.rcn.org.uk/professional-development/publications/pdf-006506 (See pages 32–34 for a comprehensive list of resources, including travel risk assessment and management templates, which can also be downloaded from items no. 1 and 2 at https://www.janechiodini.co.uk/tools/.)

Public Health England – *Immunisation Against Infectious Disease* (the 'Green Book'): https://www.gov.uk/government/collections/immunisation-against-infectious-disease-the-green-book (The online version must be used, and individual chapters are updated regularly.)

Public Health England – The UK Malaria Prevention Guidelines: https://www.gov.uk/government/publications/malaria-prevention-guidelines-for-travellers-from-the-uk

Resources essential for nurses new to travel health: https://www.janechiodini.co.uk/tools/new-to-travel/

Links to prescribing for travel health FAQs, a travel health service, vaccine storage resources, general immunisation, female genital mutilation and travel and more: https://www.janechiodini.co.uk/help/

Royal College of Nursing (Public Health Forum) – Travel health resources: https://www.rcn.org.uk/clinical-topics/public-health/travel-health

Royal College of Physicians and Surgeons of Glasgow, Faculty of Travel Medicine: https://rcpsg.ac.uk/travel-medicine/home

National Online Travel Health Websites and Helplines for Healthcare Professionals

Health Protection Scotland – TRAVAX (subscription login required if not practising in Scotland): https://www.travax.nhs.uk/

Public Health England (NaTHNaC) – TravelHealthPro: https://travelhealthpro.org.uk/

Malaria Reference Laboratory email service (for healthcare professionals only) on complex malaria queries, information: https://www.gov.uk/government/publications/malaria-risk-assessment-form

Key Resources for Vaccines and Immunisation Training

Public Health England – Immunisation Collection (includes links to Vaccine Update and the Green Book): https://www.gov.uk/government/collections/immunisation

National Minimum Standards and Core Curriculum for Immunisation Training for Registered Healthcare Practitioners: https://www.gov.uk/government/publications/national-minimum-standards-and-core-curriculum-for-immunisation-training-for-registered-healthcare-practitioners

NaTHNaC – Yellow Fever Training: https://nathnacyfzone.org.uk/managing-your-yfvc#Training

Health Protection Scotland – Yellow Fever Training: https://www.hps.scot.nhs.uk/web-resources-container/yellow-fever-training-programme/

Electronic Medicines Compendium (details of all the Summary of Product Characteristics (SmPC) of vaccines and malaria chemoprophylaxis): https://www.medicines.org.uk/emc/

NaTHNaC – Factsheets for individual diseases and details of the relevant vaccines: https://travelhealthpro.org.uk/factsheets

Travel vaccine chart tool – Item no. 3: https://www.janechiodini.co.uk/tools/

Travel vaccine chart tool – General immunisation resources: https://www.janechiodini.co.uk/help/immunisation-resources/

Useful Travel Health Sites for the General Public

Fit for Travel: https://www.fitfortravel.nhs.uk/home

TravelHealthPro: https://travelhealthpro.org.uk/

Foreign and Commonwealth Office: https://travelaware.campaign.gov.uk/

NHS Choices: https://www.nhs.uk/live-well/healthy-body/before-you-travel/

Traveller advice resources: https://www.janechiodini.co.uk/help/tar/

International resources

Centers for Disease Control and Prevention (CDC) – The Yellow Book 2020 (Health Information for International Travel): https://wwwnc.cdc.gov/travel/page/yellowbook-home

World Health Organisation – Travel Page https://www.who.int/ith/en/

REFERENCES

British Medical Association. (2018). *Focus on travel immunisation.* https://www.bma.org.uk/advice/employment/gp-practices/service-provision/prescribing/vaccination/travel-immunisation

Chiodini, J. H., Anderson, E., Driver, C., Field, V. K., Flaherty, G. T., Grieve, A. M., Green, A. D., Jones, M. E., Marra, F. J., McDonald, A. C., Riley, S. F., Simons, H., Smith, C. C., & Chiodini, P. L. (2012). Recommendations for the practice of travel medicine. *Travel Medicine and Infectious Disease, 10*(3), 109–128. https://www.sciencedirect.com/science/article/abs/pii/S1477893912000671

Department of Health and Social Care. (2012). *Statement of financial entitlements (Amendment No. 2). Directions 2012.* https://www.gov.uk/government/publications/the-statement-of-financial-entitlements-amendment-no2-directions-2012

Global Polio Eradication Initiative. (2019). *IHR public health emergency of international concern. Temporary recommendations to reduce international spread of poliovirus.* http://polioeradication.org/polio-today/polio-now/public-health-emergency-status/

National Travel Health Network and Centre. (2016). *Conditions of designation for yellow fever vaccination centres, 2016.* https://nathnacyfzone.org.uk/managing-your-yfvc#Conditions_of_Designation

National Travel Health Network and Centre. (2019a). *Children factsheet.* https://travelhealthpro.org.uk/factsheet/82/children

National Travel Health Network and Centre. (2019b). *Factsheet: Travelling to visit friends and relatives.* https://travelhealthpro.org.uk/factsheet/91/travelling-to-visit-friends-and-relatives

National Travel Health Network and Centre. (2019c). *Philippines: Falsified rabies vaccines and rabies immunoglobulin – Update.* https://travelhealthpro.org.uk/news/440/philippines-falsified-rabies-vaccines-and-rabies-immunoglobulin-update

National Travel Health Network and Centre. (2019d). *Rabies factsheet.* https://travelhealthpro.org.uk/factsheet/20/rabies

National Travel Health Network and Centre. (2019e). *Turkey vaccine and malaria recommendations.* https://travelhealthpro.org.uk/country/227/turkey

National Travel Health Network and Centre. (2019f). *Yellow fever vaccination recommendations: Persons aged 60 years or older.* https://nathnacyfzone.org.uk/news/85/yellow-fever-vaccination-recommendations-persons-aged-60-years-or-older

NHS England. (2019). *Interim findings of the vaccinations and immunisations review – September 2019.* https://www.england.nhs.uk/publication/interim-findings-of-the-vaccinations-and-immunisations-review-september-2019

NHS England & British Medical Association. (2020). *Investment and evolution: Update to the GP contract agreement 2020/21–2023/24.* https://www.england.nhs.uk/publication/investment-and-evolution-update-to-the-gp-contract-agreement-20-21-23-24/

NHS Health Scotland. (2019). *Vaccine transformation programme – Travel vaccinations and travel health advice.* http://www.health-scotland.scot/health-topics/immunisation/vaccination-transformation-programme

Nursing and Midwifery Council. (2018). *The Code: Standards of conduct, performance and ethics for nurses and midwives.* https://www.nmc.org.uk/standards/code/

Public Health England. (2013). *Immunisation against infectious disease. 'The Green Book'.* https://www.gov.uk/government/collections/immunisation-against-infectious-disease-the-green-book

Public Health England. (2017). *Vaccine update, Issue 273.* https://assets.publishing.service.gov.uk/government/uploads/system/uploads/attachment_data/file/669418/VU_273_December2017.pdf

Public Health England. (2018). *Immunisation training standards for healthcare practitioners.* https://www.gov.uk/government/publications/national-minimum-standards-and-core-curriculum-for-immunisation-training-for-registered-healthcare-practitioners

Public Health England. (2019). *Guidelines for malaria prevention in travellers from the UK 2019.* https://assets.publishing.service.gov.uk/government/uploads/system/uploads/attachment_data/file/833506/ACMP_Guidelines.pdf

Public Health England, Medicines and Healthcare Products Regulatory Agency, National Travel Health Network and Centre, & Health Protection Scotland. (2019). *Yellow fever vaccine: Stronger precautions in people with weakened immunity and those aged 60 years or older.* https://travelhealthpro.org.uk/media_lib/mlib-uploads/full/2019-11-21-yellow-fever-vaccine-precautions-letter.pdf

Royal College of Nursing. (2018). *Competencies: Travel health nursing: Career and competence development.* https://www.rcn.org.uk/professional-development/publications/pdf-006506

Warrell, D. (2012). Animal attacks, rabies, venomous bites and stings. In R. Dawood (Ed.), *Travellers' health – How to stay healthy abroad* (pp. 176–201). Oxford University Press.

World Health Organisation. (2020). *Coronavirus disease (COVID-19) pandemic.* https://www.who.int/emergencies/diseases/novel-coronavirus-2019

20

THE FUTURE OF GENERAL PRACTICE NURSING

SUSAN F. BROOKS

INTRODUCTION

To explore the issues affecting the initial and ongoing professional development of general practice nurses (GPNs), this chapter will consider the context of healthcare in the United Kingdom and the requirements for various GPN roles.

The trajectory of growth of knowledge and skills will be explored, from early-career challenges for GPNs through to roles that encompass advanced practice, leadership and education. This will touch on many of the subjects covered in earlier chapters of the book but will hopefully enhance thinking about the possibilities for the future of general practice nursing and the exciting opportunities for this fast-moving area of healthcare.

THE CONTEXT FOR CONTINUOUS PROFESSIONAL DEVELOPMENT IN THE HEALTHCARE SECTOR OF THE UK

The context for GPN professional development is one of ongoing change when considering how the National Health Service (NHS) and the private sector organise healthcare provision. There are changes towards adopting more integrated approaches and across historical patterns of roles and responsibilities. However, openness to this change is required, along with sustained funding and innovation, described in the NHS Long Term Plan (NHS England, 2019a) and following years of austerity and difficulty in resourcing public services. In addition, a key driver for change in the role

of the GPN profession is the shifting demographic, which includes people with longer life expectancy in the UK, who have more complex and varied healthcare needs, and rising expectations and demand for support (Davies, 2019). The climate of increased demand alongside the reduction in the supply of suitably qualified healthcare professionals (Majeed, 2017) has created the need for all healthcare professions, including GPNs, to rethink their roles and competencies to meet service users' needs and work within a multidisciplinary team of healthcare and social care workers (Department of Health (Northern Ireland), 2016; NHS England, 2019d).

Similarly, the Scottish government (2018) has discussed a transformational change agenda where GPNs act as key practitioners with pivotal roles in integrated community nursing teams. In Wales, there has been an emphasis on the development of GPN roles, with the expectation that training opportunities will help equip nurses for integrated and partnership work arrangements (Primary Care One, 2019).

Clusters of healthcare providers, federations and super-partnerships, such as sustainability and transformation partnerships (STPs), could be in a better position to respond to the rising demands of their local populations from a healthcare and social care perspective. This will require multidisciplinary collaboration and investment in the workforce, including in GPNs, as numbers of general practitioners continue to fall (Majeed, 2017; NHS England, 2016).

Spending on primary care needs to reflect the government's emphasis on care being accessed as close to home as possible, along with a preventative and empowering approach to equip the population to care for itself more effectively (NHS England, 2019d). GPNs have key roles to play in this new environment, and the development of expertise in clinical and adjunctive areas, such as leadership and education, is a challenge to be addressed against these changes in healthcare.

The lack of a standardised route in general practice nursing across the UK (unlike the specifications to become a general practitioner (GP)) means that recruitment of both new and experienced nurses must be underpinned by the provision of continuous professional development (CPD), which has been successfully developed in certain areas, such as the Midlands, Scotland and Yorkshire (Aston, 2018). However, the details of what is required by GPNs to meet the clinical needs of patient populations are an area of debate, and there is an additional challenge regarding who should fund their training and academic development (Oxtoby, 2018). A Queen's Nursing Institute (QNI, 2015) survey reported that only 57.3% of nurses always received support for professional development from their employers, with 53% of employers taking full responsibility for payment to support CPD. It may be that there is a potential dissonance for some budget holders in general practice regarding the needs of newly qualified GPNs, juxtaposed against the advanced skills development being requested by more experienced nurses whom practices may wish to retain. Sustainability for service provision could be argued to require both areas of investment, but this remains challenging for many practice managers, clinical commissioning groups (CCGs) and general practitioner partners. However, the Royal College of Nursing (RCN, 2018b) is clear about the three categories of CPD in the UK:

- Statutory – required for compliance with specific legislation, such as moving and handling training
- Mandatory – essential to the nature of the role, such as infection control updates
- Developmental – individually determined for personal or workforce requirements and including advanced and specialist practice qualifications

It is evident that there is much that can be identified as required and optional routes under the umbrella of CPD for GPNs. Perhaps a more relevant question is how to provide and encourage access to more than what is statutory and mandatory to meet the needs of local population groups and how to provide logical and fulfilling career trajectories for GPNs from the beginning of their careers to retirement.

EARLY PREPARATION FOR GPN ROLES

The role of the GPN has witnessed significant changes in recent decades with the alteration in thinking to promote this as a first choice of career for newly qualified nurses (Duncan & Hayes, 2017), which is a long way from previous descriptions of GPNs as the unsung heroes and invisible clinicians. Change has occurred in the way GPNs are managed, often by senior nurses rather than the previous expectation that GPNs could be solely managed and mentored by GPs and/or practice managers, and thus their careers would largely reflect what the employers were able to provide in terms of training and development (QNI, 2015).

Variation in the expectations and preparation for the GPN role in general practice have contributed to a potential undervaluing of this route as a career choice, although much has been invested to counter this disparity. For example, The General Practice Forward View (NHS England, 2016) referred to nationally funded support for GPNs, although evidence for this has continued to be mixed across the United Kingdom (Oxtoby, 2018). More recently, Health Education England has commissioned Skills for Health to create a core capabilities framework for primary care and general practice nursing, which will be a welcome benchmark of standards to promote excellent care for service users and to help to structure the development of GPNs (Health Education England (HEE), 2021). In addition, higher education institutions have developed partnerships for undergraduate placements in community-based units such as general practice and walk-in centres, and the focus of teaching and learning activities is not exclusively on acute and care provision in hospitals (HEE, 2017).

Integrated care with improved communication between healthcare and social care professionals can be engendered through the ethos of multi-professional education in core subjects. This could result in less silo working as healthcare undergraduates from a wide range of backgrounds learn to understand their similarities and unique approaches to care provision. Some areas have seen that new interdisciplinary forums are starting to communicate at the local level, resulting in improved outcomes, understanding and respect, as well as learning from models of good practice. A generic goal is surely for the reduction of the frustration of service users when co-ordinated care is lacking between GP practices and other services, including community nursing services, accident and emergency (A&E), ambulance services, care homes and mental health and social care teams (Aston, 2018).

A standardised route into GPN roles could be classed as professional preparation, but the umbrella of CPD still applies when considering that all GPNs are qualified nurses and therefore require initial and ongoing development to meet the requirements of the role. There is variation across the four countries of the United Kingdom, with the best practice of full induction or introductory courses with agreed competencies for new GPNs still not being mandatory (Duncan & Hayes, 2017). NHS England (2019b) has produced a General Practice Nursing Induction Template, with Action 4 of the GPN 10-point plan recognising the need to establish a national standard that will benefit all nurses making the transition into general practice (p. 3):

> Work with commissioners and the Royal Colleges to ensure all nurses new to general practice have access to an approved employer-led induction programme and a continuous professional development (CPD) plan that includes the GPN foundation or fundamentals standards.

The emphasis on induction as well as CPD is encouraging, but establishing a standardised competency framework for GPNs has not been an easy task. The checklist approach could be viewed as being relatively superficial – for example, the elements of the list that could be interpreted as requiring considerable study within a CPD framework, such as the following (NHS England, 2019b):

> Comprehensive Health Assessment – including history taking, clinical examination and nursing diagnosis.

However, employers are encouraged to create a bespoke checklist with common 'national' elements that can be adapted to suit local areas. The development of voluntary standards of education for GPNs new to the role is a welcome publication from the QNI (2020) providing clarification regarding what is an induction-level competency and what is part of CPD and professional development. This has partly been informed by the changes in the Nursing and Midwifery Council (NMC) standards for education and training (NMC, 2018a), which detail enhanced assessment skills. Higher education institutions are working on their curricula to incorporate these elements that were previously part of post-registration training.

GPN OPPORTUNITIES IN EDUCATION AND RESEARCH

Student nurses began to have access to practical placements in general practice during their undergraduate programmes over 10 years ago, and it could be argued that this may be one of the most logical developments in terms of recruitment of GPNs (HEE, 2017). Further, this is responsive to the Five Year Forward View challenge (NHS England, 2014) to increase recruitment, retention and return to practice into this area. However, the situation may not be so positive when the broader picture of the GPN workforce is examined, revealing the estimated imminent retirement of a third of the practice nurse workforce by 2020 (Eveleigh, 2019) and much dissatisfaction with the pressure of the workload (Davies, 2019). An additional issue is the lack of men recruited into GPN roles and the scarce current research to discover why this is the case (Duncan & Hayes, 2017).

Solutions to this crisis have been focussed on recruitment, new ways of working and retention of experienced practitioners. One key element of all these solutions is education, and the recent changes to the standards for education and training (NMC, 2018a) and the standards for supervision and assessment (NMC, 2018b, 2018c) have altered the landscape and refocussed emphasis on shared responsibility for the supervision of students in practice. GPNs can fully embrace these changes by accessing training for the roles of practice supervisor and practice assessor (NMC, 2018b), acknowledging that many excellent mentors have previously supported learners in general practice. The opportunity for developing the abilities of GPNs as educators is not to be missed (Aston, 2018), and they have much to pass on and help empower both students and those more recently employed in general practice (NHS England, 2018). Key to the NMC Code (2018c, p. 10) is the requirement for all registered nurses and midwives to fulfil their roles to 'support students' and colleagues' learning to help them develop their professional competence and confidence'. One of the recommendations from HEE's (2017) general practice nursing workforce development plan cites the need for GPN educator roles to be developed to cover all CCG areas and to include promoting mentor training (now practice supervisors and assessors) for all GPNs, including sign-off mentor roles.

However, Eveleigh (2019) writes about the urgent need to increase retention and the enticement back of previously employed GPNs to return to general practice, rather than awaiting newly qualified nurses and slowly evolving models for training. And this directs focus towards the imperative for continuous investment in professional development.

It could be argued that this must include more than the revalidation process (NMC, 2019), which includes a basic level of development requiring 35 hours of relevant CPD (20 hours participatory), with five pieces of feedback and five written reflective accounts, which are mandatory, along with confirmation by another registrant, albeit this has improved and standardised the benchmark from the previous post-registration education and practice standards for remaining on the nursing and midwifery register (Ipsos MORI, 2019; NMC, 2019).

Interestingly, the report from Ipsos MORI (2019) indicated that over half of registrants completed more than 60 hours of CPD in the 3-year period before submitting their revalidation application, far more than the minimum 35 hours required. However, it could be more difficult for registrants to find CPD opportunities that are relevant to their scope of practice. The application of this statement to general practice would require greater analysis of the data and is likely to be a variable picture across the countries and regions making up the United Kingdom. HEE's (2019) commitment of £50 million as a workforce development fund to help employers develop their existing workforce in 2019/20 is still being actioned

and was notably not for basic CPD, such as mandatory training. However, the NMC's commitment to changing behaviour to emphasize the importance of listening and responding to service users is an important sea change when considering the GPN and professional development.

Previous influencers on career trajectories may not have included the population receiving care and health services (Ipsos MORI, 2019). As with all changes, the embedding and application into action may take longer to actualise when the paucity of funding for GPNs is considered. There could be a lack of clarity from nurses and those who conduct appraisal and personal development planning to really respond to the findings emerging from the revalidation process. There is much work to be done in order for all GPNs to receive appropriate and timely access to training and development (Oxtoby, 2018).

Online resources are increasing in number and quality to meet the needs for CPD and are becoming a vital means to facilitate development by widening accessibility and reducing the costs of face-to-face learning opportunities. An example of this is the Advanced Practice Toolkit (eLearning for Health, 2019) developed from a collaboration between NHS Improvement, NHS England, NHS Employers and HEE. Similarly, NHS Education for Scotland (2018) has produced excellent resources for GPN learning and development, with an important emphasis on clinical updates and links to the latest evidence-based research. Additional sources of professional development include commercially sponsored study days and conferences. These may be of variable quality and value, but they can provide the adjunctive benefit of networking, participatory learning and informal support systems when GPNs meet each other outside their usual workplaces, increasing wellbeing and productivity and innovative practice (RCN, 2018a). Critics of some forms of CPD provision cite the lack of robust assessment strategies as one of their major limitations (RCN, 2018a), and there is a notable challenge in aligning credits and qualifications from different institutions, private providers and online learning platforms. The effectiveness of CPD in its many forms is a contentious issue, with many evaluations being self-reported and therefore difficult to assess for validity and reliability. However, there is an unequivocal impetus for

GPNs to access high-quality and relevant educational opportunities for development and to take roles as educators themselves to supervise, challenge and assess practice in the workplace and in higher education institutions.

The evidence base for practice has long been valued, and the aim to close the so-called theory–practice gap is an ongoing challenge for evolvement in healthcare. GPNs have not always seen research as a focus of CPD for developing expertise. Nevertheless, HEE has started to promote clinical academic career pathways (HEE, 2017), and the National Institute for Health Research (NIHR) (2021) has an active primary care sector where, in 2018/19, the NIHR Clinical Research Network (CRN) involved 38% of general practices in England. Similarly, the Scottish government (2017) identified the need for nurses to continue their involvement in the vibrant research community, and in Wales, the government has increased support for general practice surgeries to become research active through investment by Health and Care Research Wales (Welsh Government, 2019). GPNs have a key role in understanding and participating in research projects through recruiting, collecting data and being involved in the research community to influence and improve care and services. CPD to encourage this is vital but is not always readily available compared with some of the clinical competency and skills-based resources for developing the GPN workforce.

In England, practices that engage with research activities receive payments, dependent on the level of involvement, and this may incentivise contribution and drive CPD training for GPNs (Royal College of General Practitioners (RCGP), 2018).

ADVANCED PRACTICE – GENERALISTS AND SPECIALISTS

Career development is an interesting challenge for GPNs when many of their roles have been based in the treatment room and involve carrying out a variety of care processes for a wide range of people who are living with increasingly complex conditions (Duncan & Hayes, 2017). The RCGP (2013) sought to encourage generalist training programmes for practice nurses and encouraged the development of services that can, in theory, be culturally responsive, flexible and relevant to the patient population and its local demographic identity. The RCGP (2013, p. 19) also noted that 'practice teams will require the skills and expertise of nurses, physician assistants and other professionals who have undergone specific vocational training in community-based settings and are trained for their generalist role, which will complement that of the expert generalist physician'.

Some have interpreted the generalist role to mean that GPNs should develop their skills in the management of commonly presenting but undifferentiated conditions, often spending hours of their working week seeing people who would previously have seen a medical GP (NHS England, 2019b). The investment in GPNs to deliver this level of service is a challenge under current budgetary restraints, but applications for physical health assessment and nonmedical prescribing modules at higher education institutions increase each year.

Delivery of care must be set against the context of health promotion and disease prevention to continue the vision described in the Five Year Forward View (NHS England, 2014) to radically upgrade prevention and public health to close the health and wellbeing gap and to reduce the burden of avoidable ill health. Thus it would seem logical to acknowledge the commonality of the required knowledge and skill base for GPNs among all other healthcare professions and ensure that CPD always includes a preventative focus (NHS England, 2018).

An example of this could be the involvement of GPNs in the Diabetes Prevention Programme, a nationally funded and commissioned programme, and, more recently, the Diabetes Remission Clinical Trial (DiRECT) (Lean et al., 2019), whereby targeted funding is being considered for the next few years for a small number of sites to test and refine an enhanced weight-management support offering for those with a body mass index (BMI) of 30+ with type 2 diabetes or hypertension.

Interestingly, the Career Pathway for General Practice Nursing in Northern Ireland (Northern Ireland Practice and Education Council for Nursing and Midwifery, 2019) includes specific guidance in health promotion within the framework covering clinical, leadership, research and education. And in Scotland, NHS Education for Scotland (2018) seeks to co-ordinate access to quality, accessible and locally relevant information, support, education and representation for general practice nursing, thereby reducing isolation and improving the quality of service delivery.

The key issues to be addressed that relate to GPN career progression and provision of integrated services for the population of the UK are summarised in the NHS Long Term Plan Implementation Framework (NHS England, 2019c) to address the new service model for the 21st century and include primary and community care with integrated care services that are delivered by workers who are suitably prepared and sustained to fulfil and flourish in their roles.

One of the 10 action points from the general practice 10-point action plan (NHS England, 2018, p. 19) is to 'increase access to clinical academic careers and advanced clinical practice programmes, including nurses working in advanced practice roles in general practice'.

This has been recognised as career development for many years, and some GPNs have taken on extensive academic and practical teaching and learning opportunities as advanced nurse practitioners with qualifications in history taking and physical assessment, management of long-term conditions and non-medical prescribing (NHS England, 2019b).

The consensus regarding the requirement for Level 7, master's level study or equivalent (NHS England, HEE, & NHS Improvement, 2017), has been a potential barrier to some but an enabler to others as they seek to develop this strand of their advancing role as a GPN educator. Because education is identified as one of the key pillars of advanced practice (NHS England, HEE, & NHS Improvement, 2017), the development of skills in facilitating learning and assessment must be a challenge accepted by GPNs. Similarly, leadership skills need to be developed, including the ability to analyse and apply relevant theory from the literature, in order that innovative development of teams will occur to improve the skill mix and specialisation through integration of medical and nonmedical health professionals (NHS England, HEE, & NHS Improvement, 2017).

In academia, programmes to support nurses new to general practice have sometimes struggled to resource the teaching and learning opportunities, possibly as a result of the paucity of GPNs who enter university teaching roles (Aston, 2018). This is a challenge to the current and future workforce of GPNs. This is a challenge to the current and future workforce of GPNs, but support for development has been emphasised in the NHS People Plan 2020/2021 (NHS England, 2020) with refocus on CPD provision following the crisis of the Covid-19 pandemic, including backfill for the service, increased access to elearning and blended approaches to degree and higher level studies.

GPNS AS LEADERS AND STRATEGISTS

Working as a GPN in general practice may not seem to be an obvious clinical area for the development of leadership skills. Teams are often small, and opportunities can be limited for taking on strategic roles with the practice or the wider structure of the CCG. However, the development of integrated teams working across traditional practice boundaries may signal a change and open doors for potentially influential leaders from within the GPN workforce who understand the key issues for nurses.

The NHS Leadership Academy Bespoke Rosalind Franklin leadership programme has been commissioned as part of the GPN 10-point plan programme (NHS England, 2018) and seeks to provide guidance and inspiration for some who have been able to access this excellent resource. Some would argue the imperative to challenge outdated views that assume that GPs deliver all services in general practice, whilst GPNs remain invisible as a vital part of the growing multiprofessional team that includes physiotherapists, paramedics and pharmacists.

Advanced practice has certainly identified leadership and management skills as core to the pillars required for a master's level award in this area (NHS England, HEE, & NHS Improvement, 2017). And recent initiatives embed this thinking, such as the QNI's (2021) Aspiring Leaders Programme that includes intensive input regarding the growth of individual leadership and a deep understanding of the primary care network at a local and strategic level. The task to complete this programme is a quality-improvement project proposal to improve care or services for patients. These are exciting and tangible developments for some GPNs to excel in leadership roles with appropriate and inspirational training and support.

The media needs to reflect these developments of nurses in key positions of influence, both locally and nationally. Raising the profile of nurses and nursing as part of the 'We Are The NHS' campaign (Public Health

England, 2021) is a welcome and more accurate portrayal of the wide range of roles and expertise.

CPD that is quality assured, locally relevant and encompassing of new means of digital consulting is identified as a key factor for GPNs and healthcare support workers in general practice in Section 3 of the General Practice Nursing Workforce Development Plan from the HEE (2017). Davies (2019) points out that recent cuts to HEE's budget have resulted in a significant lack of investment in ongoing learning and development for nurses and how e-learning options should not be the main means of CPD for a patient-led service. In addition, there are questions regarding how the NHS Long Term Plan Implementation Framework will translate using the needs STPs and integrated care systems (ICSs) that are currently creating their 5-year strategic plans by November 2019, covering the period 2019/20 to 2023/24 (NHS England, 2019c).

SUMMARY

Undisputed is the necessity of CPD for GPNs to increase their knowledge, skills and satisfaction in their roles, but the funding of quality-assured opportunities for early-career nurses and those with substantial experience needs to be addressed. The NHS needs to retain and recruit nurses for all areas of service provision, and general practice should not be neglected if patients and their families are to benefit from excellent care for this and coming generations. The development of voluntary standards of education (QNI, 2020) is seen as progress towards making explicit the expectations for a Level 5 registered nurse new to general practice nursing. Best practice is the goal of the initial preparation and ongoing progression of GPNs in their vital role in primary care. This will include being watchful of the NMC's review of Specialist Practitioner Qualifications, which includes GPNs. The domains of clinical care, leadership and management, facilitation of learning and evidence and research and development apply to CPD as well as initial preparation and provide structure for career progression and excellence to provide the best possible service for our communities:

Let us never consider ourselves finished nurses. We must be learning all of our lives.

(attributed to Florence Nightingale from the 1800s)

REFERENCES

Aston, J. (2018). The future of nursing in primary care. *British Journal of General Practice, 68*(672), 312–313.

Davies, N. (2019). Bridging the CPD gap. *Independent Nurse*. https://www.independentnurse.co.uk/professional-article/bridging-the-cpd-gap/221152/

Department of Health (Northern Ireland). (2016). *Health and wellbeing 2026 – Delivering together*. https://www.health-ni.gov.uk/publications/health-and-wellbeing-2026-delivering-together

Duncan, D., & Hayes, S. (2017). Developing the role of the GP nurse. *Independent Nurse*. http://www.independentnurse.co.uk/professional-article/developing-the-role-of-the-gp-nurse/155185/

eLearning for Health. (2019). *Advanced clinical practice toolkit*. https://www.e-lfh.org.uk/programmes/advanced-clinical-practice-toolkit/

Eveleigh, M. (2019). *Nurses need a reason to 'return to practice'.* https://www.nursinginpractice.com/views/nurses-need-a-reason-to-return-to-practice/

Health Education England. (2017). *The general practice workforce development plan*. https://www.hee.nhs.uk/sites/default/files/documents/The%20general%20practice%20nursing%20workforce%20development%20plan.pdf

Health Education England. (2021). *General practice nursing*. https://www.hee.nhs.uk/our-work/general-practice-nursing

Ipsos MORI Social Research Institute. (2019). *Evaluation of revalidation for nurses and midwives: Year three report*. https://www.nmc.org.uk/globalassets/sitedocuments/annual_reports_and_accounts/revalidationreports/ipsos-mori-revalidation-evaluation-report-year-3.pdf

Lean, M., Leslie, W., Barnes, A., Brosnhan, N., Thom, E., & McCombie, L. (2019). Durability of a primary care-led weight-management intervention for remission of type 2 diabetes: 2-year results of the DiRECT open-label, cluster-randomised trial. *The Lancet Diabetes and Endocrinology, 7*(5), 344–355.

Majeed, A. (2017). Shortage of general practitioners in the NHS. *British Medical Journal, 358*, Article j3191. https://doi.org/10.1136/bmj.j3191

National Institute for Health Research (NIHR). (2021). *Primary care specialty profile*. https://www.nihr.ac.uk/documents/primary-care-specialty-profile/11603

NHS Education for Scotland. (2018). *Coordinated learning and development network for general practice nursing* [Newsletter]. https://www.scotlanddeanery.nhs.scot/media/197761/gpn-newsletter-summer-2018-003.pdf

NHS England. (2014). *Five year forward view*. https://www.england.nhs.uk/wp-content/uploads/2014/10/5yfv-web.pdf

NHS England. (2016). *General practice forward view*. https://www.england.nhs.uk/wp-content/uploads/2016/04/gpfv.pdf

NHS England. (2018). *General practice – Developing confidence, capability and capacity. A ten point action plan for general practice nursing*. https://www.england.nhs.uk/wp-content/uploads/2018/01/general-practice-nursing-ten-point-plan-v17.pdf

NHS England. (2019a). *NHS long term plan*. https://www.longtermplan.nhs.uk/

NHS England. (2019b). *General practice nursing induction template*. https://www.qni.org.uk/wp-content/uploads/2019/05/General-Practice-Nursing-Induction-Template.pdf

NHS England. (2019c). *NHS long term plan implementation framework.* https://www.longtermplan.nhs.uk/wp-content/uploads/2019/06/long-term-plan-implementation-framework-v1.pdf

NHS England, Health Education England, & NHS Improvement. (2017). *Multi-professional framework for advanced clinical practice in England.* https://www.lasepharmacy.hee.nhs.uk/dyn/_assets/_folder4/advanced-practice/multi-professionalframeworkforadvancedclinicalpracticeinengland.pdf

NHS England. (2020). *Online version of the People Plan for 2020/2021.* https://www.england.nhs.uk/ournhspeople/online-version/

Northern Ireland Practice and Education Council for Nursing and Midwifery. (2019). *Career pathway for general practice nursing in Northern Ireland.* https://nipec.hscni.net/download/professional_information/resource_section/general_practice_nursing/documents/GPN-Career-Pathway-2019.pdf

Nursing and Midwifery Council. (2018a). *Part 1: Standards framework for nursing and midwifery education.* https://www.nmc.org.uk/globalassets/sitedocuments/education-standards/education-framework.pdf

Nursing and Midwifery Council. (2018b). *Part 2: Standards for student supervision and assessment.* https://www.nmc.org.uk/globalassets/sitedocuments/education-standards/student-supervision-assessment.pdf

Nursing and Midwifery Council. (2018c). *The code. Professional standards of practice and behaviour for nurses, midwives and nursing associates.* https://www.nmc.org.uk/globalassets/sitedocuments/nmc-publications/nmc-code.pdf

Nursing and Midwifery Council. (2019). *Revalidation.* http://revalidation.nmc.org.uk/

Oxtoby, K. (2018). *CPD funding for practice nurses – Why is it so variable?* https://www.nursinginpractice.com/professional/training/cpd-funding-for-practice-nurses-why-is-it-so-variable/

Primary Care One. (2019). *Developing primary care in Wales.* http://www.primarycareone.wales.nhs.uk/home

Public Health England. (2021). *NHS recruitment. We are the NHS.* https://campaignresources.phe.gov.uk/resources/campaigns/77-nhs-recruitment-/overview

Queen's Nursing Institute. (2015). *General practice nursing: A time of opportunity in the 21st century.* https://www.qni.org.uk/wpcontent/uploads/2016/09/gpn_c21_report.pdf

Queen's Nursing Institute. (2020). *The QNI standards of education and practice for nurses new to general practice nursing.* https://www.qni.org.uk/wp-content/uploads/2020/05/Standards-of-Education-and-Practice-for-Nurses-New-to-General-Practice-Nursing.pdf

Queen's Nursing Institute. (2021). *Aspiring leaders programme.* https://www.qni.org.uk/explore-qni/leadership-programmes/aspiring-leaders/

Royal College of General Practitioners. (2013). *The 2022 GP. A vision for general practice in the future NHS.*

Royal College of General Practitioners. (2018). *Clinical research for GP practices.* https://www.rcgp.org.uk/clinical-and-research/about/clinical-news/2018/june/clinical-research-for-gp-practices.aspx

Royal College of Nursing. (2018a). *Improving continuing professional development: How reps can make a difference in the workplace.*

Royal College of Nursing. (2018b). *Investing in a safe and effective workforce: Continuing professional development for nurses in the UK. A policy report.*

Scottish Government. (2017). *Nursing 2030 vision: Promoting confident, competent and collaborate nursing for Scotland's future.* https://www.gov.scot/binaries/content/documents/govscot/publications/strategy-plan/2017/07/nursing-2030-vision-9781788511001/documents/00522376-pdf/00522376-pdf/govscot%3Adocument/00522376.pdf

Scottish Government. (2018). *Transforming nursing, midwifery and health professions' (NMaHP) roles: Pushing the boundaries to meet health and social care needs in Scotland. Developing the general practice nursing role in integrated community nursing teams.* https://www.gov.scot/publications/developing-general-practice-nursing-role-integrated-community-nursing-teams/

Welsh Government. (2019). *Health and care research Wales.* https://www.healthandcareresearch.gov.wales/

INDEX

Note: Page numbers followed by '*f*' indicate figures, '*t*' indicate tables, and '*b*' indicate boxes.